MANAGING QUALITY

A Guide to System-Wide
Performance Management
in Health Care

MANAGING QUALITY

A Guide to System-Wide
Performance Management
in Health Care

Jacqueline M. Katz, RN, MS
Vice President
Division of Continuing Education and Training
Mosby–Year Book, Inc.
St. Louis, Missouri

Eleanor Green, RN, BSN
President
Frederick Nursing Consultants
Frederick, Maryland

SECOND EDITION

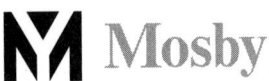 Mosby

St. Louis Baltimore Boston Carlsbad Chicago Naples New York Philadelphia Portland
London Madrid Mexico City Singapore Sydney Tokyo Toronto Wiesbaden

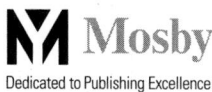

Mosby

Dedicated to Publishing Excellence

A Times Mirror
Company

Publisher: Nancy L. Coon
Editor: N. Darlene Como
Developmental Editor: Dana L. Knighten
Project Manager: Mark Spann
Production Editor: Jennifer Doll
Designer: Judi Lang
Manufacturing Supervisor: Linda Ierardi

SECOND EDITION
Copyright © 1997 by Mosby–Year Book, Inc.

Previous edition copyrighted 1992

Printed in the United States of America
Composition by Shepherd, Inc.
Printing/binding by Maple-Vail

Mosby–Year Book, Inc.
11830 Westline Industrial Drive
St. Louis, Missouri 63146

Library of Congress Cataloging in Publication Data

Katz, Jacqueline.
     Managing quality: a guide to system-wide performance management
in health care / Jacqueline M. Katz, Eleanor Green. --2nd ed.
          p.   cm.
     Includes bibliographical references and index.
     ISBN 0-8151-4973-5
     1. Nursing services--Evaluation.   2. Medical care--Evaluation.
I. Green, Eleanor.   II. Title.
     [DNLM: 1. Nursing Services--organization & administration--United
States.   2. Quality Assurance, Health Care--United States.   3. Task
Performance and Analysis.   4. Data Collection.   5. Program
Evaluation.   WY 100 K195m 1996]
     RT85.5.K38   1996
     362.1'73'0287--dc20
DNLM/DLC   96-15639
for Library of Congress   CIP

97 98 99 00 01 / 9 8 7 6 5 4 3 2 1

To
Jay and Bunky
Two husbands who set the standard
against which all other husbands are measured.

Preface

When we first conceived the idea of writing a book based on our consultative work with many divisions of nursing across the country, we had no idea how successful it would be. The first edition of *Managing Quality* quickly became known as the "red book," and it was used by hundreds of nurses to make the transition from QA to CQI.

In the midst of this transition, a new era of capitation and managed care dawned. Suddenly health care organizations were reorganizing themselves for capitation; money was scarce and many organizations were faced with threats to their survival. Many questioned the value of continuous quality improvement and began battening down the hatches against the revolutionary crisis of cost containment that was fomenting on the horizon.

The revolution within the health care industry escalated into a crisis and reality forced traditional, costly paradigms to shift rapidly in the direction of practicality and reduced spending. One of the greatest paradigm shifts has been away from CQI and toward performance improvement with an emphasis on outcomes. CQI fell by the wayside as health care organizations began to understand that measurable outcomes can be achieved only through performance.

We discovered that all outcomes—good and bad—are derived from performance in three distinct areas of a health care organization: service, practice, and governance. Those of you who were students of the first edition will recognize this expanded trifocus.

We now know that survival in today's health care environment requires a much broader approach. We found, through our consultative efforts, that a multidimensional, complex health care organization understood and easily adapted to a trifocus approach to performance management, when we implemented the concept of measurement in the three areas of service, practice, and governance. We were able to refine the concept further through the development of three programs: (a) the performance awareness program, (b) the performance measurement program, and (c) the performance improvement program. Together, these three programs make up the performance management system described in this book.

Because costs are the driving force behind today's health care crisis, we have created concrete strategies for costing out processes that permit an organization to know where its resources are being spent.

The famous coach Vince Lombardi says that timing is everything! The time has come for us to share, once again, the work that we have done with organizations throughout the country to develop this new, step-by-step, organization-wide approach. As we began to prepare for the revision of the "red book," we realized that we have reengineered the processes of achieving value in health care by refining our model, "THE BLUEPRINT for Performance Management," from one specific discipline to an organization-wide approach.

We were gratified to witness our practice model, which is based on business principles rather than the traditional nursing principles, survive the fusillade of the health care revolution with its basic structure intact. We refined processes in the model, solidified the importance and use of outcomes in measurement, and expanded our emphasis on cost; however, the basic construct, concept, and tenets on which the model was built are still sound. The fact that THE BLUEPRINT has been employed successfully in so many health care settings as the organizing framework for their performance management systems has reinforced to us the applicability of this model in any setting, regardless of the size or complexity of the organization.

This second edition takes the foundational work of the "red book" and refines it through the benefit of our additional field experience with a variety of accreditation systems, practice arenas, and disciplines. The book's new title, *Managing Quality: A Guide to System-Wide Performance Management in Health Care*, reflects this refinement to an organization-wide approach. So does the new cover design, which retains the original red yet adds other colors and elements for a new look.

Health care organizations throughout the world have successfully piloted and used our strategies and tools. They have been proven to be both effective and easy to use, and we think you will find them to be immediately useful in your day-to-day activities. We believe that this book will assist top, middle, or front-line management to focus on priorities within health care organizations, and we hope that the tools and techniques within its pages will enable practitioners to identify the critical processes that will have the greatest impact on outcomes.

This book is divided into six parts. Part One describes the major changes in the pursuit of quality in health care and the impact of managed care on performance. Chapter 1 focuses on trends in quality in health care. Chapter 2 redefines quality in a managed care environment. Chapter 3 presents an organizational model, THE BLUEPRINT for Performance Management.

Part Two outlines a structure for organization-wide performance management. Chapter 4 defines the responsibility and accountability of the CEO for an organization-wide performance management system. Chapter 5 describes a council structure to support implementation of THE BLUEPRINT.

Part Three defines the steps for creating an organization-wide performance awareness program. Chapter 6 provides tools for identifying the organization's customers and delineating the scope of service, practice, and governance. Chapter 7 highlights the identification and prioritization of key functions and critical processes. Chapter 8 emphasizes the importance of development and dissemination of structure, process, and outcomes standards.

Part Four is devoted to the creation of an organization-wide performance measurement program. Chapter 9 details how to design organization-wide performance measures, and Chapter 10 focuses on setting statistically based performance targets. Chapter 11 presents the tools for collecting and organizing data. Chapter 12 concentrates on evaluating process variation.

Part Five outlines the steps for creating an organization-wide performance improvement plan. In Chapter 13 we discuss the role of the organization-wide improvement plan. Chapter 14 focuses on action and documenting organizational improvement. Chapter 15 emphasizes the importance of communicating results.

Part Six, which contains Chapters 16, 17, and 18, applies the concepts of performance awareness, performance measurement, and performance improvement to the perform management system itself.

It is through the kindness and cooperation of many health care organizations that we have been able to engage in the piloting and testing of a performance management system—the results of which are published in this book. We have made an attempt to provide the latest information on how to implement an organization-wide performance management system. Because information about this subject can be a bit dry, we have chosen to introduce each chapter with an enlightening quote and a relevant story, anecdote, or joke. The world's most revered teachers were great storytellers. We hope that you will enjoy the levity and that the message of the stories will help you to better understand the thrust of the chapters.

This book provides you with all the elements necessary for implementing a successful performance management system that meets accreditation requirements. If you are new to performance management, the book will guide you through the process step by step. If you already have a system in place, you can use the book as a benchmark to improve or streamline your current approach. Regardless of your previous experience, we think you will find the tools in this book useful to help you tame the paper tiger and reduce the frustration of developing a "from scratch" performance management system.

It continues to be our intent as educators, authors, and consultants to provide a simple, realistic approach to developing a performance management system that is cost-effective, easy for staff to live with, yet comprehensive enough to meet accreditation requirements. Good luck!

Jackie and Ellie

Acknowledgments

Many people have played many different and important roles in the development and publication of this book. Our special thanks go to:

Darlene Como, for providing us the opportunity to publish our work.

Dana Knighten, for keeping us on track—if not on schedule.

Jenny Doll, for making the editing process so much fun.

The many hospitals who believed in us and piloted our ideas and projects during the development phase and continue to support this work.

Bronson Medical Hospital in Kalamazoo, Michigan, for helping solidify a tool for easy computation of the cost of nonconformance.

Living Centers of America, in Houston, Texas, a corporation of more than 300 long-term care facilities in 16 states, who successfully reengineered their entire company for shared leadership based on the principles of THE BLUE-PRINT. Special thanks to Edward Kuntz, CEO; Keith Krein, the Medical Director; and Barbara Baylis, the Corporate Performance Management Director, for providing us the opportunity to implement our concepts.

Ellie's children: Sheri and Robert Forquer, for always saying, "Of course you can, Mom!" Scott, for being my [Ellie's] cheering section.

Jackie's children: Lauren, for perspective; Meryl, for reflection; and Evan for just being.

Our parents, Melvin and Ann Kedzior and Bill and Evelyn Postlewait, for being lifelong, untiring supporters of their daughters' projects, whatever these projects have been or may be in the future.

Madeline Green, who is the world's most patient and loving mother-in-law, for keeping up with the washing, cooking, and mending, while the computer occupied Ellie's full-time attention.

Ellen Katz, whose inner strength is a constant source of inspiration.

Ellie's best friends, Marilyn and Lois, who have been patiently waiting for manuscript completion so that Ellie could once again "come out and play" (go shopping).

Finally, we express a special thanks to our best friends and husbands, Jay and Lloyd, who tolerated our hours of telephone consultation and filled in for us with our personal responsibilities so that we could finish this work.

Contents

MANAGING QUALITY

A Guide to System-Wide
Performance Management
in Health Care

Part One

INTRODUCTION TO ORGANIZATION-WIDE PERFORMANCE MANAGEMENT

Chapter 1

In Pursuit of a Definition of Quality

> **Styles stipulation:**
> **"As a word gains in popularity, it loses in clarity."**
> Margretta M. Styles

COSTELLO: Hey, Abbott, tell me the names of the players on our baseball team so I can say hello to them.

ABBOTT: Sure, Now, Who's on first, What's on second, I-Don't-Know on third . . .

COSTELLO: Wait a minute.

ABBOTT: What's the matter?

COSTELLO: I want to know the names of the players.

ABBOTT: I'm telling you. Who's on first, What's on second, I-Don't-Know on third . . .

COSTELLO: Now, wait. What's the name of the first baseman?

ABBOTT: No, What's the name of the second baseman.

COSTELLO: I don't know.

ABBOTT: He's the third baseman.

COSTELLO: Let's start over.

ABBOTT: Okay. Who's on first . . .

COSTELLO: I'm asking *you* what's the name of the first baseman.

ABBOTT: What's the name of the second baseman.

COSTELLO: I don't know.

ABBOTT: He's on third.

COSTELLO: All I'm trying to find out is the name of the first baseman.

ABBOTT: I keep telling you. Who's on first.

COSTELLO: I'm asking YOU what's the name of the first baseman.

ABBOTT (*Rapidly*): What's the name of the second baseman.

COSTELLO (*More rapidly*): I don't know.

BOTH (*Most rapidly*): Third base!!

COSTELLO: All right. Okay. You won't tell what's the name of the first baseman.

ABBOTT: I've *been* telling you. What's the name of the second baseman.

COSTELLO: I'm asking *you* who's on second.

ABBOTT: *Who's* on *first.*

COSTELLO: I don't know.

ABBOTT: He's on third.

COSTELLO: Let's do it this way. You pay the players on this team?

ABBOTT: Absolutely.

COSTELLO: All right. Now, when you give the first baseman his paycheck, who gets the money?

ABBOTT: Every penny of it.

COSTELLO: *Who?*

ABBOTT: Naturally.

COSTELLO: *Naturally?*

ABBOTT: Of course.

COSTELLO: All right. Then Naturally's on first . . .

ABBOTT: No. Who's on first.

COSTELLO: *I'm asking you!* What's the name of the first baseman?

ABBOTT: And I'm telling you! What's the name of the second baseman.

COSTELLO: You say third base, I'll . . . (*Pause*) Wait a minute. You got a pitcher on this team?

ABBOTT: Did you ever hear of a team without a pitcher?

COSTELLO: All right. Tell me the pitcher's name.
ABBOTT: Tomorrow.
COSTELLO: You don't want to tell me now?
ABBOTT: I said I'd tell you. Tomorrow.
COSTELLO: What's wrong with today?
ABBOTT: Nothing. He's a pretty good catcher.
COSTELLO: Who's the catcher?
ABBOTT: No, Who's the first baseman.
COSTELLO: All right, tell me that. What's the first baseman's name?
ABBOTT: No, What's the second baseman's name.
COSTELLO: I-don't-know-third-base.
ABBOTT: Look, it's very simple.
COSTELLO: I know it's simple. You got a pitcher. Tomorrow. He throws the ball to Today. Today throws the ball to Who, he throws the ball to What, What throws the ball to I-Don't-Know, *he's* on third . . . and what's more, I-Don't-Give-A-Darn!
ABBOTT: What's that?
COSTELLO: I said, I-Don't-Give-A-Darn.
ABBOTT: Oh, he's our shortstop.*

The historical development of quality in health care reads somewhat like the above Abbott and Costello routine. Although consumers and providers agree that quality is a major issue in health care, nobody is quite sure "who's on first."

One of the important challenges facing health care today is to define *quality*. Individual definitions are numerous, and one can easily be confused by the verbiage. Ask any health care practitioner what is meant by the term and he or she may have difficulty putting the concept into words. Describe for that practitioner a patient situation, however, and he or she can easily point out the factors that indicate quality care or the lack of it.

This chapter provides a historical perspective on the quality phenomenon, both in industry and in health care. It provides the context for understanding how we have gotten to the current conventional wisdom about quality.

Quality in health care has been affected by the retrenchment that has occurred throughout American industry over the past decade. Like other businesses, health care has been harmed by the upheaval of its economic base. The combination of the Tax Equity and Fiscal Responsibility Act (TEFRA) and prospective payment has shaken the foundation of the health care industry; moreover, the nation's medical bill rose to $615 billion in 1989, a 10.8% increase. In 1993 the health care share of the national economy hit 14.4% of gross domestic product ($903.3 billion).[1] Higher labor costs, failure of the government's efforts to curtail costs by limiting reimbursement, and a growing number of uninsured Americans are wreaking havoc in the

industry. At the same time the demand for quality services is greater than ever.

As a major American industry, health care has now begun to study the strategies used by other businesses to foster both excellence and economic survival. These methods are exerting a significant effect on how the health care industry looks at quality.

QUALITY IN BUSINESS

Concepts of quality that initially brought about a restructuring of health care were grounded in the works of industrial experts such as Fiegenbaum, Crosby, Juran, and Deming. The importance of quality in business first began to be appreciated in the 1940s and 1950s. Initial efforts focused primarily on the manufacturing sector; the need for quality in the service industry was later recognized.

In 1951 Fiegenbaum defined quality straightforwardly as the capability of a product to fulfill its intended purpose, produced with the least possible cost.[7] A complementary relationship between quality and cost was thus established early on.

Perhaps the three best-known quality leaders who have had the most significant impact on business today are Philip Crosby, Joseph Juran, and W. Edwards Deming.

Philip Crosby acknowledges the importance of the relationship of quality and cost but broadens the definition to include conformance to requirements; that is, quality is achieved through compliance with defined specifications or standards. Poor quality results from nonconformance. In Crosby's view, quality is not synonymous with luxury or goodness. A product or a service that conforms to its specifications demonstrates quality, whatever the product. "Quality is an achievable, measurable, profitable entity once you have commitment and understanding and are prepared for hard work."[4] Crosby emphasizes the need to do things right the first time. His work is based on 14 steps, which are summarized in the box on p. 5.

Juran developed a three-part approach to quality: quality planning, quality control, and quality improvement. Quality planning involves determining who the customers are and what their needs are, then developing products based on those needs and designing processes to produce those products. Quality control is the evaluation of performance to identify discrepancies between actual performance and goals. Quality improvement establishes an infrastructure and the project teams to carry out process improvement. Juran strongly emphasizes the use of statistical analysis in the quality control stage.[12]

W. Edwards Deming helped the Japanese to rebuild their economy after World War II. His techniques

---

*From Einstein C: *The fireside book of baseball*, New York, 1956, Simon & Schuster.

CROSBY'S 14 STEPS

1. Management commitment
2. The quality improvement team
3. Quality measurement
4. The cost of quality
5. Quality awareness
6. Corrective action
7. Zero defect planning
8. Supervisor training
9. Zero defects day
10. Goal setting
11. Error-cause removal
12. Recognition
13. Quality councils
14. Do it over again

DEMING'S 14 POINTS

1. Create constancy of purpose for service improvement.
2. Adopt the new philosophy.
3. Cease dependence on inspection to achieve quality.
4. End the practice of awarding business on price alone—make partners out of vendors.
5. Constantly improve every process for planning production and service.
6. Institute training and retraining on the job.
7. Institute leadership for system improvement.
8. Drive out fear.
9. Break down barriers between staff areas.
10. Eliminate slogan, exhortations, and targets for the work force.
11. Eliminate numerical quotas for the work force and numerical goals for the management.
12. Remove barriers to pride of workmanship.
13. Institute a vigorous program of education and self-improvement for everyone.
14. Put everyone to work on the transformation.

From Walton M: *The Deming management method*, New York, 1986, Putnam.

became the standard in Japan; the success of Japanese business and its dominant economic position is often attributed to his influence. His strategy centers first and foremost on the development of quality and its continual improvement. The idea underlying his 14-point system is to do things right the first time, with emphasis on meeting both company and customer expectations as the primary source of quality improvement. Deming's 14 points are summarized in the box on the right.

The Disney Company exemplifies Deming's commitment to internal and external customers in creating quality service. The Disney culture has three focal points: its customers (guests), its employees (cast members), and its managers. Guests will receive only the sort of treatment management desires, provided the cast members receive the same sort of treatment. In orientation, new recruits learn to deal with fellow cast members as guests.

Meeting customer expectations of quality is defined as follows by Dr. Irving G. Synder, Jr., Vice President and Director of Research and Development for Dow Chemical USA: "This is what quality is all about: the customer's perception of excellence. And quality is our response to that perception."[23] Allen Jacobson, Chairman and CEO of 3M, agrees. The 3M company defines quality as a business management process to achieve consistent conformance to customer expectations. This philosophy is the basis for the company's total quality management (TQM) system.[18]

Deming's focus on continual improvement is evident in the Japanese concept of *Kaizen*—a continual improvement process involving everyone in a personal quest for excellence.[14] It is based on the belief that we must constantly improve and develop more efficient systems that will produce a higher quality at lower cost.[17] Continual improvement is a recurring theme in contemporary industrial definitions of quality.

In addition to Crosby, Juran, and Deming, many business experts have begun to express concern that quality cannot be reduced to a mere definition. Rather, quality is the embodiment of shared values and vision, and as such it requires a new paradigm for defining itself.

Harvard's David Garvin has summarized eight key dimensions that define quality. He suggests that rather than attempt to be "number one" in all aspects, the organization should focus on a few of these dimensions. According to Garvin, the key dimensions of quality are as follows:

- Performance, or the primary operating characteristics of a service
- Features, or the secondary characteristics that supplement the service's basic functioning
- Reliability, or the probability of malfunction or failure within a specified period of time
- Conformance, or the degree to which a service meets preestablished industry standards
- Durability, or the amount of use one gets from a product/service before it physically deteriorates

- Serviceability, or speed, courtesy, competence, and ease of repair; responsiveness
- Aesthetics, or how a product/service looks, feels, tastes, sounds
- Perceived quality, or what the customer thinks is quality[9]

In his book *Managing for World-Class Quality*, Edwin Schecter states that achieving quality performance requires a clear sense of what quality is. He continues by defining quality according to the following characteristics:

1. Conformance: meeting or exceeding the minimum standards
2. Fitness for use: performing the task as advertised
3. Reliability: performing the intended function in the specified environment for the prescribed period of time
4. Yield: the percent of the product/service that conforms to specifications at each evaluation point
5. Customer satisfaction: the customer's perception of value; meeting customer expectations[26]

Defining quality by specific characteristics enables one to convert quality goals into measurable indicators of performance.

The latest twist on the quality definition comes in the form of a lesson sorely learned by industry. It seems that as the total quality management movement escalated into a national battle cry, the idea of "doing" quality became the mission of many companies. The process of quality became an end rather than a means to an end. Inflated quality departments grew larger and larger. The pursuit of quality became a mechanistic exercise that proved meaningless to customer satisfaction. According to Schecter, "Quality that means little to customers usually doesn't produce a payoff in improved sales, profits, or market share. It's wasted effort and expense."[26]

Quality bureaucracies emerged and red tape multiplied. Doing flowcharts and cause-and-effect diagrams became more important than analyzing them to improve outcomes. Emphasis was on monitoring and evaluating processes that did not necessarily improve outcomes or that were not necessarily important to the customers.

One casualty of quality "out of control" was the Wallace Company, which won the Malcolm Balridge National Quality award in 1990. Two years later the company filed for Chapter 11. Another 1990 Balridge award winner, Federal Express, identified speed of delivery as a key variable for improvement. They stressed speed over accuracy. The number of misdirected packages soared, resulting in an increased cost

of $50 per package to correct the mistakes, not to mention the adverse effects of lost packages on customer satisfaction.[26]

Today's quality slogan is "return on quality" (ROQ). The emphasis of this quality/cost duality is on customer satisfaction and financial payoff. It involves developing strategies that take the cost out of making systems and services better.

Although the quality pioneers always advocated a bottom line orientation to quality, the confusion came in its application. Many companies confused process with outcome. Quality became its own reward. Doing things quicker, better, and faster did not necessarily result in better sales, greater profits, or increased customer satisfaction. Also, the cost of maintaining the quality program was not recouped by increased revenues. Industry had created a monster, and those proponents of quality as the panacea of industry's woes began to look askance at the whole approach to quality improvement. Many were ready to toss out the baby with the bathwater, and rumors started flying that quality was not working.

Return to quality refocuses thinking about quality improvement to measuring and improving processes that produce tangible customer benefits, while lowering costs or increasing revenues. It forces an assessment of preconceived beliefs and a willingness to re-engineer entire processes.

For example, one of the cornerstone tenets of United Parcel Service's (UPS) approach was the belief that on-time delivery was their customers' chief priority. As a result, systems were designed to improve delivery times. Time and motion studies had figured the average time it took for elevator doors to open in certain buildings and how long it took for people to answer their doorbells. The drivers' seat corners in the delivery trucks were shaved off to improve speed. All these things were done in an effort to deliver all next-day packages by 10:30 AM. However, speed was not what customers valued most. What they really wanted was more face-to-face time with the drivers, which was diametrically opposed to the exacting time schedules to which the drivers were expected to adhere. A retooling of the entire delivery process has occurred, and although this has cost millions of dollars, the company has generated tens of millions of dollars in return within the first year of operating within the new process.[26] A key point to remember from this example is that it takes money to improve quality, so the return on investment for process improvement has to justify the expense related to improving the process. Otherwise, quality measurement and improvement activities become a financial drain rather than a solution.

APPLYING BUSINESS CONCEPTS TO HEALTH CARE

The confusion about quality in industry is evident in the number of theories about it. Although the primary focus of each theorist may differ, there appear to be similarities in all of the theories that have applications to health care.

The first is that quality can be defined and measured. It may be defined on the basis of specifications on the company's side and on the basis of expectations on the customer's side. These specifications take into consideration the customer's needs and wants. In applying business principles of quality to health care, certain problems have evolved. Defining quality according to customer expectations is controversial. A poll conducted for the magazine *Hospitals* revealed that a patient's satisfaction with the hospital experience represented more than half of the overall evaluation of the quality of care provided. Concern on the part of staff had the greatest influence on the patient's overall rating. Although patients are capable of evaluating the quality of the hotel services provided (e.g., whether food is served at the proper temperature and whether the staff is courteous), they are less capable of evaluating whether the correct IV fluid is dripping at the appropriate rate.[10]

> *The perspective of the customer is very important but it may not be as important in the health care delivery process as the measurable quality of the delivery processes that provide care during a customer's service episode.[24]*

Second, quality is dynamic—it is not simply achieved and then disregarded. Quality develops from continual improvement. Tom Peters says that all quality is relative. "Each day, each product or service is getting relatively better or relatively worse, but it never stands still."[23] This is particularly true in a service business such as health care, where it is not possible to accumulate an inventory of services.

Third, quality involves a competitive edge. Philip Crosby states, "Quality is free. It's not a gift but it is free. What costs money are the unquality things—all the actions that involve not doing jobs right the first time."[4] Quality and cost go hand in hand. Quality is the primary source of cost reduction; however, the reverse of that statement is not true. Cost-reduction campaigns do not usually lead to improved quality and they usually do not result in long-term lower costs.[22]

Fourth, quality has to do with doing the "right" things right. It is estimated that poor quality accounts for 40% of the cost of people and assets in a service firm.[22] As a result, almost every other person is working on fixing something that should have already been done rather than accomplishing a new task. There is no excuse for failure to do things right the first time.

Peters describes the need for quality obsession.[22] Whether or not it is possible to achieve 100% quality in a service program, not striving for 100% results in mistakes. Approach each patient as 100% and the variation will consist of justifiable outliers, those patients who would have ended up with a C-section or a cutdown despite our best efforts rather than resulting from our mistakes. In health care, part of the answer to labor shortages may lie not in hiring more staff or developing new levels of personnel, but in refocusing efforts toward achieving zero deficits. Hospital administrators are now beginning to appreciate that a significant amount of the labor cost is related to the tremendous amount of rework that goes on.

Fifth, quality relates to outcomes. The late Ray Brown, hospital administrator and past president of the American Hospital Association, said, "Doing something may be confused with getting something done."[2] The focus of all quality efforts must be on the results produced. Emphasis is on what is achieved, not solely on what is done. Management guru Peter Drucker supports this idea. "Quality in a product or service is not what a supplier puts in. It is what the customer gets out and is willing to pay for."[6] This approach also emphasizes a results orientation.

Robert Kemmel, Vice President of Corporate Marketing and Communications at Albert Einstein Health Care Foundation, states that in the year 2000 there will be 40% fewer hospitals because of the retrenchment that will occur because of the new focus on outcomes: "Does the patient become healthier as a result of the care provided?"[13] All the measurement in the world is a waste of time if it does not result in improved clinical outcomes.

Sixth, quality is everyone's responsibility. Peters and Waterman advocate a strong sense of personal accountability among all employees. The attitude that "each member is the company" must prevail.[23] Dennis O'Leary, President of the Joint Commission on Accreditation of Healthcare Organizations (JCAHO), states that there is a long tradition of giving no more than lip service to quality. "Quality . . . is everybody's business—not simply that of the quality assurance office."[20] Commitment must be made at the executive level and permeate the organization. It must be at the top of everyone's agenda, foremost in everyone's mind. As the current Ford Motor Company slogan puts it, "Quality is job one."

Seventh, quality and costs are irrevocably linked. Quality improvement can be the key to controlling expenses and generating revenues, but the process of quality improvement itself can be an enormous profit drain if it is not controlled and/or if the organization is improving the wrong processes.

Eighth, quality and performance are synonymous. Garvin defined performance as the primary operating characteristics of a product or service. What has evolved in health care is less emphasis in defining quality and a more concentrated attempt to define the dimensions of performance.

DEFINITIONS OF QUALITY IN HEALTH CARE

Just as the definition of quality in business has evolved, so too has the definition of quality in health care. Initially, definitions of quality in health care tended to focus on the technical aspects of quality. The National Association of Quality Assurance Professionals described quality as levels of excellence produced and documented in the process of patient care, based on the best knowledge available and achievable at a particular facility.[15]

The Joint Commission defines quality as "the degree to which patient care services increase the probability of desired outcomes and reduce the probability of undesired outcomes given the current state of knowledge."[8] The Joint Commission outlined 12 factors that determine the quality of patient care and recently redefined these factors as dimensions of performance. These factors and their definitions are outlined in the box below.

Differences among institutions regarding factors contributing to quality were shown in a survey conducted among 663 CEOs. In hospitals with more than 400 beds, the medical staff tended to be ranked as most significant; in hospitals with 200 to 400 beds, the nursing staff was more likely to be ranked as most significant. Overall, nursing care was mentioned as one of the three most significant factors in 97.3% of the responses. Clinical skills of the medical staff ranked second (96.4%) and employee attitudes ranked third (93.3%).[16]

The pursuit of an all-embracing definition of quality has been elusive. Donabedian suggests that no one definition will suffice, and proposes three definitions: (1) the *absolutist* definition considers the possibility of benefit and harm to health as valued by the practitioner, with no attention to cost; (2) the *individualized* definition focuses on the patient's expectations of benefit and/or harm and other undesired consequences; and (3) the *social* definition includes the cost of care, the benefit/harm continuum, and the distribution of health care as valued by the population in general.[5] C. Duane Dauner, President of the California Hospital Association, states, "It can no longer simply be defined by what technology is available. The challenge facing providers is to balance human values, technological resources, quality of life and innovation with economic reality, to provide the best possible care."[19]

DEFINITIONS OF THE DIMENSIONS OF PERFORMANCE

Appropriateness: the degree to which the care/intervention provided is relevant to the patient's clinical needs, given the current state of knowledge

Availability: the degree to which the appropriate care/intervention is available to meet the needs of the patient served

Continuity: the degree to which the care/intervention for the patient is coordinated among practitioners, between organizations, and across time

Effectiveness: the degree to which the care/intervention is provided in the correct manner, given the current state of knowledge, in order to achieve the desired/projected outcome(s) for the patient

Efficacy: the degree to which the care/intervention used for the patient has been shown to accomplish the desired/projected outcome(s)

Efficiency: the ratio of the outcomes (results of care/intervention) for a patient to the resources used to deliver the care

Respect and caring: the degree to which a patient, or designee, is involved in his or her own care decisions, and that those providing the services do so with sensitivity and respect for his or her needs and expectations and individual differences

Safety: the degree to which the risk of an intervention and the risk in the care environment are reduced for the patient and others, including the health care provider

Timeliness: the degree to which the care/intervention is provided to the patient at the time it is most beneficial or necessary

---

From *The measurement mandate,* Chicago, 1993, The Joint Commission on Accreditation of Healthcare Organizations.

It does not appear that a universal definition of quality is forthcoming. Nevertheless, even in the absence of a formal definition, a patient or provider can certainly identify its absence—substandard care or less-than-optimal results. Three or more attempts at venipuncture and hot meals served cold exemplify substandard care. Pressure sores and postoperative infections are examples of poor outcomes.

Defining quality performance through measurable dimensions enables organizations to make those dimensions explicit through clearly written standards.

STANDARDS DEFINE QUALITY/PERFORMANCE

The quality of care that is expected from a health care facility is made explicit by written standards that direct the way the service is to be provided and the results that should be achieved from that service. Standards, therefore, define quality. A standard is a written value statement of rules, conditions, and actions in a patient, staff member, or the system that are sanctioned by an appropriate authority.

There are four components to this definition of a standard. The first is that the standard is written. Holding staff accountable for unwritten or word-of-mouth standards is like trying to pin Jell-O to the wall . . . virtually impossible! The standards adhere to current acceptable levels of practice and are presented in a form that is easily understood by those who are expected to conform to them.

Second, standards define a set of rules, actions, or outcomes. Rules constitute the structure of the service, actions are the process of how the service is carried out, and outcomes define the results of the services. Structure standards define the rules under which the service must be delivered; for example, all patients transported by wheelchair or gurney must have a seat belt in place. Structure standards are nonnegotiable and nonmodifiable.

Process standards define how the service is to be carried out. Examples of process standards include the practice guidelines, procedures, and plans that direct service delivery. Process standards are modifiable based on the individual practitioner's analysis of the situation at hand. For example, a process standard might suggest that peripheral IV sites be rotated every 72 hours. On assessment of Mrs. Jones, an 85-year-old patient with inadequate veins, the nurse determines that her IV is patent and there are no signs of phlebitis or infection after 3 days; weighing these facts, the nurse decides not to rotate the IV site but rather to maintain the current site and monitor it closely.

Outcome standards define both the desired results to be achieved and the undesirable results to be avoided. They are part and parcel of every process

standard. The service provided must lead to a clearly defined and measurable outcome. Process and outcomes are inseparable, just like cause and effect.

The third critical component is that standards are written for consumers, staff members, and systems. Quality must permeate the organization. Standards must state what consumers are to receive, how staff members are to function, and how the system is to operate. These three components are integrally linked. The finest clinical standards will not facilitate quality if staff members are not competent to carry them out, or if there are not enough staff members to comply.

Finally, the standard must be approved by an authority. An authority is a group or individual empowered to enforce the standard and to hold staff members accountable. Without proper sanctioning the standard may be ignored. There are many sources of sanctioning. Hierarchical approval is the most common; however, a significant and powerful source of sanctioning comes from the individuals who are expected to uphold the standard in their day-to-day practice. The endorsement and support of staff are critical to both implementation and measurement of standards. Compliance with standards is more likely if those involved feel that the standards are achievable and especially if it is a standard they play a role in setting.

FROM QUALITY ASSURANCE TO QUALITY IMPROVEMENT

In the beginning was the word, and the word was quality assurance (QA).

Coyne and Killien describe QA as a process for evaluating patient care in a particular setting by developing standards of care and implementing mechanisms for ensuring that the standards are met.[3]

According to the Joint Commission, QA was initially defined as the process for objectively and systematically monitoring and evaluating the quality and appropriateness of patient care, for pursuing opportunities to improve patient care, and for resolving identified problems.[8] *Appropriateness* referred to the extent to which a particular procedure or treatment is efficient, is clearly indicated, is neither excessive nor deficient, and is provided in a setting best suited to the patient's needs.[21]

In its current *Lexicon*, the Joint Commission defines *quality assurance* as

1. Designing a product or service and controlling its production so well that quality is inevitable
2. In health care, the activities and programs intended to guarantee or ensure quality of patient care[11]

Quality control is defined as

1. The process by which actual performance is measured, the performance is compared with goals, and the difference is acted upon
2. The use of statistical methods to measure quality[11]

Quality improvement is defined as

1. The process of attaining a new level of performance or quality that is superior to any previous level of quality
2. The attainment of a new level of quality that is superior to any previous level of quality[11]

Quality management is defined as the process by which people are mobilized to achieve quality goals.[11]

Traditionally, quality assurance focused on finding problems and fixing them. It was based on the old adage, "If it ain't broke, don't fix it." If the results of the monitoring activities did not indicate a problem, health care professionals congratulated themselves on a job well done and moved on their merry way in search of new problems to tackle. Traditional QA was steeped in quality control methodology and focused on volume indicators, counting and sorting deficiencies. So, if the side rails were up and all the crash carts had been checked each shift, health care was in compliance and all was right with the world. It soon became apparent that this approach to problem identification did not necessarily ensure quality, and a shift in philosophy and methodology began to emerge.

In the late 1980s, the Joint Commission expressed that, although quality couldn't be ensured, it could be measured, and if it could be measured, it could be improved. This could be accomplished by identifying key indicators of quality within a service, monitoring those indicators, and measuring the quality of outcomes. To improve the quality of those outcomes, it would be necessary to identify the key processes leading to those outcomes. By focusing improvement efforts on those key processes, the quality of the outcomes achieved would ultimately be improved as well. Thus began the movement from quality assurance to quality improvement, from a hunt-and-seek approach to problem identification to a proactive approach to process improvement. The "If it ain't broke, don't fix it" mentality converted to "Even if it ain't broke, it can still be improved."

We are suggesting in this text that an additional step is needed to move the thinking as well as the jargon forward. If it is accepted that quality is defined by how well an organization performs, the attempts to improve the quality of performance would be termed *performance improvement*. It is our opinion, however, that attempts at improvement are doomed to failure if a more holistic definition of performance is not adopted.

Performance must be managed if an organization is to survive and ultimately thrive in the chaotic seas of health care.

OUR DEFINITION OF PERFORMANCE MANAGEMENT

Performance management is a system composed of an orderly series of programs designed to define, measure, and improve organizational performance. It is the system for ensuring conformance with requirements, that is, that staff are in compliance with the written standards. In other words, it is the system for ensuring that what was specified actually occurs, that things turn out as intended—every time.

Performance management uses the tools of statistical process control to form the basis for decisions about change. It incorporates the processes of performance awareness, performance measurement and performance improvement.

Performance awareness involves assigning responsibility for performance management, defining key processes and desired outcomes, and educating the responsible parties about their roles in the performance management system. Performance measurement involves collecting performance data and compares the actual results with projections. Finally, performance improvement includes the plan to improve the dimensions of performance, the implementation of the improvement plan, and the communication of the results of the plan's implementation.

Trudy, the bag lady in Jane Wagner's *The Search for Signs of Intelligent Life in the Universe*, states, "I worry whoever thought up the term 'quality control' thought if we didn't control it, it would get out of hand."[27]

Performance can get out of hand if it is not managed properly. Managing performance successfully requires mechanisms to define and revise standards and to inform those affected by the standards about them. It requires mechanisms for the systematic and continuous measurement of those standards and mechanisms to improve performance. Most of all, performance management requires the judicious deployment of fiscal, human, and material resources.

To effectively display resources to manage performance, the organization must refocus its thinking and retool its structure and its operating systems.

This chapter has provided some background on quality in health care. It paves the way to redefine quality in the environmental context of managed care. Chapter 2 addresses the impact of a regulated health care model on traditional quality approaches and describes current initiatives to improve health care performance within a capitated system.

REFERENCES

1. Anderson R: Atlas of the American economy, *Congressional Quarterly*, Washington, D.C., 1994, Elliot & Clark Publishing.
2. Brownisms: words of wisdom on management style, *Hospitals*, p 88, December 5, 1989.
3. Coyne C, Killien M: A system for unit-based monitors of quality of nursing care, *J Nurs Admin*, 17(1): 26-32, 1983.
4. Crosby PB: *Quality is free*, New York, 1979, New American Library.
5. Donabedian A: *The criteria and standards of quality*. In Donabedian A, editor: *Explorations in quality assessment and monitoring*, vol 2, Ann Arbor, Mich, 1982, Health Administration Press.
6. Drucker PF: *Innovation and entrepreneurship*, New York, 1985, Harper & Row.
7. Fiegenbaum AV: *Quality control*, New York, 1951, McGraw-Hill.
8. Fromberg R, editor: *Monitoring and evaluation in nursing services*, 1986, Joint Commission on Accreditation of Hospitals.
9. Garvin DA: Competing on the eight dimensions of quality, *Harvard Bus Rev*, pp 101-109, Nov/Dec 1987.
10. How consumers perceive health care quality, *Hospitals*, p 84, April 5, 1988.
11. Joint Commission on Accreditation of Health Care Organizations: *Lexicon dictionary of health care terms, organizations, and acronyms for the era of reform*, Chicago, 1994, JCAHO.
12. Juran JM: *Juran's quality control handbook*, ed 4, New York, 1988, McGraw-Hill.
13. Kemmel RB: Agreeing on a definition of quality care may be healthcare's biggest challenge, *Modern Healthcare*, p 37, March 24, 1989.
14. Kerfoot K, Rohe D: KAIZEN: innovations for nurse managers to improve productivity, *Nurs Econ* 7(4): 228-230, July-August 1989.
15. Kibbie PE, editor: *Quality assurance, utilization and risk management: a study guide*, 1986, National Association of Quality Assurance Professionals.
16. Koska M: Quality—thy name is nursing care, CEOs say, *Hospitals*, p 32, February 5, 1989.
17. Masaaki I: *KAIZEN: the key to Japan's competitive success*, New York, 1986, Random House.
18. Melum M, Siniores M: The next generation of health care quality, *Hospitals*, p 80, February 5, 1989.
19. *NEWS*. California Hospital Association, Sacramento, 18(21), September 12, 1986.
20. O'Leary D: President's column, *Joint Comm Perspect*, 8(1/2): 2-3, 1988.
21. Patterson CH: Standards of patient care: the Joint Commission's focus on nursing quality assurance, *Nurs Clin North Am* 23(3): 625-637, 1988.
22. Peters T: *Thriving on chaos*, New York, 1988, Alfred A Knopf.
23. Peters T, Waterman R: *In search of excellence*, New York, 1982, Harper & Row.
24. *Productivity and performance management in health care institutions*, 1989, American Hospital Publishing.
25. Quality: how to make it pay, *Business Week*, p 54, August 8, 1994.
26. Schecter E: *Managing for world-class quality*, Milwaukee, 1992, Quality Press.
27. Wagner J: *The search for signs of intelligent life in the universe*, New York, 1986, Harper & Row.

Chapter 2

Redefining Quality in a Managed Care Environment

Nobody likes change but a wet baby.
Roy Blitzer

It is a well-known fact that horses, confronted with a life-threatening stable fire, cannot easily be made to leave the comfort and familiarity of their environment. The very sights, smells, and sounds of the fire, which others recognize as signals to abandon the stable, compel the terrified animals to cling to familiar surroundings. Unless led to safety, these animals will perish, incapable of making the move necessary to save their lives.

The fire of reform has been ignited in the health care industry, and there are a lot of frightened health care professionals out there who are clinging to smoking stalls. Like their equine counterparts, these professionals and the industry as a whole can survive only by abandoning traditional practices.

One of the key strategies in shifting the health care paradigm is the switch from fee-for-service to capitation. A major result of managed health care is the restructuring of traditionally held views and rituals related to health care delivery. Although attempts by the federal government to legislate health care reform "fizzled," the proverbial snowball has been pushed from the top of "The Hill" and it has been gaining momentum ever since, flattening obstacles in its path. Many experts now believe that by the time health care reform is finally legislated, the industry itself will have effected more dramatic change than legislation ever could.[1]

In health care today, changes are occurring at breakneck speed both from within the industry itself and as a result of external pressures. The incentives are changing and there is little time to adjust. Survival depends upon adaptability to change. This chapter explores some of the forces acting upon health care and their impact on quality.

MANAGED CARE DEFINED

"Managed care is a system of cost containment programs . . . It consists of the systems and mechanisms utilized to direct access to the wide range of services and control costs within the health care delivery system . . ."[16]

Managed care is based on a system of capitated costs rather than the traditional cost-based fee-for-service delivery model. Capitation limits the amount of money that a payer will pay for a specific health care service or procedure or a specific episode of illness. This payment mechanism minimizes financial incentives to increase services. Managed care is a system based on providing the highest quality health care services to the largest number of recipients for the lowest possible cost. Managed care is based also on principles related to the care of aggregate populations; "pooled risk" and the importance of outcomes.

The managed care organization (MCO) uses group demographic and financial analysis to calculate for a specific group of people, such as an employee group, what the average cost of providing health care services would be by diagnoses and usage trends. Then it is determined what percentage of the cost the company pays per employee and what percentage the employee pays. The number of individuals enrolled in the plan are referred to as "covered lives."

Providing care for a covered life means that the managed care company allots a set dollar amount per year to pay for that person's health care costs. If the person's health care costs are less than that amount, the managed care company makes money on that covered life. If the costs are more than the allotment, then the company incurs a loss on that covered life. Hopefully the gains outweigh the losses, and with creative budgeting, purchasing, and service delivery, the managed care company makes a profit on providing health care.

Based on the use of cost-containment programs that include guidelines and criteria for health care delivery, managed care incorporates a variety of models and techniques for achieving a quality/cost balance. These include health maintenance organizations (HMOs), preferred provider organizations (PPOs), direct contracting (in which an employer contracts directly with a hospital or other health care facility), bill audits, utilization review, preadmission authorization, concurrent review, retrospective review, second surgical opinions (SSOs), independent medical examinations (IMEs), and case management.[16] The hope is that by shifting from fee-for-service to capitation, providers will have greater incentives to consider variables such as appropriateness and cost when prescribing care.

Employers bear much of the financial burden of rising health care costs, and in this new model they are becoming increasingly involved in cost-reducing activities. Larger employers are turning to self-insurance as a means to control costs, while smaller employers are forming coalitions to purchase health care services more reasonably. This means that more and more the purchaser of health care services is taking an active role in defining what quality is.

Russ Coile recently identified the top 10 trends for the era of capitation. These include the following:

1. State health reform. State legislatures are addressing the health care issue, with at least 20 states enacting some type of reform legislation in 1995.
2. Statewide networks of integrated delivery systems (IDSs). Providers and payers are building these systems to provide the full range of health care services.
3. Independent Physician Organizations (IPOs). Physicians are banding together and forming independent organizations to give them more

clout when negotiating with hospitals and health systems.
4. Types of IDSs: Insurer-led networks, staff model (employed physicians), hospital hub, and spoke regional system. Thomas P. Weil of Bedford Health Associates predicts that almost every hospital in America eventually may be affiliated with a regional network.
5. Community Health Information Networks (CHINs). The information superhighway will link regional and state IDSs. More than 40% of U.S. hospitals are forming CHINs or plan to join one.
6. Provider-sponsored HMOs. Providers are realizing that there are three types of options in the managed care marketplace: HMO owner, HMO partner, and HMO vendor.
7. Global capitation. This type of reimbursement, which covers *all* services, not just primary care and gate keeping, will become the dominant form of provider reimbursement. Providers will accept the full risk for primary care, specialist care, hospitalization, and provision of tertiary services. They will most likely subcontract (subcapitate) for the remaining types of services across the continuum of care.
8. For-profit deal making. Now that national health care reform poses no threats to corporate profits, Coile predicts ongoing mergers and mega-deals among the for-profit organizations.
9. Stage 3 of managed care. As those populations who have not traditionally been enrolled in HMOs succumb and with the traditional target population's enrollees over 100 million, managed care penetration will reach record levels.
10. Payer-provider mergers. These mergers are the last step in full integration. Every IDS must have a financing mechanism that links providers with consumers. By combining reimbursement infrastructures and claims management, the IDSs can potentially reduce their costs by almost 10%.[3]

MANAGED COMPETITION

Managed competition has arisen out of the managed care environment. It refers to the competition generated by the various providers of managed care services. Coined in the late 1970s by Alain Enthoven, the term initially was used to describe agencies that served as brokers. These brokers would examine all the health provider possibilities and negotiate with the various providers to assist the patient in obtaining the best care at the best cost. Today, health insurance purchasing cooperatives (HIPCs) are serving as brokers to small employers and individuals.[8] "Managed competition introduces new criteria for health care decision making and price evaluation and puts control back in the hands of the purchaser."[16]

THE IMPACT OF MANAGED CARE

Health care reform has propelled a domino effect throughout the industry, causing multiple shifts from traditional health care practices. These shifts include

- Revenue to cost center
- Illness response to health promotion
- Hospital-based acute care to ambulatory-based acute care services
- Discipline focus to patient focus
- Episodic to seamless care

Revenue to Cost Centers

Acute care organizations are shifting from revenue centers to cost centers. Traditionally, filling hospital beds made money. However, in a managed care world, a full house is considered a major financial liability. The emphasis is on keeping patients out of the hospital, or if that is not possible, at least to minimize the number of days of hospitalization. Although this drive to reduce length of stay is not new to the industry, the resultant oversupply of hospital beds with subsequent downsizing of staff and closing of not just units but hospitals themselves had not been fully anticipated. "Rightsizing and cost reduction activities are a direct result of managed care with the planned outcomes of reduced lengths of stays and reduced admissions."[22]

Restructuring has struck fear in the hearts of the most venerable institutions and the hardiest of health care professionals, because the effort can often result in a major downsizing project. This fear can paralyze an organization at any or all levels, from the boardroom to the bedside. Maslow's hierarchy kicks in and all efforts are focused on survival.

Edwards and Horn fear that a bottom line approach, often administered by corporate executives who know little or nothing about health and/or care, will have an adverse effect on public health and welfare. They believe that as long as hospital trustees focus on "outperforming" their competitors (market penetration and margin) rather than serving the needs of the community, the health care crisis will continue to spiral out of control.[9]

Low occupancy rates, competitive insurance bidding, high debt service, expensive capital budgets, high labor costs, and large Medicare/Medicaid populations are spawning a financial crises. Knee-jerk reactions for institutions "circling the drain" include closing units, staff layoffs, early retirement programs, and down substitution of care provision. Consolidation through mergers and partnerships has provided some relief for many overextended institutions. Columbia Health Care Corporation merged with Hospital Corporation of America in 1994. This merger consummated a growth curve for Columbia from 12 hospitals in 1991 to 192 in 1994, and the number continues to grow.[15]

Illness Response to Health Promotion

The second major shift is from an illness response system to a health promotion approach. It has been catalyzed by financial liability for covered lives. Those who have been "around the block" in health care have seen an ebb and flow in the emphasis on wellness. However, the financial incentive has never been there before. Now it is. Reducing costly medical care through health awareness and education, screening, and early interventions is a major thrust of capitated care. Thus the health care industry is in the throes of a proliferation of companies aimed at providing services and products ranging from worksite wellness programs to health promotion multimedia kits. The race to provide consumer education is on and the track now resembles the start of the Boston marathon. Issues relating to performance, appropriateness, and demand will determine how many make it to the finish line.

Hospital-Based Acute Care to Ambulatory Acute Care

The third shift involves the move from hospital-based acute care to providing acute care delivery in ambulatory settings. This shift is the result of attempts to reduce the cost of providing medical care. Home care has been targeted as a viable form of providing acute care services, once again spawning a bevy of specialty service companies, providing a range of services from home infusion therapy to hospice services. This shift has also hastened the development of many freestanding ambulatory centers providing acute care, urgent care, surgical procedures, and emergency services. The number of ambulatory surgery centers (ASCs) has more than doubled in just the last 10 years. Other cost-reducing efforts include attempts to redirect patients to appropriate level and type of health care services. Telephone triage and telephony services are surfacing in attempts to discourage inappropriate use of emergency rooms or to reduce unnecessary office visits.

Reducing inappropriate use of high-cost health care professionals is another tactic being implemented. Although it has always been a basic tenet of good management to deliver services through the least costly, most qualified employee, this has not always happened in health care. The use of unlicensed assistive personnel, nurse practitioners, and physician's assistants is gaining acceptance throughout the country.

Discipline Focus to Patient Focus

The fourth shift is one of changing the focus from a discipline driven system to one that is patient focused. Although the intent of health care services has been improved patient outcomes, the proliferation of medical and allied health specialities has contributed to fragmentation of patient care services. Attempts are being made to refocus services on the patient. Many hospitals have addressed the need for customer-driven service, primarily through customer satisfaction analysis and guest relations programs. Clinically, however, efforts to develop interdisciplinary approaches to patient care have been slow to happen. The recent efforts of the Agency for Health Care Policy and Research in the interdisciplinary development of practice guidelines have done much to pave the way for this type of collaboration.

Picker Institute, a not-for-profit affiliate of Beth Israel Hospital in Boston with support from the Commonwealth Fund, defines seven patient care dimensions that dominate one's experience in health care. These include the following:

- Access to care
- Respect for patients' values, preferences, and expressed needs
- Communication between patients and providers
- Physical care, comfort, and alleviation of pain
- Emotional support
- Involvement of family and friends
- Transition and continuity[2]

Many institutions are beginning to develop these types of patient-focused indicators. However, there is still much work to be done in many organizations. Thomas L. Delbanco, MD, Beth Israel Hospital's director of general medicine and primary care, believes that few hospitals are equipped to support patient-centered care.[2]

Proponents of patient-centered care also believe that re-engineering may in fact be stymieing efforts. The truth is probably somewhere in between. Customer satisfaction must coexist peacefully with financial constraints. This can be achieved through a change from episodic care to a carefully managed continuum of patient care services.

Episodic to Seamless Care

The final major shift that has resulted from capitation is the restructuring of care delivery from episodes of care to a seamless continuum.

A component-based, or episodic, approach to quality and cost containment cannot work in managed care. It is too fragmented, consuming valuable resources in often redundant services. What is necessary is an approach that looks at providing seamless health care services.

Seamless service in a managed care environment can be defined through some type of disease management approach, particularly in the chronic disease arena. Disease management is an approach that integrates the components of health care to provide better care at less cost. Disease management attempts to integrate guideline use, outcomes management, and performance improvement. "Disease management applies the principles of continuous quality improvement to the whole spectrum of care for a particular condition, including outpatient, inpatient, and ancillary services. By persuading physicians to follow practice guidelines, measuring the results, and feeding those results back to the doctors, health plans, and medical groups hope to reduce variations in care and produce better outcomes."[24]

Disease management "represents the continuing evolution of managed care, from reviewing components of utilization to developing a broader perspective of what happens to patients as they move through the health care system."[24] Rather than managing episodes of care, which may ultimately result in higher long-term costs, a disease management approach applies the principles of performance improvement to the entire spectrum of care for a specific disease.

Rather than trying to improve quality across service lines, a disease management approach focuses on the patient and attempts to improve quality along disease-specific lines. Diseases that are the most expensive to treat and that involve wide practice variations have been the first under scrutiny. It is the Pareto principle exemplified and a basic principle of most quality improvement efforts. By focusing on the few disorders that generate most of the service utilization, better results can be obtained more cost-effectively. Chronic problems such as diabetes, asthma, and hypertension are getting priority attention. The focus of programs aimed at these disorders is to help patients manage their conditions and stay out of the hospital.

Although support for disease management is growing rapidly, there currently exists little hard core data that shows it saves money. However, that data is being compiled by a variety of proponents.

Using the Health Plan Employer Data and Information Set (HEDIS) 2.0 performance criteria compiled for 90 of the 139 health plans that serve GTE corporation, Dwight McNeill, a manager at GTE, ranked the plans and found that those in the top quartile had lower premiums and lower price increases last year than those ranked further down. The Mayo Clinic guideline on urinary tract infections saved $60,000 during a 6-month trial of 35,000 patient visits. Harvard Community Health Plan (HCHP) reduced its hospital admission rate for pediatric asthmatics by 25% and for adults by 10% by using an asthma management plan.[21]

Concerns have been expressed that in the short term, disease management may actually increase costs because of the elimination of practice variance and the identification of previously misdiagnosed and/or inappropriately treated patients. The industry is not waiting for proof that disease management is cost-effective. Many HMOs are already in the process of implementing or considering the development of disease management systems. These include Health Partners in Minneapolis, Group Health Cooperative of Puget Sound in Seattle, the Lovelace Health System in Albuquerque, HCHP in Massachusetts, and Kaiser Permanente's northern California division.

INTEGRATED DELIVERY SYSTEMS

As stated previously, inherent in any disease management system is the basic assumption of a continuum of services. These services are being provided through integrated delivery systems.

Many of the past problems with health care systems stemmed from fragmentation of services, duplication, gaps in coverage, and care continuity. Integration is a vital key to resolving these problems within the delivery system. Mergers and alliances aimed at integration of provider organizations and networks are a daily occurrence in an attempt to design one-stop, one-shop health care. An integrated delivery system is one that provides all types and levels of health care services within the same health care plan. Those services include everything from preventive screening to acute care, critical care, home care, subacute care, long-term care, and hospice.

Delivery system integration is coming from both the demand and the supply side. Purchasers, such as employers, purchasing alliances, insurance companies, HMOs, and other payers, as well as providers, such as hospitals, physicians, multiprovider networks, HMOs, and PPOs, are pushing for integration. As HMOs, PPOs, and integrated delivery systems (IDSs) compete for more of the prepaid health care market, seamless, gap-free delivery systems that provide A to Z health care services are beginning to emerge. These systems will provide not only primary and secondary services but also tertiary, community, and home care as well.[4]

Systems are looking for cost-effective ways of providing services for "covered lives" regardless of the cause. "Cost effectiveness activities are part of a new culture in which every member of the organization is committed to finding ways to reduce costs and add value, while we focus on continually improving the quality of patient care and our patient/family satisfaction."[22]

This integrated approach strives not only to evoke higher customer satisfaction but also to give the provider a "leg up" in the managed competition arena.

THE GOVERNMENT'S ROLE IN QUALITY

The government plays a powerful role in structuring the community of professional, industry, purchaser, and consumer groups interested in quality. By promoting and regulating disclosure, government can create dialogues between hospitals and purchasers. Stephen Jencks suggests that the government may shape hospital accountability by (a) mandating uniform performance measurement and disclosure, (b) replacing emphasis on minimum standards with emphasis on improvement, (c) changing the structure of certification requirements, (d) requiring participation in performance improvement activities, and (e) funding new performance improvement structures.[11]

"As the language of 'quality' has shifted from quality assurance to quality improvement to performance management, the role of the government has also shifted . . . Strategies include not only stimulating a market force for improvement by publishing performance information but also providing technical assistance and nonpublic information."[11]

In 1989 Congress passed the Omnibus Reconciliation Act (OBRA). Part of this legislation created the Agency for Health Care Policy and Research (AHCPR) as the eighth agency of the federal government Dept. of Public Health. AHCPR serves as the federal government's linchpin for health services research. It was designed to expand the work of its predecessor, the National Center for Health Services Research and Technology Assessment.

AHCPR's mission is to enhance the quality of patient care services through improved knowledge that can be used in meeting society's health care needs. The impact of this agency on performance is felt by the setting of professional practice standards by spearheading the development of clinical practice guidelines; by researching medical effectiveness through the agency's Medical Treatment Effectiveness Program (MEDTEP); and through the development of Patient Outcome Research Teams (PORTS), multi-disciplinary task forces that define and evaluate patient outcomes for specific disorders that result from variations in practice patterns.

During the 1980s Medicare's PROs dominated quality assurance and were based primarily on the "bad apple" theory. The major current government effort in technical assistance is the Medicare Health Care Quality Improvement Program (HCQIP). It attempts to emphasize professional review rather than performance improvement by focusing on processes of care instead of on negative outcomes.

Although private groups such as the Joint Commission and the National Committee on Quality Assurance can establish performance measures and offer accreditation to health care facilities, only the government can require those facilities to collect data and disclose performance measurements. State governments license hospitals, whereas the federal government is responsible for setting standards for its entitlement programs, such as Medicare and/or Medicaid. However, the federal government's efforts are akin to licensure. Since few hospitals can financially forego Medicare participation, compliance with these government standards are critical for fiscal survival. So far the federal government has not mandated collection and disclosure, but Medicare does require submission of billing data that have been used to compute standardized mortality measures.

"Almost certainly, the next few years will see a growing governmental role in standardizing and using quality performance measures. This role will likely be part of a public-private partnership that will evolve . . . over the coming decade."[11]

In 1986 the National Association of Health Data Organizations (NAHDO) was established to support state data organizations (SDOs) and to promote the development and enhancement of publicly accessible databases at the state level. The term *state data organization* refers to the state agencies that, at a minimum, are mandated to maintain statewide hospital use, hospital financial databases, or both. By early 1994, 38 states had invested in data collection, analysis, and dissemination on the use, cost, effectiveness, and performance of hospitals.[10]

A hospital discharge database, the most common type, includes demographic, clinical, identifier, and billing and payer data for each patient's hospital stay. Although hospitals collect these data for administrative purposes, the data also provide information on service use, charges, and organizational performance.

The typical report produced by an SDO includes hospital-specific experience by diagnosis or diagnosis-related group (DRG) and surgical procedure by volume of services/procedures and total charge. Standard reports include

- Charge and volume of services/surgical procedures by hospital
- Patient origin studies by geographic area
- Length of stay, occupancy, and number of admissions.[10]

Although many states have focused on basic data, such as all payer hospital discharge data, others, such as Iowa and Pennsylvania, have mandated collection under commercial systems that adjust for differences in risk. Others, such as New York, have developed their own systems.

Many states treat average performance rather than best achievable performance as the reference standard, and no known governmental group to date has used its data to establish benchmarks or best achievable performance levels.

ERISA

Although many states are interested in implementing health system changes, their efforts, for now at least, have been constrained by the 1974 Employee Retirement Income Security Act (ERISA). This act prohibits states from regulating the health-benefit plans of companies that self-insure.

Whereas the states feel that ERISA will stifle their reform efforts, employers contend that ERISA has enabled them to develop innovative health benefits programs. Also, many employees feel that state control of self-funded health plans may increase costs. The box on p. 18 summarizes the opposing perspectives of business and states. Congress faces a dilemma as it tries to reconcile the differences related to ERISA between states and the business community.

ERISA exempted employers' self-insured benefits plans from state oversight. This became problematic as the number of self-funded programs dramatically increased during the last decade.

> Today roughly half of all employees in the U.S. are covered under self-funded ERISA qualifying plans. As the self-insurance movement has gained momentum, its ERISA protection has been upheld in the courts, including the Supreme Court. But as the volume of ERISA case law grows, so does the conflicting nature of the results with sometimes desperate decisions.
>
> Conflict over ERISA's impact on managed care also has heated up as that industry has grown. ERISA has left self-insured employers free to enter into a variety of arrangements with the managed care industry virtually without state regulation.[19]

Some skeptical health care professionals feel that ERISA's preemption of state laws will enable fraudulent self-insured plans to "siphon off millions through excessive administrative costs, unauthorized participants or outright embezzlement and the state laws don't apply!"[7]

Leah Curtin, in a recent editorial, quotes the FBI director who told Senate committee members that drug dealers in California and southern Florida have switched to health care fraud schemes because they can make as much or more money and there is far less chance of being caught.[7]

TWO PERSPECTIVES

Businesses and States See the Health-Care Provisions of ERISA from Very Different Vantage Points

From employers' vantage point, the statute

- Eliminates inconsistencies among state laws and the overlap of federal and state statutes that regulate benefit plans, thus relieving purchasers and providers of a tangle of compliance responsibilities.
- Creates a stable and consistent foundation for employer innovations in managing benefits and containing costs.
- Reduces the cost of regulation for purchasers, providers, and taxpayers.
- Gets around such state-erected obstacles as benefit mandates and managed care laws that could hinder development of cost-effective benefit plans and organized delivery systems.
- Precludes barriers to the free movement of health care goods and services in interstate commerce.

From the states' point of view, however, ERISA

- Allows self-insured firms to conduct health-benefit programs with virtually no federal or state oversight or regulation.

- Undermines proper legal redress for plan enrollees who allege denial of covered care.
- Raises costs for small businesses that cannot afford to self-insure, by reducing the community pool and hindering health reforms.
- Thwarts state efforts to contain costs and expand affordable care to the uninsured because it undermines insurance reform, community rating, and efforts to raise revenues to pay for expanded coverage.
- Prevents state or federal efforts to create a meaningful national package of standard or minimum benefits.
- Keeps states from collecting complete and uniform data on claims, utilization, and medical outcomes.
- Precludes employer mandates as a means to bring about universal coverage.
- Hamstrings state efforts to oversee health-care delivery.
- Defeats initiatives that would impose state tort or contract law on the relationship between self-funded plans and beneficiaries.

Critics of ERISA also cite that recent lawsuits attempting to broaden the reach of ERISA by making a violation any state law that imposes costs in health providers and thus higher costs for self-funded employers. One could interpret that broadening to include any state law that would increase the expenses of an MCO as an ERISA violation.

Twenty-eight states to date have passed any willing provider (AWP) laws that require MCOs to contract with any provider willing to abide by the terms the MCOs impose. It is sort of like an equal opportunity law. Self-insured employers contend that these laws impede the MCOs' ability to contract with the most cost-effective providers and essentially violate the ERISA law. This battle is being waged in courtrooms around the country.

Whether ERISA is part of the problem or the solution remains to be seen. Either way, by tackling ERISA, Congress could play a major role in the future direction of health care delivery.[19]

DEVELOPMENT OF REPORT CARDS

With annual spending for health care approaching $1 trillion, the public cry for accountability is finally being heard. However, no voice is louder than that of employers, many of whose health expenditures now exceed their gross profits. As a result, providers are feverishly attempting to prove the quality of their delivery systems. Many are seeking objective performance measures or indicators, also called *report cards.*

"Performance measures are 'in'—whether they reflect outcomes, selected processes, patient satisfaction, functional status, or yet-to-be-determined measurement dimensions. A variety of environmental, political, and professional factors will keep performance measures 'in' for the foreseeable future (read: at least a decade and probably many decades)."[16]

The requirements for a useful report card are the following:

- reliability
- relevance
- prediction
- definitions
- improvement utility[17]

There are many advantages to the report card system. These include that report cards

- help purchasers and providers decide where to "shop" for high-value care.
- hold providers accountable for outcomes and cost.
- document trends in outcomes and cost.
- identify areas of provider strength and opportunities for improvement.
- identify benchmarking sources.[17]

An inherent disadvantage is the retrospective nature, which limits report cards' predictive value. Other disadvantages relate to the state of the science itself.

The number of agencies developing report cards is growing. Perhaps the three largest projects related to performance measure development are the Consortium Research on Indicators of System Performance (CRISP), the Health Plan Employer Data and Information Set (HEDIS), and the Joint Commission's Indicator Measurement System (IMSystem).

CRISP

CRISP links measurement standards to the qualitative themes expressed in an organization's mission statement. It is composed of 23 vertically integrated health care systems formed for the purpose of testing and refining a set of system-level performance measures. The project was launched in 1991 to ensure the performance accountability of large vertically integrated systems. A conceptual framework and 91 indicators were developed that were performance-based and quantitative. These indicators were organized around a "generic" mission statement (see box below) in an effort to link performance measurement to stated goals for which a system should be "willingly" held accountable.[18]

Within each area of system mission, three or four performance attributes and specific numeric indicators were defined. Eighteen volunteer systems began using the indicators in 1992.

HEDIS

In November 1993 the National Committee for Quality Assurance (NCQA) released a document titled *The Health Plan Employer Data and Information Set Version 2.0 (HEDIS 2.0)*. This document outlines a core set of health plan performance measures. Selection for inclusion in HEDIS 2.0 was based on three criteria:

1. relevance and value to the employer community
2. reasonable ability of health plans to develop and provide the requested data in the specified manner
3. potential impact on improving patient care and reducing morbidity and mortality.

By recommending standardized definitions and specific methodologies, HEDIS enables plans and employers to trend health plan performance and use them comparatively. Ongoing updates of HEDIS are indicated by changes in its numbering (2.5, 3.0) and continue to refine and expand the measures.

Many of the performance measures cover a broad spectrum of subjects, including prevention, acute illness, chronic illness, mental health, and substance abuse. Many of the measures address public health concerns such as childhood immunization; medical processes for which there is a known relationship between process and outcome, such as annual eye care for diabetics; and clinical areas of concern to the employer community, such as mental illness. For each quality measure, two measurement strategies are recommended: chart review and administrative data.

In addition to the technical quality measures, access to services and enrollee satisfaction were considered. A section is also devoted to specifications and formats for reporting descriptive information on a health plan's membership and its utilization of services. HEDIS requests that health plans report summary financial statistics, such as plan revenues, reserves, short-term liquidity, and capital structure.[5]

IMSystem

The Joint Commission's (JCAHO) IMSystem is a performance measurement system that attempts to integrate standards and performance measures into a substantive evaluation process. This system is designed to become an integral part of the JCAHO's accreditation process. The system will include a variety of performance measures, not merely those developed in the first phase of their own indicator development process. There has been a shift in focus from JCAHO indicator development to the testing of performance measures developed by others for possible inclusion in the IMSystem.[20] The IMSystem includes not only the indicators developed by the JCAHO (see indicator boxes in Chapter 9), but also those of other organizations meeting preset criteria for indicators.

CRISP'S GENERIC MISSION STATEMENT

To enable a given population to **maximize its present and future health** and provide tangible **benefit to the community,** the health system will provide the **highest quality service** to **prevent episodes of illness** and **provide coordinated episodes of care** in a way that **satisfies and delights both clients and system staff,** with **efficient use of resources, appropriate facilities and labor capacity,** and **financial performance** to maintain and improve the above activities, while continuing to **support research and education.**

From Nerenz DR, Zajac BM, Rosman HS: Consortium research on indicators of system performance, *The Joint Commission Journal on Quality Improvement* 19(12): 577-585, 1993.

Additional Report Card Efforts

In addition to these, there are others who have initiated work in the arena of performance measurement. For example:

- The Health Care Financing Administration (HCFA) is investigating the feasibility of developing a report card for Medicare MCOs.
- The Managed Health Care Association's (MHCA) Outcomes Management Systems Project is a nationwide collaboration between 13 major employers and 16 managed care companies. It uses quality measures from the Health Outcomes Institute.
- The AHCPR is exploring the potential for developing a report card for the nation's health care delivery system.

The box below lists some of the individual states that have developed some type of report card.

Managed care organizations have picked up the gauntlet and joined the battle cry for comparative

STATE-SPECIFIC INITIATIVES IN REPORT CARDS

- **California:** Issued its first hospital outcomes report in December 1993. Updates will be developed.
- **Florida:** Health care reform initiative includes performance reports.
- **Iowa:** Released its first hospital outcomes report in 1992.
- **Maryland:** The Maryland Quality Indicator Project (MQIP) began in 1985 as a pilot study for seven hospitals. The inpatient and ambulatory measurement program has grown to include over 950 hospitals nationwide and overseas.
- **New England:** The Harvard Community Health Plan, a coalition of payers and providers, released its first report on HEDIS performance measures in 1994, comparing care delivered by 15 health plans providing care for over 3 million enrollees.
- **Ohio:** Cleveland Health Quality Choice, a coalition of employers and health care providers, began releasing severity-adjusted reports on mortality, length of stay, and patient satisfaction for 29 hospitals in the greater Cleveland area. In June 1994 they released the third report on hospital outcomes and efficiency.
- **Pennsylvania:** Pennsylvania Health Care Cost Containment Council (PHC4) has released four hospital-specific reports on mortality and other outcomes.

data. In November 1993 the Northern California Region of Kaiser Permanente released its report card, offering more than 100 quantitative indicators of clinical and service performance. Other managed care groups that have released quality data include Group Health Cooperative of Puget Sound, Harvard Community Health Plan, and Methodist Hospital of Minneapolis.

The list of individual states, organizations, and MCOs that are compiling data is growing steadily. However, some questions still remain to be answered, such as these:

- Should quality be measured at the level of MDs, of hospitals, of systems, of plans, or of communities?
- By "quality" do we mean the competent execution of critical processes or the improvement of a person's health and well-being?
- Is clinical quality consistent with the patient's perceptions of quality (satisfaction)?
- Is the improvement of quality primarily the responsibility of the government, the health plan, the MD, or the facility?
- Will greater consumer information about quality actually change purchasing decisions or how people select doctors or hospitals?
- Are the internal objectives of quality improvement compatible with the marketplace and governmental demands for accountability?[13]

The development of report cards is "a positive response to legitimate customer needs and requirements for comparative information on quality and costs."[17]

Nelson[17] lists the following concerns that report cards

- cause consumers to be misled.
- are used as an approach for finding "bad apple" providers.
- include data because it is available rather than because it provides quantifiable answers to critical questions.
- show that improvements are needed but do not show how to make improvements.
- can be unreliable: without independent, impartial third party analysis, results can be manipulated to achieve a competitive edge.
- add unnecessary costs.

An additional concern relates to data reliability issues, e.g., variation in the interpretation of indicator definitions and the need for clearer definitions and inclusion and exclusion of criteria so that comparisons may be made on comparable data.

BUSINESS COALITIONS IN HEALTH CARE

"As early supporters of publicly sponsored databases, they [coalitions] were in the forefront of collecting comparative information on hospital performance."[5]

The development of business coalitions in health care has emerged as another major managed care trend. These coalitions initially developed in the late 1970s and early 1980s in response to spiraling health care costs. As nonprofit community-based membership organizations, health care coalitions attempt to manage the cost and quality of health care. In these organizations, employers work with other employers and health care providers. They engage in data collection and reporting activities, purchasing, and education. Some are involved in selective contracting for hospital, physician, prescription drug, and other ancillary services.[6]

The National Business Coalition on Health (NBCH), founded in 1989, serves as a coalition of coalitions with the major mission of facilitating communication and sharing among coalitions on issues related to specific projects, public policy and management.

The major efforts of the coalitions have focused on quality data projects, such as that of the Cleveland Health Quality Choice Program. This program using the Community Health Management Information Systems (CHMIS), an effort funded by the John A. Hartford Foundation, includes electronic transaction systems that link purchasers and payers to expedite benefit eligibility and claims payments. It also includes an information highway to disseminate clinical information and a data repository where employers, providers, insurers, consumers, and the government can access provider performance data. States implementing CHMIS include Iowa, Minnesota, New York, Ohio, Vermont, and Washington. Numerous other states are developing variations of this system for their own use.

Group purchasing activities are another of the functions of coalitions. More than 24 cities, including Milwaukee, Detroit, Chicago, Denver, and Birmingham, are involved in some type of group purchasing.

The third major area of activity involves education, specifically consumer education regarding quality of care. Coalitions in cities such as St. Louis and Seattle have developed consumer education programs that are being adopted nationally.[6]

The future of coalitions is uncertain. Group purchasing activities could end as large employers are required to buy care either on their own or through state-established health purchasing alliances, or they could be strengthened by offering a viable alternative to publicly established purchasing alliances.

Direct Contracting

Direct contracting is a strategy that is gaining in popularity. Anecdotal evidence indicates this strategy can reduce costs. In 1997 the Business Health Care Action Group (BHCAG) in Minneapolis will launch one of the most ambitious direct contracting programs in the nation. Direct contracting bypasses the mega-managed care firms and deals directly with the providers. "This has the potential to completely change the way health care is delivered in Minneapolis and in any other area where there is a mature managed care market," according to Mark Skubic, vice president of public policy and government relations for Health System Minnesota.[25]

Opponents of direct contracting argue that if a group of providers agrees to be responsible for a given set of health care services, then the group is acting as an insurer. Insurance regulators are concerned about an unauthorized group assuming risk and not complying with insurance regulations. The providers counter that they are not pooling risk as an insurance company would but rather are providing specific services requested by employers.[21]

Business and Health Magazine conducted a survey in 1994 on the subject of direct contracting with employers and health plans. Sixty-six hospitals responded.

Fifty-seven percent (57%) of the surveyed hospitals had direct contracts with employers, up from 36% of respondents to a similar study in 1993. Only 13, however, had direct contracts with business coalitions and 16 with other health care buyers, including labor unions and third-party administrators.[14]

There are four major types of direct contract payment arrangement capitation: DRG-based (diagnoses-related group–based) fixed rates, per-diem rates, and straight discounts on billed charges. In this study approximately 77% chose discounts, probably the least effective tool for holding down costs.

Although the most popular choice, discounts can expose an employer to unlimited fee-for-service charges, with no control on volume of services and no way to prevent having the discount based on inflated prices.

"A DRG arrangement doesn't limit volume, either, but at least it fixes the price of each service or procedure. Capitation puts a ceiling on an employer's total health care costs and per diems make costs more predictable."[14]

Despite increasing use, direct contracting is still new enough that many employers are just beginning to learn how to interpret and use hospital quality data. In this survey, only a handful of hospitals had received a request from an employer regarding their data on quality, and none had expressed skepticism regarding the ability of employers, business coalitions, or even insurers to interpret performance data. Providers suggest that the requesting payer meet with the provider to review the significance of the data.

Whichever way one chooses to approach this argument, the concepts of cutting out the middleman and employers contracting with providers are trends to watch.

FORECASTING THE FUTURE OF QUALITY IN MANAGED CARE

The quality gurus agree that quality is not an isolated department as it had been in the past. Nor is it the sole responsibility of the front-line worker. Rather, trends indicate that responsibility for quality in the future is shared by both front-line personnel and management.

When asked about the future of quality, Philip Crosby stated that quality will become an integral part of what managers do for a living. "Executives have to worry about only three things: finance, quality, and relationships."[1] He believes that while management has always been concerned with cost, it has taken a more functional approach to quality and relationships, relegating these issues to a specific department, such as the quality department or the human resources department.

Fiegenbaum also discusses the transformation taking place in the executive leadership of quality. He predicts an emphasis on affordable quality. He describes the need for a shift from a "we'll make it right" approach, and he believes that warranties will not work anymore. Given today's convenience-oriented society, the mere promise of fixing poor products or service is no longer valued. The customer wants it "right" the first time, every time.

In his final public speaking appearance at the American Society of Quality Control Annual Quality Congress, J.M. Juran discussed the upcoming century of quality. He suggested the following to meet the challenges of the 21st century:

- The entire managerial hierarchy must be trained to manage for quality.
- The upper managers must personally take charge of managing for quality, much as they have long done in managing for finance.
- The business plan must be enlarged to include quality goals.
- Managing for quality must be integrated into managing the business.
- Quality improvement must become an ongoing process, year after year.
- New measures must be created to enable upper managers to follow the progress of parameters such as customer satisfaction, competitive quality,

performance of business processes, and cost of poor quality.
- Members of the work force must be given the training and empowerment needed to enable them to participate widely in job planning and improvement.
- The reward system must be revised to take into account the changes in job functions and responsibility.[12]

Although there is nothing earth-shattering about this list and although we have heard many of these ideas before, the challenge is to do all of this in a time of turmoil in health care. Balancing the business goals and needs of today while positioning the organization for tomorrow is not a task for the weak-hearted.

Many initially looked to the quality movement as the quick fix. Many paid lip service to quality improvement efforts but never changed the culture of the organization to reflect a lifelong commitment to improving the organization's performance. Stratton states, "The common practice is to compare financial performance with quality."[23] When they do not improve together, the value of quality is quickly dismissed.

There are those who have questioned whether the quality movement will survive capitation. The traditional approaches to quality assurance cannot. Managed care is here to stay. What is needed to survive in a managed care world is managed performance. Managed performance revolves around critical processes and cost. It is the fiscal responsibility and accountability as well as performance responsibility and accountability through which an organization provides value-driven service.

This paradigm of managed care has opened numerous opportunities for the development of new approaches to health care delivery. What is needed is a mechanism to monitor these new approaches that is itself seamless as the delivery system it serves. As was mentioned earlier in this chapter, many of the past problems with the health care system stemmed from fragmentation, redundancy, and gaps in coverage and in service continuity. The same can be said of the traditional approach to quality.

Just as integration is vital to resolving service delivery problems, so too is it vital to resolving the problems that exist in administering that service delivery. Chapter 3 describes an integrated approach to performance management for the new era of health care business.

REFERENCES

1. Axland S: Forecasting the future of quality, *Quality Progress,* 26(2): 21-25, 1993.
2. Bell CW: Crusade continues for patient-centered care, *Modern Healthcare,* p 25, May 29, 1995.

3. Coile R: Health care 1995: top 10 trends for the ERA of capitation, *Aspen Publishers Special Report,* Bowie, Md, 1995, Aspen Publishers.

4. Coleman J: Integration trends are reshaping MCOs—and may change CMs as well, *The Case Manager,* pp 34-37, Jan/Feb/Mar 1995.

5. Corrigan JM, Nielsen DM: Toward the development of uniform reporting standards for managed care organizations: the health plan employer data and information set (version 2.0), *The Joint Commission Journal on Quality Improvement,* 19(12): 566-575, 1993.

6. Cronin C: Business coalitions in health: their activities and impact, *The Joint Commission Journal on Quality Improvement,* 20(7): 376-380, 1994.

7. Curtin LL: Doctor Godfather, *Nursing Management,* 26(8): 7-8, 1995.

8. Custer WS: Health care reform: managed competition and beyond, *EBRI Issue Brief,* 135: 4-7, 1993.

9. Edwards DS, Horn PA: War on many fronts troubling trends in health care delivery, *J Nurs Adm,* 25(5): 5-7, 1995.

10. Epstein MH, Kurtzig BS: Statewide health information: a tool for improving hospital accountability, *The Joint Commission Journal on Quality Improvement,* 20(7): 370-375, 1994.

11. Jencks SE: The government's role in hospital accountability for quality care, *The Joint Commission Journal on Quality Improvement,* 20(7): 364-369, 1994.

12. Juran JM: The upcoming century of quality, *Quality Progress,* 27(8): 29-37, 1994.

13. Lansky D: Health care quality: all dressed up with nowhere to go in quality improvement in health care: the year behind, the year ahead, *The Joint Commission Journal on Quality Improvement,* 21(1): 32-33, 1995.

14. Leavenworth G: Direct contracting, *Business & Health,* pp 31-32, Feb 1995.

15. Lutz S: Industry follows, fears the leader, *Modern Healthcare,* p 23, 1994.

16. Mullahy CM: *The case manager's handbook,* Gaithersburg, Md, 1995, Aspen Publishers, Inc.

17. Nelson EC et al: Report cards or instrument panels who needs what, *The Joint Commission Journal on Quality Improvement,* 21(4): 155-166, 1995.

18. Nerenz DR, Zajac BM, Rosman HS: Consortium research on indicators of system performance, *The Joint Commission Journal on Quality Improvement,* 19(12): 577-585, 1993.

19. O'Keefe AM: Will ERISA's wall come tumbling down? *Business & Health,* pp 35-40, Feb 1995.

20. O'Leary DS: President's column, *Joint Commission Perspectives,* 14(5): 2-3, 1994.

21. Scott L: Disease management faces obstacles, *Modern Healthcare,* pp 30-33, June 12, 1995.

22. Sovie M: Tailoring hospitals for managed care and integrated health systems, *Nursing Economics,* 13(2): 72-82, 1995.

23. Stratton B: Why you can't link quality improvement to financial performance, *Quality Progress,* 26(2): 5, 1993.

24. Terry K: Disease management, *Business & Health,* pp 65-72, April 1995.

25. Weissenstein E: Cut out the middleman, *Modern Healthcare,* pp 28-30, July 3, 1995.

Chapter 3

THE BLUEPRINT for Performance Management

*If you always do what you've always done,
you'll always get what you've always gotten.*
Jay Katz

The classic book by Ayn Rand, *The Fountainhead*, portrays architects as a group of traditionalists whose creativity is constrained by their inability to let go of the past. The book describes professionals receiving accolades for creating buildings that are clones of those of ancient Greece and Rome. Only one architect, Howard Roark, creates bold, innovative designs. The profession, however, does not recognize the value of Roark's talent and rejects his work. The climax comes when Roark secretly agrees to design, free of charge, a low-income housing project. He receives a promise that the project will be built **exactly** as designed with no changes to his specifications.

As the project proceeds, alterations are made to Roark's design to conform with surrounding buildings. Appalled and embarrassed by the finished project, Roark reduces the building to a heap of rubble in a spectacular dynamite blast. The book concludes with Roark's arrest and dramatic trial in which he successfully defends his actions.

This story could just as easily have been scripted about the status of the quality movement in health care today. Just as the architects in *The Fountainhead* could not conceive of a building without historical influence, the traditionalists in health care are often hesitant to accept new ideas that deviate from "the

way we've always done it here." New approaches to performance management are often molded into the accepted ways of doing things, just as Roark's buildings were redesigned with pediments, cornices, and cherubs.

Frequently, an organization will superimpose one performance improvement project onto an existing one. For instance, we have encountered many institutions that have tried to piggyback a performance improvement program onto an existing quality improvement program. Others have interspersed and overlapped customer service initiatives, employee satisfaction studies, restructuring and reengineering projects concurrently with no interface among the efforts. Many times these efforts can be working at odds with each other and with the ultimate mission and goals of the organization. This fragmentation provides shifting sand upon which to build a successful enterprise.

The key to achieving true quality in health care lies in the ability of an organization to design and implement a new paradigm, managed performance. Quality is defined by performance dimensions. Gone are the days of grappling with the quality/cost dilemma. It does not exist anymore. The *managed* in *managed care* refers to attempts at controlling costs while maintaining a level of performance that meets customer expectations. This objective is synonymous with managed performance. The framework of managed performance is an effective performance management system. "Performance is viewed as the all-important concept underlying the survival and viability of an organization in a competitive environment."[1]

Performance can be defined as the application of inherent and/or learned capabilities that enable an individual, group, or organization to carry a process through to completion according to its specifications. Capabilities refer to essential knowledge, skills, and attitudes. Performance management is a standards-based approach to the reduction of process variance and the improvement of process capability. Process variance is the inevitable differences among individual outputs of a process, whereas process capability refers to the measured built-in reproducibility of the outcome of a process.[4] In other words, a performance management system focuses on the awareness, measurement, and improvement of critical capabilities.

In 1994 McDonald, Thuld, and Smith analyzed 437 companies, comparing those who had performance management systems and those who did not. They found companies that used performance management systems had greater profits, better cash flow, stronger stock market performance, greater stock value, and higher productivity than those who did not.[6a]

Risher believes that this new paradigm is "leading us from the old military model toward an enlightened, empowered philosophy (most organizations fall somewhere in the middle of this spectrum)."[8] Experience confirms that peak performance in health care requires all employees at all levels doing their jobs differently and better than they ever have. This means that peak performance becomes an organizational priority that is communicated throughout the organization. Although the system will play out differently in different organizations, the purpose is singular: to improve organizational performance by helping individuals improve their performance.[8] This chapter describes one such performance management system: THE BLUEPRINT for Performance Management.

COMPONENTS OF PERFORMANCE MANAGEMENT

An effective performance management system is composed of two critical components and three major programs. The two components include standards/specifications and scope. The three programs include performance awareness, performance measurement, and performance improvement.

Standards

A performance management system is built upon clearly defined standards. A *standard* is a written value consisting of the rules that apply to key processes, the processes themselves, and the results that can be expected when those processes are enacted according to specifications.[5] There are three types of standards: structure, process, and outcomes.

Structure standards outline the legal parameters that govern performance expectations of both the organization and its employees. They include the mission, philosophy, goals, policies, and job descriptions of an organization.

Process standards outline how the performance capabilities of the organization and its employees are operationalized. Process is how one gets from "here" to "there." Procedures, practice guidelines, plans, and documentation are process standards. Clearly defining the types of processes and the actions involved in each is the first step in eliminating process variation.

Outcome standards define the results that can be expected if a process is carried out according to its specifications. They are used to benchmark performance.

The development of these three types of standards are discussed fully in Chapter 8.

Scope

The second critical component of an effective performance management system is scope. Scope is the range of performance that the performance management system controls. Many organizations limit their measurement efforts to the clinical domain and have focused on staff performance as the chief cause of problems. As the science of performance management evolves, however, more and more we have come to appreciate that the system is often the culprit. The results of analyzing the root causes of problems throughout the 1980s led many quality professionals to develop a truism called the 85/15 rule. The rule reflects evidence clearly indicating that errors are caused by people problems only about 15% of the time. More than 85% of the time, the root cause is found in organizational systems, processes, or structure.[2]

For example, an infection control department discovered a sudden, dramatic increase in urinary tract infections in catheterized patients. Alarmed, the administration devoted time, money, and staff to remedying the "poor nursing care." After weeks of investigation of the nursing staff, however, no breach of practice could be located. Further review uncovered that the "sterile" urinary catheters, in their unopened state, were contaminated and were the source of the infections.

Sometimes the cause of a less-than-optimal outcome lies in the customer. "Bad" anatomy and noncompliance are two patient-related causes of poor performance.

Given the fact that the root of performance problems may lie in the customer, the staff, or the system, the scope of the performance management system should include all three.

Health care is a service delivery business and the scope of any business includes

- Someone to receive the service: the customer
- Someone to deliver the service: the employees
- Someone to manage the service: the managers[5]

Therefore, it makes sense that in creating performance awareness and measuring and improving performance, a tri-focus approach is needed.

This tri-focus approach represents three distinct yet interrelated domains of the business: the service domain, the practice domain, and the governance domain. The service domain focuses on the customer; the practice domain focuses on the employees; and the governance domain focuses on the administration, or governance, of the business.

Attempts to reduce process variation and improve process capability must by necessity include all three domains. New tools such as the cause and effect diagram (explained in Chapter 11) are useful to ensure a tri-focus approach to process variation analysis.

Performance Management System

There are three important programs associated with a performance management system: performance awareness, performance measurement, and performance improvement. To be truly comprehensive, a performance management system includes all three. This was one of the reasons that the traditional approach to quality assurance was doomed. Measurement alone is insufficient to improve performance. It is like a coach who looks only at the stats, without analyzing the play-by-play and devising a counterattack. The stats alone never helped a losing team improve their game.

To omit one of the three programs seriously hinders the ability of the organization to affect its performance level. Many organizations have instituted activities in all of these areas. Unfortunately, the attempts are often fragmented. The key to an effective performance management system lies in having all three programs. Just like the steel girders, wooden studs, concrete, and bricks needed to work in unison to create a magnificent edifice, these three programs must come together to create a meaningful performance management system. Figure 3-1 diagrams the relationship among

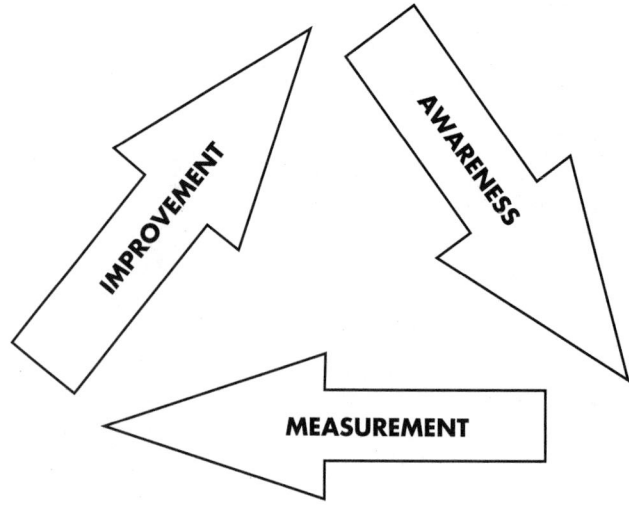

Figure 3-1   Three programs of a performance management system.

awareness, measurement, and improvement. Although we describe these as separate programs conceptually, in actual practice they blend together to form a seamless continuum.

Performance awareness

Before any measurement can occur, there must be something to measure. The performance awareness program consists of a number of important steps:

1. Identification of the customer(s) and the scope of services provided by the organization (department)
2. Identification and prioritization of key functions and critical processes
3. Development and dissemination of structure, process, and outcome standards

The performance awareness program serves as the basis for defining performance expectations. It begins with a clear definition of whom the organization is serving. It includes all customers of the organization, both internal and external. There are a number of tools that are helpful to implement this program. These include such tools as the flowchart, key process matrix, and indicator development form.

Once the customer base has been defined, the organization outlines the scope of its major services and the key functions that it performs within those services. Processes for each function are defined and prioritized. It is then that performance standards/specifications can be set for critical processes.

Once the performance standards have been defined, the staff members of the organization are educated regarding the standards/specifications and their role in fulfilling those performance standards. Peters suggests that quality must be at the top of every agenda. It must be made visible and each individual must be held accountable for it.[7] From the chairman of the board to every volunteer, the commitment to quality performance begins by understanding performance expectations.

In the performance awareness program, the individuals affected by the standards and those who are expected to implement them are involved in defining them. Performance awareness includes not only the internal customers but also the external ones. Informing patients, for example, about the performance standards provides the patients with a realistic picture of what types and levels of service to expect from the organization.

It is during this program that all personnel are made aware of the role of standards in achieving performance targets and the importance of complying with written standards. Crosby suggests that we dispel the myth that quality means goodness or luxury. He believes that it means conformance to requirements.[3] It is during the performance awareness program that those requirements are defined and communicated to all involved in delivering health care services.

Performance measurement

Once standards have been written and everyone is made aware of them, their implementation begins. It is then that the performance measurement program begins. During the performance measurement program, the question "Are we performing according to expectations?" is answered. Performance measurement is the process of quantifying performance relative to a defined goal.[7] Performance measurement validates an acceptable level of performance or it identifies variation in service delivery/outcomes. Through evaluation of variance, opportunities to improve service delivery/outcomes are identified.

"Measurement can guide steady advancement toward established goals and identify shortfalls or stagnation. . . Measurement becomes a waste of time with little or no organizational value when an organization measures items that have no influence on organizational success. The result is a bean counting approach that focuses on irrelevant details."[9]

There are three types of measurement: performance analysis, satisfaction analysis, and technology analysis. These types occur in each domain: service, practice, and governance.

Performance analysis includes the measurement of specific indicators of performance. It is achieved through the use of performance measurement studies that incorporate statistical process control tools. These measurement studies may be organization wide or unit based in origin. They may occur in any or all domains.

"Satisfaction analysis is the customer's evaluation of the value of the service provided."[5] It includes input from both internal and external customers. The types of tools utilized can include patient satisfaction surveys and interviews, climate surveys, focus groups, and administrative surveys.

"Satisfied patients are more compliant, demonstrate increased adaptive skills and are more likely to stay with and recommend their health care provider. Patient satisfaction measurement furnishes a means of proving quality of care delivery to payers and improves an agency's bottom line."[9]

Much work is being done in the development of standardized satisfaction indicators. For example, Press, Ganey Associates recently conducted a survey of more than 7000 home health agency clients to determine the top 10 patient satisfaction issues for home health agencies. The box below lists their findings.[11]

Technology analysis includes research and product evaluation. Research is an evaluative function that occurs in all three domains. Conducting research or utilizing the results of research enables the organization to expand existing scientific knowledge upon which to base decisions. Product evaluation encompasses the routine equipment evaluation in the attempt to improve the resources that the health care workers use to deliver services. The use of a new type of urinary catheter or laser may have a profound impact on the level of performance.

TOP 10 PATIENT SATISFACTION ISSUES FOR HOME HEALTH AGENCIES

1. Agency is responsive to requests to change nurses or aides.
2. Family is kept informed about treatment.
3. Family is involved in planning home health services.
4. Nurses show concern for client's comfort.
5. Aides show concern for client's comfort.
6. Nurses contact client when they will be late or absent.
7. Nurses teach client self care.
8. Nurses' strong technical skills.
9. Initial plan of health care or treatment meets client's needs.
10. Helpfulness of the person who makes initial arrangements for service.

From Top 10 patient satisfaction issues, *Home Health Digest*, 1(2): 4, 1995.

"Where payers used to decide whether or not to pay for a product based upon a 'gut feeling,' they are now looking for demonstrated proof that the product adds value."[6]

The steps involved in this program include

1. Designing performance measures
2. Setting performance targets
3. Collecting and organizing data
4. Evaluating variation

The critical element of this program is the need for it to be statistically based. There are many tools available to assist during the measurement program. These are the tools of statistical process control and include histograms, pareto charts, run charts, control charts, and cause and effect diagrams. These are the tools necessary to measure the level of performance and compare it with established norms.

Performance improvement

Crosby states "It isn't what you find, it's what you do about what you find. All the planning, inspection, testing, measuring and other activities . . . are a waste of time if they don't lead to preventing the recurrence of a problem."[3] In the performance improvement program, the question "How can we improve the level of performance?" is asked. This program is the response system. "It is how we strive to make our service smarter, less costly, better and faster." The old approach to quality improvement was a seek-and-repair mentality. The new thrust of performance improvement is adding to something that is already good.

Once an organization has identified and corrected its problems, the attention turns to process innovation. Once an opportunity for improvement has been identified, the improvement program kicks in, and through the process of action planning, a strategy is devised. The steps involved include

1. Creating a process improvement team
2. Developing and implementing an improvement plan
3. Assessing and documenting improvement
4. Communicating results

There are many tools that facilitate the work involved in this program. These include such tools as the tree diagram, affinity diagram, interrelationship diagram, prioritization matrices, matrix diagram, process decision program chart, activity network diagram, action plans, and progress records.

It is in the improvement program that the results of scientific research are of critical value. "Using the research findings of others or implementing in-house studies can lend critical support to desired changes in practice, thus ensuring a scientific basis for change rather than an intuitive one."[5]

Performance improvement occurs through teams and is manifested in process simplification and work redesign. This involves a process analysis, not simply to validate that the process achieves the desired outcomes but to identify quicker, easier, and simpler ways of performing the process without affecting the outcome. Clean versus sterile dressings save time and money. As long as there is no adverse effect on the incidence of wound infections, the advantages to the organization of this change can be substantial.

This book is organized into units that discuss how to develop and implement these three programs.

INTEGRATING STANDARDS, DOMAINS, AND PROGRAMS

The following examples demonstrate how a tri-focus approach to standards development, dissemination, measurement, analysis, and improvement would affect some specific key issues in health care.

Impaired professionals may be a problem population with which an organization is confronted. It is a practice issue; therefore, it is within the **practice domain.** If handled improperly, this issue can have a serious effect on process variation and capability. In the **performance awareness program, standards** are written regarding the structure, processes, and outcomes expected. These might include hiring policies related to impaired professionals and types of patients or situations from which these individuals are restricted or practice guidelines related to monitoring of the individual's performance. Communication of these standards forms the basis of the relationship between an impaired professional and the organization. The ongoing performance of the affected individuals is measured as a part of the **performance measurement program.** As part of the **performance improvement program,** an employee development plan for continued progress may be developed and implemented, or the original policies and procedures may be redesigned.

Budgeting is a critical process of the fiscal function and as such falls under the **governance domain. Standards** related to the budget function would include policies related to the budget process, such as job description requirements for the individuals responsible for preparing, administering, and reviewing the budget and procedures and practice guidelines related to budget preparation. Fiscal outcomes are set as financial targets. The development of these standards occurs during the **performance awareness program.** Also at this time, training related to budget preparation may occur as part of a management development training program. The **performance measurement program** enables the organization to measure its progress compared with the financial performance targets that have been set. Results of this analysis may indicate the need to design a strategic plan to correct spending if the budget is not meeting its margins. Should a variation exist, all three domains must be evaluated to determine the cause of the variance. Perhaps the organization is admitting sicker patients with more complications that require longer lengths of stay and greater resource consumption. Perhaps the staff members are squandering resources or using them inappropriately. Perhaps within the organization itself, capital expenditures were poorly planned or there has been an inordinate amount of unplanned overtime or agency staff required. Then, during the **performance improvement program,** action plans are developed to address all of the significant root causes.

In each of these examples, **standards** drive the system. Using a tri-focus approach, the three programs, **performance awareness, performance measurement,** and **performance improvement** are implemented.

The three programs described above are inextricably linked. Successful measurement is impossible without well-defined specifications upon which to base your study. It is likewise futile to improve something you have not evaluated. When all three programs are in place and functioning interdependently, written standards are in place upon which to measure performance. Performance data can be drawn from those standards and the results can be analyzed to determine actual performance compared with desired performance. Then performance improvement efforts can be directed toward reducing process variation and improving process capability. This usually involves reexamining the current standards and modifying them as indicated.

To ensure that the performance management efforts of the organization are integrated and that the system is performing as intended, a model is helpful.

THE BLUEPRINT FOR PERFORMANCE MANAGEMENT

Just as a blueprint is essential to constructing a complex building, so a blueprint is necessary to construct a comprehensive performance management system. THE BLUEPRINT (Figure 3-2) is a model that provides an integrating framework for managing performance within an organization.

Vertically, each **domain** is represented. There are three vertical tracks. The first vertical track represents the service domain. The middle track represents the practice domain and the third track, the governance domain. Clearly delineating each domain has distinct advantages. First, appropriate standards may now be written specifically for each domain. This brings organization and direction to standards development. Second, performance measurement activities may now be directed toward each specific domain so that performance improvement activities can be identified in each and appropriate resources allocated for their completion.

Using this approach ensures that standards development, performance measurement, and improvement activities will focus not only on customer services but also on the practice and governance variables that affect results in the service domain.

Horizontally, the model reflects the various types of standards—structure, process, and outcomes—and defines the specific formats of each.

Figure 3-3 represents a three-dimensional view of the model depicting the tri-focus approach to standards development and evaluation.

Basic Principles of THE BLUEPRINT

There are five underlying principles of THE BLUEPRINT.

Service is outcome focused. "Everything that happens in a quality system must be a result not a reaction."[3] Although much emphasis is placed on reducing process variation and improving process capability, one must not forget that the ultimate goal of a performance management system is the service outcomes of the organization. Patient outcomes are the results of clinical processes. "The services provided are the means to an end, not the end itself."[5]

Bedside-based accountability is essential. Individuals within the organization are held accountable for their role in achieving outcomes. Accountability refers to the individual's answering to someone or something outside himself/herself for his/her actions. Meeting performance expectations is the responsibility of every member of the health care team, whether or not he or she is involved in direct patient services. Thus each person must see his or her responsibility for performance and be held accountable for it. "Opportunities to abdicate accountability upward or laterally must be eliminated."[5]

Shared decision making must occur. For a performance management program to work, decisions must be made at the appropriate level of expertise. Individuals, departments, and organizations have defined scopes of authority regarding decision making. Each, however, is not autonomous but rather interdependent with the degree of decision making authority clearly defined. This concept is called *shared leadership* and is explored fully in Chapter 5.

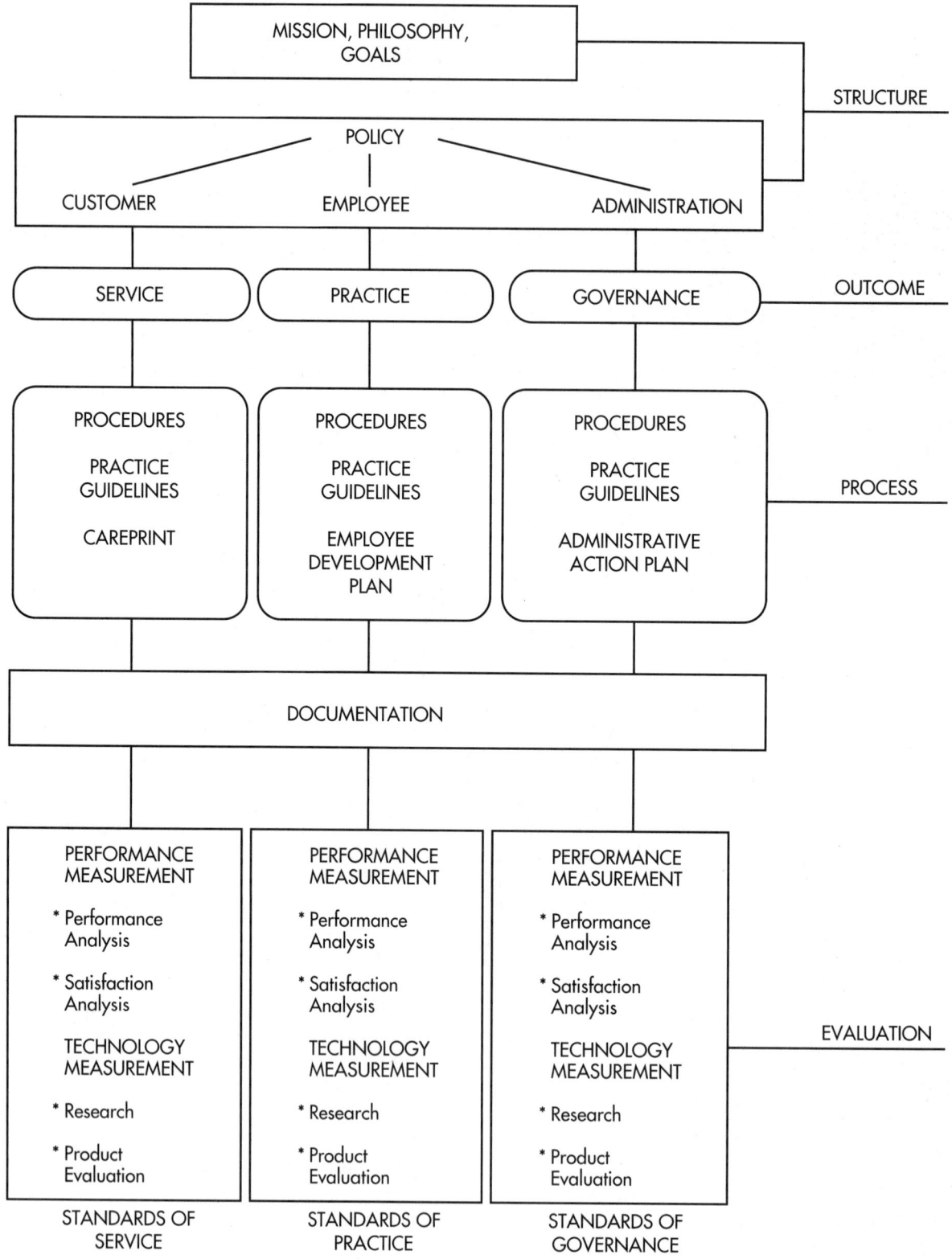

Figure 3-2   THE BLUEPRINT for Performance Management (Copyright Katz and Green, 1995).

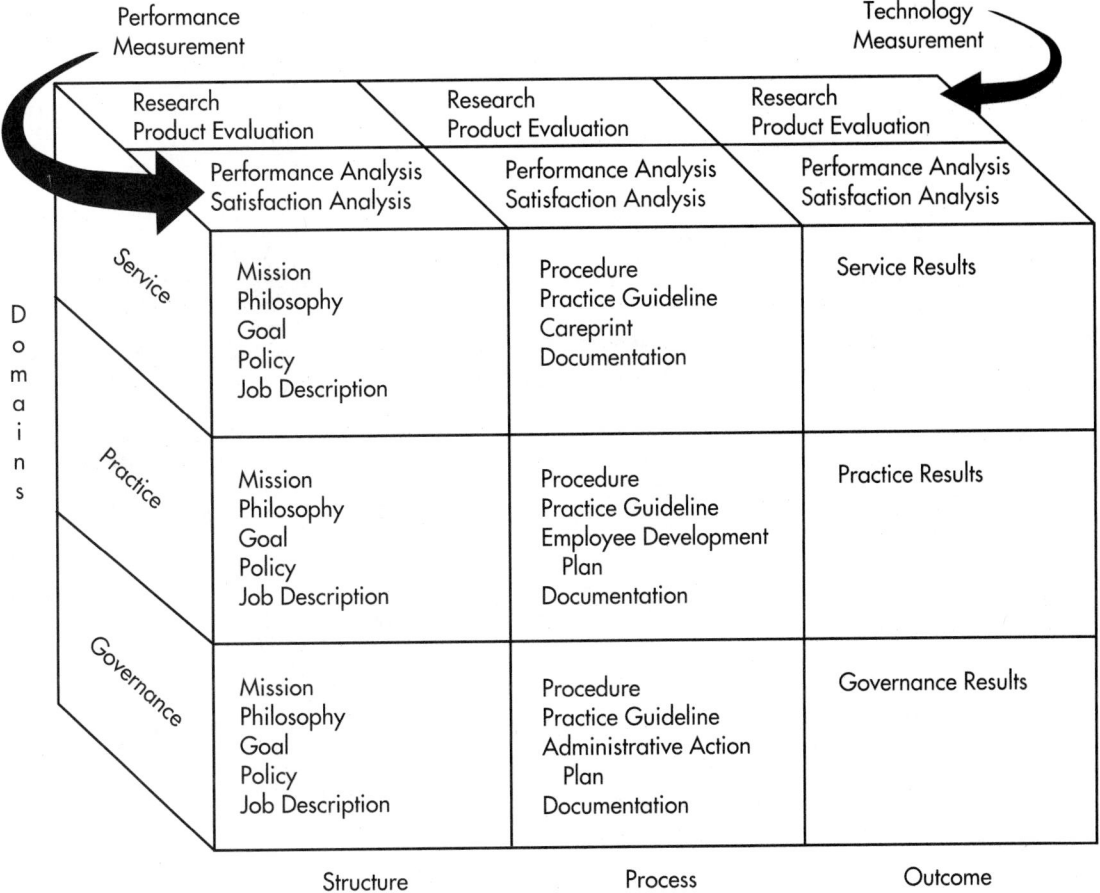

Figure 3-3 BLUEPRINT paradigm (Copyright Katz and Green, 1995).

Management by crisis is eliminated. This model advocates a proactive, preventive approach to insuring peak performance. Using the tools of statistical process control to track and trend processes increases the predictive ability of the organization relative to those processes. Process capability focuses on the ability of the organization to produce the outcomes it desires, each time, every time. This level of confidence in its processes and results increases the organization's competitive edge.

"The 'knee jerk' reaction to constant problems is replaced with a logical, well thought out priority focus. The result is a system that is in control of its resources and its future."[9] When the day-to-day brush fires arise, instead of becoming a major tangent, they are a minor diversion, to be managed without losing sight of the critical performance improvement efforts.

Organizations must be value-driven for survival. Customers are looking for the best value in health care, whether the customer is the individual patient, the third-party payer, or the federal government. Value means the best buy for the dollar. A value-driven organization strives for the most affordable, highest quality health care. To do this and stay in business, the orga-

nization must look at performance variables, cost, and satisfaction factors. As a business, it is not reasonable to provide all of the services in 5 days that once were provided during a 10-day length of stay. Or is it? Were all of those services truly necessary? Could those services be provided at home as easily and safely as in the hospital? Will cutting those services harm the patient outcomes in any way?

To protect the rights of the individual from unproven, potentially harmful early discharges, for example, some professional associations are championing minimum acceptable lengths of stay. Maryland in fact was the first state to pass a law related to a minimum length of postpartum stay. Value closely balances the scales between cost and quality.

Advantages of THE BLUEPRINT

The key to survival in the "jungle" of managed care today is the development of a value-driven organization with an exceptional outcomes record. THE BLUEPRINT attempts to organize the journey through that jungle by providing a step-by-step approach to a comprehensive performance management system.

Tom Peters believes that the winners of tomorrow will deal proactively with chaos. THE BLUEPRINT provides a proactive approach to reducing process variation and improving process capability.

Just as all performance must be judged using a tri-focus approach, the advantages of THE BLUEPRINT have a threefold impact:

For the Customer
1. Increased continuity and consistency in service delivery
2. Specified outcomes for the services provided
3. Improved satisfaction with the services provided

For the Staff
1. Increased participation in decision making
2. Increased autonomy and control of practice
3. Increased accountability

For the Organization
1. Increased control of department functions
2. Increased coordination of services
3. Improved use of resources (human, fiscal, and material)

THE BLUEPRINT is an outcome-focused, proactive model for managing performance within organizations by developing the organizational structure and operating systems necessary to manage the business of health care.

"Strong leadership is the key to high performance. Someone has to articulate the vision and sell it to the organization."[8] Chapter 4 focuses on organizing for peak performance. It emphasizes the role of the CEO in performance management and describes a system for including and empowering "stakeholders" in decisions affecting performance.

REFERENCES

1. Bennett AC, Tibbitts SJ: *Maximizing quality performance in health care facilities*, Rockville, Md, 1989, Aspen Publishers.
2. Clemmer J: *Pathways to performance*, Rocklin, Calif, 1995, Prima Publishing.
3. Crosby PB: *Quality is free*, New York, 1979, New American Library.
4. Juran JM, Gryna FM: *Juran's quality control handbook*, ed 4, New York, 1988, McGraw-Hill.
5. Katz JM, Green E: *THE BLUEPRINT for Quality Management: The Agenda for the Future*. In Schroeder P, editor: *The encyclopedia of nursing care quality*, vol 2, Gaithersburg, Md, 1991, Aspen Publishers.
6. Last JV, Nash OB: Developing health care products in a managed care environment, *The Journal of Outcomes Management*, 2(1): 18-21, 1995.
6a. Performance management, *Harvard Business Review*, May/June 1995, pp 11-12.
7. Peters T: *Thriving on chaos*, New York, 1988, Alfred A Knopf.
8. Risher H: Defining the role of outcomes data in measuring and managing hospital performance, *The Journal of Outcomes Management*, 2(1): 5-11, 1995.
9. Rose KH: A performance measurement model, *Quality Progress*, 28(2): 63-66, 1995.
10. Reference deleted in pages.
11. Top 10 Patient Satisfaction Issues, *Home Health Digest*, 1(2): 4, 1995.

Part Two

STRUCTURING FOR ORGANIZATION-WIDE PERFORMANCE

Chapter 4

Responsibility and Accountability for Organizational Performance: The Role of the CEO

> *The buck stops here.*
> **Harry S. Truman**

When Harry Truman was President of the United States, he kept a sign in the Oval Office that read, "The buck stops here." In assigning responsibility for quality in today's complex health care systems, there must be a place where the buck stops and accountability for quality is acknowledged. In the past the department of nursing has served as the place where the "quality buck" stopped.

The *quality* interest of the chief executive officer (CEO) and other top managers of many health care organizations was formerly brief and cyclic. It revolved around the 3-year cycle of survey visits. If the organization fared well in the state, government, or independent agency survey process, management sighed with relief and put the quality program on the back burner for another 3 years. If the organization fared poorly in the survey, "heads rolled." The heads that rolled were usually those of various people under the control of the department of nursing, such as the quality assurance coordinator.

One CEO of a health care organization that fared poorly in a recent accreditation survey reasoned, "If our QI Coordinator had been doing her job right we would have been viewed in a more favorable light by the survey team."

THE BUCK STOPS

In the previous example, it did not cross the CEO's mind that if *he* had been doing *his* job right, his organization would have been viewed in a more favorable light! "Both Dr. Deming and Dr. Juran, two of the early pioneers of the modern quality movement, are very clear about the CEO's role in designing the organization's structure so that it will be conducive to performance improvement. Deming states in *Out of Crisis* that the 'support of top management is not sufficient.' They also must *get involved*; they must act."[2]

Dr. Juran uses "The Quality Trilogy" to describe management's process improvement role. In Juran's *Quality Control Handbook*, he describes the activities of management as: "1) *quality planning*, the 'activity of developing products and processes required to meet customers' needs'; 2) *quality control*, the 'process used by operating forces as an aid to meeting the product and process goals based on the feed-back loop'; and 3) *quality improvement*, 'to attain levels of performance which are unprecedented—levels which are significantly better than any past level.'"[7] "From this we see that top management must be involved to make improvements in performance, and that involvement must be both structural and behavioral."[10]

No longer does the responsibility and accountability for performance improvement lie within the department of nursing nor is it the responsibility of employees with "quality" in their employment position titles. Furthermore, it is no longer *directed* by the department of nursing. The buck now stops with the CEO!

Although nursing continues to be a major player in health care organizations' performance improvement programs, and quality professionals continue to gather and analyze data, the responsibility and accountability for an organization-wide performance management system lies with the CEO.

SHIFT FROM QA TO PM

Traditionally, planning and organizing a quality assurance (QA) program of a health care organization has been the responsibility of the department of nursing. It has now become the responsibility of the CEO, because the priorities of the health care industry have shifted dramatically. This shift also has created a parallel and necessary shift in the significance of health care organizations' quality programs to (a) manage cost containment, (b) avoid litigation, (c) create alliances between organizations, (d) move into a managed care arena, and (e) justify staffing ratios and mix. These changes to the quality focus of health care organizations are beyond the scope of the nursing department's mission. Furthermore, the department of nursing's employees do not have the business knowledge and experience or scope of authority necessary to carry out the current quality mandates. However, the CEO has been educated, trained by job experiences, and has the scope of authority to carry out the organization-wide quality mission. Leadership of the organization's performance management system has, therefore, become part of the CEO's job description.

This shift in quality priorities within the health care industry also has driven a vocabulary change to reflect the new methods being used to continually assess the complex major functions of today's health care organizations. (For a list of functions see the box on p. 49 in Chapter 5.) The term *quality assurance* has become obsolete because the term indicates an end—i.e., *we have achieved quality!* The term *quality* should be a means, not an end. Furthermore, the term originally was associated with the percent of errors tolerated at the end-of-line production. For example, "We will tolerate a two percent error rate out of every hundred widgets that we manufacture." In the early days of QA, health care organizations counted how many "bad things" happened to patients divided by the total number of things done to patients. For example, the total number of medication errors was divided by the

total number of medications administered; the results were called volume indicators.

The trouble with this rationale became apparent as health care became more technologically sophisticated, workers became more stratified, and patient diagnoses became more complicated. Variations in service, practice, and governance were impossible to correct when data simply was reflective of "how many negative occurrences happened this month." What the health care industry desired was evidence of a continual performance improvement of all processes of service, practice, and governance within each health care organization, regardless of the number of negative occurrences.

Accreditation agencies responded by rewording accreditation requirements to reflect the new focus. The new term is *performance management (PM)*, which reflects the present philosophy of constantly seeking better ways of delivering service, practice, and governance to all customers. Underlying the new philosophy is the concept of never being satisfied with present processes or outcomes but continually seeking ways to improve.

It also became apparent to the health care industry that "without a solid foundation of continuous improvement, long-term profitability cannot be achieved, trust relationships with customers cannot be built, and the hearts of employees cannot be fully engaged."[3]

COLLAPSE OF HIERARCHICAL MANAGEMENT STYLE

"If you take a frog and put it in a shallow pan of scalding water, it will jump out. If the same frog is put in tepid water over a low flame, it will sit calmly and gradually boil to death."[3] In other words, the health care crisis has been boring, quiet, and slow to "boil." There is such resistance to change and such reluctance to face crises that many health care organizations have slowly "boiled to death" and no longer exist.

John Stepp says that

> as business people became aware of the slipping American economy during the 1980s, management had three basic reactions: (a) keep the old system intact—tighten the screws, (b) play along with a few new things, but not go too far because who knows what may happen in terms of our own power, perks and rewards, to (c) "Look, we live in a new world with new requirements, and the old ways are no longer working, and we've got to fundamentally rethink what we're doing and why we're doing it."[3]

THE ROLE OF THE CEO

What, exactly, is the role of the CEO? The CEO is responsible and accountable for *total* organizational performance. One of the distinguishing features of this role is that the CEO must secure results through the efforts of other people. He or she is accountable for organization-wide performance, and the only way to achieve it is by harnessing the efforts of other people. The CEO's job now relies on the job of every other employee; it cannot be done alone.

Traditionally CEOs were able to delegate the QA job. The change in name from *QA* to *PM* reflected the change in philosophy in the quality movement driving the health care industry. QA was a counting job and almost anybody could do it. PM is everybody's job, and it must be initiated, organized, and managed by the organization's top leader—the CEO.

Although this creates additional job responsibilities and a broader net of accountability for the CEO, it is a giant leap forward in the health care industry. The CEO's responsibility for PM proves that the job of continually improving organization-wide performance will receive top-priority attention, because it is the designated responsibility of the top leader of the organization (see the box below).

Many CEOs did not view continuous performance improvement, customer satisfaction, and continual innovation as part of their role—those responsibilities were delegated. They were trapped in the hierarchical governance management style, where their attention was occupied with budgets, alliances, and contracts and meeting local, state, and government requirements. Indeed, this was an acceptable way to do business in the health care industry—until the CEOs realized that the dramatic changes facing health care were having an enormous impact on the viability of the future of their organizations.

DO YOU KNOW WHO'S IN CHARGE?

There was an important job to be done,

and Everybody was asked to do it.

Everybody was sure Somebody would do it.

Anybody could have done it, but Nobody did it.

Somebody got angry about that,

because it was Everybody's job.

Everybody thought Anybody could do it,

but Nobody realized that Everybody wouldn't do it.

It ended up that Everybody

blamed Somebody, when actually

Nobody asked Anybody!

(Author Unknown)

From *The critical path: NASA flight projects directorate quarterly publication, A newsletter published for code 400 employees,* 3(3): 8, 1995.

The visionary CEOs began to think and plan for the future. Experimentation proved that a non-hierarchical structure enabling employees to carry out responsibilities for service, practice, and governance at the point of intervention was a more efficient and cost effective management style. Furthermore, restructuring health care organizations using a multidisciplinary framework provided for a free flow of interaction and consultation among staff across disciplines. It was obvious that this afforded the essential flexibility that enhanced the organization's service, practice and governance as well as customer satisfaction.

PERFORMANCE IMPROVEMENT FOR SURVIVAL

"The issues in healthcare delivery with their concomitant changes such as reimbursement regulation and development of networks for delivery of healthcare have profound effects on organizational structure designs."[14] As we enter the second decade of performance improvement in the United States, it is clearer than ever that a performance management program is a fundamental survival issue—companies that cannot consistently deliver a performance management system of awareness, measurement, and improvement to their customers at competitive prices will not survive in today's global marketplace.[1]

In short, *someone* must oversee a total performance management system if the organization is to survive into the next century. That person is logically the CEO—the place where the "buck" stops. The CEO now becomes the health care organization's number-one performance management leader. "It is the job of the CEO to structure or 're-structure' the organization to position it for the future."[11] The present health crisis that is being exacerbated by customer-driven demands and by imposed performance measures with emphasis on complex service, practice, and governance outcomes requires that CEOs abandon traditional hierarchical management practices. Driven by the consumers, government, insurance companies, and accrediting organizations, the health care industry has begun to adopt a fundamentally new view of health care leadership.

The former view, held by many hospital CEOs, was that quality was simply a control issue and anyone who could count could do the quality job. Although he was speaking of industry, MIT economist Lester Thurow also could have been speaking for health care organizations when he said, "Management is responsible for quality control. If American products are shoddily built, then American management is shoddy."[1] This statement can be paraphrased for the health care industry: Management is responsible for a health care organization's performance. If health care's services, practices, and governance systems are shoddily delivered, then the management of health care is shoddy.

Furthermore, the CEO, with help of the management team and representation from all departments of the organization, has the responsibility to design a system that assigns responsibility and accountability for performance. (See Chapter 5 for details on constructing such a program.) This requires seeking new ways to perform management functions.

"One of the great lessons of the American quality revolution is that leadership is the most important ingredient for launching and sustaining a quality improvement process."[11] "If the top dog and his immediate poundmates don't believe in the performance improvement program and behave accordingly, it won't happen."[13] Dr. Deming and many accrediting agencies such as the NCQA and the JCAHO place great emphasis on the leadership role of top management. Members of top management are to provide evidence of awareness, measurement and improvement of performance in every department of the health care organization that they manage.

CEO: THE NEW PM LEADER

Unless top management has a vested, ongoing interest in improvement, no lasting improvement is likely to be made. As Ray Boedecker, IBM's director of quality, put it, "When the CEO says, 'Let's go. Let's learn. Let's do it.'—that's when quality begins. It's the single most compelling, motivating factor."[1] "Accordingly, Dr. Deming has some parting advice for top managers who want to delegate quality, '. . . if *you* can't come, send *nobody*.'"[2] In other words, there is no substitute for the CEO in a health care organization. He or she *is* captain at the helm of the performance management ship and ultimately responsible for how the crew performs and where the ship goes.

Initially CEOs did not understand the need to be so intimately involved in the quality movement even though it was shaking the foundation of the health care industry to its core. But now that each organization's performance is being measured by the "dimensions of performance" and quantifiable performance measures are being developed based on these dimensions and translated into facts and figures for the purpose of reimbursement and comparative analysis, CEOs have begun to appreciate the necessity of involvement.

Organizations are diligently working to develop measures of performance. Organizations such as Joint Commission on Accreditation of Healthcare Organizations (JCAHO), are developing performance measures for acute care and extended care facilities, the National Committee for Quality Assurance (NCQA) through their Health Plan Employer Data and Information Set (HEDIS) are developing performance measures for managed care organizations, the federal government who created a Health Care Quality Improvement System (HCQIS) that are developing performance measures for Medicaid managed care organizations that are receiving government funding.[4]

For those health care organizations that seek accreditation from one of the accreditation organizations, there are some new expectations about the role of the CEO as it pertains to leadership of the performance management system. Each of the accreditation organizations expects top leadership to

(a) describe the organization's philosophy and approach to performance improvement, (b) explain the rationale for adopting this approach, and (c) discuss how the organization has tailored this approach to accommodate its mission, vision, scope of services, and culture. Additionally, the organization's leadership is expected to (a) identify those responsible for coordinating quality activities, (b) explain the relationship of the coordinating quality group to senior leadership, (c) describe any unique ways that measurement or other activities have been organized, and (d) tell how the organization is evolving from quality assurance/assessment and improvement to performance improvement.[6]

For success during the accreditation process, regardless of the organization that has been chosen to perform the survey, the CEO should use visual aids, such as flow charts, models, an organizational framework, a video presentation, or a graphic representation, in the initial presentation to the survey team. This will indicate that preparation was taken seriously and that a performance management system is so important that the CEO chooses to present it him- or herself. He or she may then explain how the organization is structured vis-à-vis performance management and how every employee fits in to the PM Program. Trying to explain the organizational performance system to a stranger is difficult. That is why we recommend that the CEO both *show* and *tell* the details of the performance management structure to the surveyor team.

This activity (the initial presentation by top leadership) "provides a basis for surveyors' document review and subsequent staff interviews."[9] Today's accrediting agencies of health care organizations have invested millions of dollars in creating performance measures and developing indicators by which to benchmark an organization's success. Most are insisting that organizations present a detailed performance management system and outline how the organization is structured to facilitate its programs. Keep in mind that the CEO may no longer present a three-page, typed, brief overview. There should be evidence of a well-developed system. Accreditation agencies are looking for proof that (a) the mission, philosophy, and goals of the organization are in place and drive the behavior of all employees and (b) that performance management system is part of every employee's daily work experience.

Regardless of how motivated a CEO might be to get started on an organization-wide performance management system, education is necessary. Many employees do not understand the fundamental principles of performance management, which include a working knowledge of statistics and statistical process control tools, in addition to a complete understanding of the team process.

Many CEOs, when questioned about a definition of performance management, often respond by saying, "shortened length of stay for the total hip patient," or "decrease in number of medication errors," or "an eight million dollar profit this year—we must be doing something right." Although these things are important, none of them, by itself, demonstrates improved performance.

What is performance? Indirectly, performance is shortened lengths of stays of patient population groups, the profit, the decrease in medication errors rate, and so on. These positive outcomes represent the *results* of a well-organized performance management system; they do not represent the system itself. The traditional quality program in the health care industry had its roots grounded in *inspection*. The new performance management system has its roots grounded in *people*.

TAKING THE PM PLUNGE

The pressure is immense for CEOs to take the plunge into the "sea" of performance management. Many CEOs are cautious. Some previously have been "burnt" by hopping on band wagons—is this another band wagon? Some question the wisdom of embarking on a large-scale performance management system of unknown cost. Some question the future viability of the health care industry as well as the duration of the now-powerful regulatory organizations. Others have heard horror stories of performance management system failures and tremble at putting themselves at risk for failure. Many believe that it is safer to "keep on doing what we've always done" so we can "continue to get what we've always gotten."[8] They believe the old adage, "Better the devil that you know than the devil that you don't know!"

The philosophy of "keep on doing what we've always done" feels safe, comfortable, and controllable. Why venture into an unknown arena where there is risk of failure? Why rock a ship, of which the CEO is captain, that has been sailing the health care seas acceptably for many years? Why not wait and see how other health care organizations fare before taking the plunge?

This attitude persists despite the multitude of success stories. It appears that the bright lights on the health care horizon are from those successful CEOs who have turned their health care organizations around—and they did it by taking the plunge into the PM sea. These CEOs are the ones who understood that a "performance management system doesn't work in bits and pieces; it's either all part of a single, defined effort or its fails."[3]

CEOs who are ready to move forward with an organization-wide performance management system face a unique concern: how does one measure tangible as well as intangible services, practices, and governance systems of a health care organization?

Unlike manufacturing, there are both tangible and intangible factors affecting the service, practice, and governance of a health care organization. How can a CEO design a tangible performance management system in a multi-faceted, complex health care organization to measure intangible performance? Everyone knows that a plan is necessary. It is understood that ". . . no company without a plan for the future . . . will stay in business."[3] How can these measures prove increased productivity, staff and patient satisfaction, and continually increasing improvement to processes while continually gaining growth and profit for the organization's stakeholders? This is a difficult task, because the health care industry not only does not have a history of efficient, cost-saving delivery of services but also has no criteria for measurement of its services.

The Marketing Science Institute, located in Cambridge, Massachusetts, undertook a research study on the measurement of intangibles in an attempt to separate manufactured goods from service delivery. Their book *Delivering Quality Service—Balancing Customer Perceptions and Expectations* constitutes the most important and widely used model of "service quality" yet developed.

There are four fundamental and universal characteristics that distinguished goods from service.

The first characteristic of service is that most services are intangible because they are performances, rather than objects. Because of this, they cannot be measured, tested, or verified in advance. . .to assure quality. When your car breaks down while you're on vacation and you call the local garage to come and fix it, you have no real way of knowing in advance how well the adventure is going to turn out.

The second characteristic of service is that those having a high labor content—are heterogeneous. The quality of the actual performance will often vary from provider to provider, from customer to customer, even from day to day. For example, American Airlines is among the best-run airlines in the world, but we know very few frequent travelers who can't come up with a horror story of lost baggage . . . The damage . . . can often be minimized by intelligent handling by the company's employees. But even that is unpredictable. Not only does employee behavior vary from individual to individual, each individual employee may not consistently repeat the same behavior.

The third characteristic of service is that the production is often inseparable from its consumption. In the process of getting a haircut, for example, the service is provided and consumed simultaneously. Its success—or quality— depends upon how well the customer has communicated his specifications to the barber and how accurately the barber has interpreted and delivered what the customer wanted.

The fourth characteristic of service is that services are perishable. They cannot be inventoried, saved, and resold later. Flights that take off with empty seats or classrooms not filled to capacity have lost their value forever. This characteristic often makes it hard for companies to manage supply and demand.[1]

It is necessary to distinguish goods from service in a health care organization, because the criteria for distinguishing goods from service will have a direct impact on (a) the way in which an organization chooses to structure itself for performance management, (b) the way outcomes will be measured, (c) the method for sharing data with other providers, (d) the type of information to be disseminated into a national data bank, (e) the manner in which satisfaction surveys will be analyzed, and, finally, (f) what factors will constitute success.

The traditional quality programs may not be imported from the manufacturing business world and pressed onto the health care industry and renamed "Performance Management Systems." The system focus, initiative, employee involvement, and the way teams function are different in the health care industry.

When a CEO looks at the characteristics of a service delivery business and applies them to health care, it becomes obvious that a quality program at Ford must be structured differently than a performance management system in a large suburban hospital. It is doubtful that "death with dignity" would ever become a customer outcome of the Ford Motor Company. However, this customer outcome is perfectly acceptable in a suburban hospital's oncology unit and all the variables have been considered and documented. It is obvious, then, that the four characteristics of a service delivery business pose unique problems for the CEO of a health care organization in terms of structuring to deliver what customers perceive to be high-performance service, practice, and governance.

RETHINKING THE ROLE OF THE CEO

The CEO's performance description includes the mandate to carry the organization into the future. This means restructuring the organization from the traditional hierarchical management style to the new shared leadership style of governance. Restructuring means starting over. It is no longer enough to shore up the existing structures but leave the shell for posterity as we do when we update and remodel a pre-Civil War mansion. Nor does it mean

tinkering with what already exists or making incremental changes that leave basic structures intact. It isn't about making patchwork fixes—jury-rigging existing processes so that, for the moment, they work better. It does mean abandoning long-established processes and looking afresh at the work required to create a health care organization's performance management system. It means asking this question: 'If I were recreating this company today, given what I know and given current technology, what would it look like?' Re-engineering a company means tossing aside old systems and starting over. It involves going back to the beginning and inventing a better way of doing work.[5]

The great mystery, of course, is how to restructure a complex, multi-faceted, busy, multi-million dollar health care organization. Where does a CEO begin? The problems multiply if the restructuring is aimed at a health care system composed of a chain of hospitals, outpatient surgeries, emergency departments, clinics, long-term care facilities, assisted living centers, and several home care agencies. However, for those organizations willing to restructure themselves the payoff is a sweet savor of success. For in spite of the temporary chaos and upheaval that accompanies any reorganization of staff authority, consolidation of departments, and the cutting of budgetary "fat," the outcome will be an organization that will continue to be profitable and deliver quality service, practice, and governance well into the future.

However, this cannot be accomplished without rethinking and examining every traditional principle of management. It is scary and uncomfortable for a CEO to restructure an organization from job titles to interdisciplinary systems, and from staffing patterns to how the performance management system itself is conducted. Although the business world is filled with instruction books on creating a quality organization, there are no rule books, guidelines, or seminars to direct a health care CEO in the nitty-gritty of restructuring his or her organization for performance management. Unfortunately, there also are no long-term health care success stories of 20 to 30 years' duration to emulate.

MOP BUCKET ATTITUDE

Health care CEOs are left to draw conclusions from the business world's success stories. One such success story about a turnaround in customer satisfaction and corporate profits captured the public's eye for a time.

Mr. Near, chairman and CEO of Wendy's International franchise, explains:

After feasting on success for more than 15 years, Wendy's Old Fashioned Hamburgers restaurants developed heartburn in the mid-1980s. Costs soared, sales dropped, and formerly enthusiastic analysts waxed gloomy about Wendy's prospects, convinced our company had lost focus.

I came on as president in 1986 and found we had indeed lost our focus—on people. We had such a fear in our hearts about numbers, about the power of computer printouts and going by the book, we'd managed to lose sight of our customers and employees both. . .

As sales fell, store labor was cut and sales fell even further. Morale took a nose dive, quality became spotty, and consistency in operations was nonexistent. . . It was time to concentrate . . . on the basics. Beginning with the most basic tenet of all: Mop Bucket Attitude, or M.B.A.

Mop bucket attitude says that all the business sophistication in the world pales before the "wisdom" of a clean floor. Fancy price-cost tabulations or quarterly earnings have no meaning to the customer, but quality food, and atmosphere do. . . We . . . decided the best way to become the customer's restaurant of choice was to become the employer of choice.

We began by raising employee training to uniformly high standards . . . then we worked to . . . give managers more control and latitude in day-to-day decisions. . . We improved base compensation, offered a package of top-flight benefits, and a cash bonus paid out each quarter. We created an employee stock option plan called "We-Share" to give our employees a larger stake in the company. . . It worked. Our turnover rate for general managers fell to 20 percent in 1991 from 39 percent in 1989, while turnover among co- and assistant managers dropped to 37 percent from 60 percent— among the lowest in the business. . .

The customers who'd deserted us began to come back. . . When we started these programs in 1987, we made just five cents a share. In 1991 . . . we reported earnings of 52 cents a share. . . Wendy's realized a 31 percent rise in earnings . . . for a profit of $52 million—its best year since 1985.[8]

Mr. Near learned that restructuring involved participation of workers and a stake in the company's success.

The Forum Corporation, a training, consulting, and research firm which has conducted extensive ongoing research on leadership over the past twenty years, traces the need for a fundamentally new view of business leadership to three sources: changing organizational structures in the modern corporation; a new, more diverse work force with rising expectations, diminished institutional loyalties, and less reverence for authority; and the modern quality movement itself, which first took root in Japan.[1]

Since Japan's quality revolution, sparked by Dr. Deming, turned that nation's industry from financial calamity into unprecedented post–World War II economic prosperity, it pays to heed the methods used to create such a change in fortune. "[T]he Japanese had concluded that innovation, the power to make decisions, and the ability to mobilize others must exist throughout the ranks of the organization. They reasoned that in a complex environment those closest to the process are best suited to make decisions and see them through."[1] Wendy's accomplished this—a partnership with employees to get the job done—by putting service first and organizational processes last. Outcomes became more important than process.

Wendy's restructured across its continuum of service—customers, workers, and the organization— in a participative, shared leadership (through stock options), and the employees responded by taking ownership of the company seriously. The basic premise is this: an owner of a business accepts the responsibility for problem-solving and for keeping customers (employees and patrons) happy across a continuum of service because each has a stake in the company's success. The employees' stake lies in steady, enjoyable employment and benefits and the patrons' stake lies in predictable, pleasant service, and enjoyable food. These stakes can only be accomplished by management and staff working together.

The same basic premise underlies shared leadership in a health care organization. It gives health care employees a stake in steady employment and patients a stake in predictable, consistent, pleasant services.

THE CONTINUUM OF SERVICE

As the CEO accepts the challenge and begins to design an organization-wide performance management system, the national movement toward a continuum of service between all health care providers must be addressed. Driven by the United States health care crisis that spawned managed care, alliances, freestanding clinics, emergency centers, and so on, a continuum of care became a necessity. In fact, JCAHO introduced it as one of the 11 organizational functions to be given assessment priority. Assessing the continuum of care is necessary because of the multiple health care providers available to each patient. In addition to the health care providers, today's patients have a variety of facilities— from those in shopping malls to those that are freestanding and located miles from an acute care hospital to home-based care and treatment. The patient may enter several different kinds of specialty health care facilities for various treatments and see numerous health care providers. However, there is a lack of a central, coordinated information center that consolidates all patients' medical records for easy access.

Compliance with the "seamless" service function is aimed at the cooperative release of information between health care providers and organizations about the patient's treatment and services received. This facilitates improved patient advice, education, and treatment options without long delays between the patient's needs and the provider's and organization's response. Such a knowledge base also could facilitate the patient's integration back into the community following hospitalization, because all agencies and support groups that could be of service to the patient are part of the information and service continuum.

The continuum of service function will also apply to standards. Health care organizations should be wary of creating internal standards to be used exclusively by the organization's staff members. Standards should now be viewed as multi-dimensional, interdisciplinary documents that serve as guidelines for coordinating and integrating all components of patient services, practices, and governance systems of an integrated health care delivery system. This calls for a new way of thinking about traditional standards development as well as a new way to create them. Standards that traditionally affected only those employees within the walls of the organization will find themselves faced with the task of creating and implementing standards that are interhospital, interfacility, interspecialty, and interprovider, as well as multi-worker. The close integration of all health care systems will require an environment of cooperation instead of competition.

Restructuring health care organizations across a continuum of service, practice, and governance requires the same type of "systems thinking" that was used by James W. Near to turn around the customer satisfaction level and the meager profits of the Wendy's International corporation. To Mr. Near, outcomes were more important than structure or process. The Joint Commission seems to agree. "We are shifting the focus from structure and process to outcomes," says Dennis O'Leary, president of the JCAHO.[13]

Focusing on customer outcomes requires restructuring traditional thought processes and seeking new methods of doing business, and providing services. It will be no easy task for those CEOs managing today's health care organizations. It will, in fact, be a difficult task, because the focus cannot be shifted within the present health care environment without a complete overhaul—in philosophy, in information management, and in cooperation instead of competition with other health care organizations.

The United States' health care system has demonstrated that the traditional hierarchical model is inefficient and costly. Management structures that make the pursuit of improved performance a part of the daily work experience of all staff members are rapidly becoming the most profitable. This means that a change in management style should be one that facilitates shared responsibility and accountability across a continuum of care for the quality of delivered services.

The continuum of care concept of providing seamless service "beyond our walls" is new and revolutionary. It means being customer-centered rather than organization-centered. But it holds the exciting possibility of tracking each individual's health care status from birth to death. Armed with this kind of data, rational predictions may then be made about planning, dispensing, and costing out health-related services to the American public.

The question now arises, "How do I begin?" THE BLUEPRINT that divides the organization into three domains provides the foundational model for the organization (see Chapter 3). It serves as the "hymnal" from which everybody within the organization sings.

Additionally, there is a council framework built on the principles of THE BLUEPRINT that provides one method for restructuring a health care organization. This is discussed in Chapter 5.

REFERENCES

1. Bowles J, Hammond J: *Beyond quality: how 50 winning companies use continuous improvement,* New York, 1991, Putnam.
2. Deming WE: *Out of crisis,* ed 2, Cambridge, Mass, 1986, MIT Center for Advanced Engineering Study.
3. Dobyns L, Crawford-Mason C: *Quality or else: the revolution in world business,* Boston, 1991, Houghton Mifflin Co.
4. Grimaldi P: Monitoring managed care's quality, *Nursing Management,* 26(9): 1995.
5. Hammer M, Champy J: *Reengineering the corporation: a manifesto for business revolution,* New York, 1993, Harper Business.
6. Joint Commission: *The complete guide to the 1995 hospital survey process,* Chicago, 1995, The Commission.
7. Juran JM: *Juran's quality control handbook,* ed 4, New York, 1988, McGraw-Hill.
8. Near JW: Wendy's successful "mop bucket attitude," *Wall Street Journal,* April 27, 1992.
9. Neuhauser D, McEachern JE, Headrick L: *Clinical CQI: a book of readings,* Chicago, 1995, Joint Commission.
10. Port O, Carey J, Kelly K, Forest S: Special report on quality: small and midsize companies seize the challenge—not a moment too soon, *Business Week,* November 30, 1992, pp 66-75.
11. The quality march: part two of a national survey of quality improvement activities, *Hospitals and Health Networks,* December 20, 1993.
12. Schrage M: Accreditation becomes battleground for defining quality health care, *The Washington Post,* pF3, April 21, 1995.
13. Senge P et al: *The fifth discipline fieldbook: strategies and tools for building a learning organization,* New York, 1994, Doubleday.
14. Yoder Wise P: *Leading and managing in nursing,* St. Louis, 1995, Mosby.

Chapter 5

Shared Leadership: Structuring for Organization-Wide Improvement

Getting good players signed up is easy.
Getting them to play together—that's the hard part.
Casey Stengel

Two workmen were struggling unsuccessfully with a refrigerator at the door of a house. Finally after a half hour of grunting and groaning, the fellow on the outside yelled to the fellow on the inside: "We're *never* going to get this refrigerator in."

"IN?" cried the fellow on the inside, "I've been trying to push it out!"[3]

These two workers exemplify a phenomenon that currently is happening in the health care industry—struggling against the unrelenting forces that are "pushing and pulling" each health care facility. Because there is no way of escape from these forces, the nation's CEOs are caught in the middle of the struggle.

"Chief Executive Officers (CEOs) of the nation's health care organizations are generally a tough lot who have accomplished much," says Scholtes, author of Joiner's *Team Handbook*.[2] Although the efforts of CEOs have been instrumental in building the best health care system the world has known, our nation's competitive edge in the health care industry still appears to be toppling. The health care industry is experiencing a difficult time of rapid change, global competition, and failing institutions. "By the end of this century, it is estimated that as many as one thousand hospitals will either merge or close."[1]

In 1993 there were over 5,400 acute care community general hospitals in the United States, which are what we normally think of when we use the term hospital. In addition, there are some 880 specialty hospitals and 300-some-odd federal facilities. These range in size from less than 20 to more than 1,000 beds. And while 60 percent are not-for-profit entities, 26 percent are operated by local governments and 14 percent are owned by for-profit corporations. Some are parts of larger chains and some are operated by religious orders.[5]

Obviously these organizations vary enormously in structure, activities, financing, and management styles of their individual CEOs and governing bodies.

Many CEOs are understandably frustrated as they try to adapt to the new health care environment and position their organizations for the future. One of the greatest problems they face is the reality of the changing customer. In researching this problem, Marc Roberts found that,

First, customers will travel about as far to buy new clothes as they will for most hospital care—farther for a suit than a T-shirt and farther for heart surgery than a diagnostic X-ray. Secondly, the same forces that have disadvantaged many stores in older urban downtown areas have had a similar effect on hospitals. The suburban middle class does not want to fight downtown traffic, poor parking, and a feeling that the neighborhood is dangerous—either to shop or to seek medical care. Moreover, today nearly half of all hospital admissions come from the emergency room, and folks do not tend to drive far for that service. In addition, more than half of all surgery was done on an "outpatient" basis, which means without an overnight stay. Again, why travel far for such a short visit?[5]

It is obvious that the rapid changes in customer demographics and the economic upheaval are two of the forces necessitating restructuring. These forces beyond the CEO's control are similar to being strapped into a seat inside a jumbo jet. As the plane descends in preparation for landing, the pilot says, ". . . ladies and gentlemen, we will be on the ground shortly." There is always a bit of a chill at these words, because all passengers know that they *will* be on the ground shortly; either safely or . . . the alternative! Many CEOs find themselves "strapped in" the chaos of today's health care industry—change and restructuring *will* occur and the CEO will "be on the ground shortly." Either safely or . . . the alternative!

The chaos is no surprise to anyone associated with the health care industry. Rapid changes as organizations restructure, reposition themselves, and jockey for a place in the future are such common occurrences in many areas that they rarely make the front page of the local newspapers. In the past in rural America, health care organizations tried to locate outside of towns, where property and taxes were cheaper. Often such health care organizations were the "only game in town" and everybody who needed hospital services drove 10 to 20 miles to receive services. Today, increasing consumer affluence has led to demands that health care services be provided in areas of convenience. This has created an entire new industry of shopping mall and corner store walk-in medical services. It also has caused some large health care organizations to rethink their futures.

For example, Lahey Clinic moved from downtown Boston to a newly built facility directly adjacent to one of the area's largest shopping centers, the Burlington Mall.[5] Now, although patients drive further for health care services, traffic problems are minimal, parking is available, crime is not an issue, and customers can "one-stop shop." They may now arrive at 8:00 in the morning and have their labs drawn, x-rays and ECGs performed, fill in the preregistration papers, walk across the sky-walk when the mall opens at 9:30 and buy a new robe and slippers at their favorite department store, eat a nice lunch at the food court, pick up a few groceries, and leave the mall by noon without ever having been outside since arrival that morning at the hospital. It is no surprise that customers would choose health care at that facility.

CEOs are finding—often through trial and error—that former governance methods no longer work. The hierarchical management approach and the chain of command style, which worked in the old environment, are obsolete today, especially in the light of expanding accreditation regulations. Meeting this demand has generated new ways to provide old services.

These multi-dimensional mega complex facilities almost seem to have a life of their own. Unfortunately, some organizations have such a long history of factious leadership under multiple CEOs that they have become almost too unwieldy to handle. The right hand has no idea of what the left hand is doing. One nurse worked for years at health care organizations without knowing who her respective vice president for Patient Care Services was or what he or she looks like. After a pause, she smiled and added, "Actually, the vice president for Patient Care Services might be a 'he' for all I know!"

Similarly, Marc Roberts found that "many health care organizations' internal structure makes them what may be the most unmanageable organizations in America.[5] Clearly, creative new management methods are needed in today's health care organizations along with the governing boards' approval to act on new business techniques.

However, many CEOs are trapped in outdated hierarchical management styles and unwieldy organizations. CEOs are not only unable to use their own creative potential to restructure their organizations, but also unable to tap the creative potential of their workers. As the winds of change blow, in order to avoid unpleasantness with the governing board, a few CEOs believe that hanging on and maintaining the status quo is the safest thing to do. If a CEO decides that maintaining status quo is the best option, he or she should visit and observe a progressive nearby health care organization. The acquisitions, mergers, alliances, networking, benchmarking, reorganizations, and restructuring blazing like wildfire through the industry may serve as a warning that change is inevitable. Those that fail to remain current with the demands of the world around them will fail.

THE NEED FOR CHANGE

CEOs who choose to remain current will recognize a need to restructure their organizations to meet the growing customer expectations and financial demands of the world around them. Many CEOs already have found that they must do things differently to survive. Competition, powered by new, wiser management styles, has never been more intense. In the past, whatever a patient needed was provided and somebody paid the bill or it was "written off." Today, many patients have no access to care, and the health care dollars are elusive and tightly controlled. This is another factor that is driving and transforming every facet of the health care industry before our eyes—from the accrediting process to the delivery of all customer services in every department.

These consumer and economic forces are making restructuring mandatory. Without restructuring it will be difficult to meet accreditation requirements or to obtain a market share of the profits and stay in business. CEOs sometimes feel like their health care organizations are trapped in a vicious cycle.

It is no longer a nicety for a visionary CEO to restructure, reshape, and reform the way his or her organization does business; it is a necessity! In most organizations CEOs hold the power for change in their hands. Whether or not the organization arrives "on the ground" safely or . . . the alternative, is largely up to the top leadership of the organization.

Occasionally change is hampered by previous experiences of either the CEO or the governing board. Some CEOs and governing boards have elected to keep the traditional, hierarchical management style because it is the less offensive and troublesome of those that have been tried. There are two major governing styles that have plagued health care organizations for the past 10 years. Both are major barriers to restructuring today. They are (1) nursing shared governance and (2) the "bottom line" management style.

Barrier #1: We've Already Tried Shared Governance!

One of the most popular as well as the most unfortunate restructuring strategies that briefly engrossed the American health care industry was called shared governance. As one CEO put it, "We've been hit by that shared governance truck and we lost a lot of money in the aftermath. I want no part of shared *anything* as long as I remain CEO. I'll never make that mistake again." Shared leadership is **not** nursing shared governance! (See Appendix 5-1 at the end of this chapter.)

The concept of nurses restructuring the division of nursing into one of shared governance blazed like a comet across the national health care skyline in the early 1980s. Many health care organizations, recognizing the need for change and listening to the rhetoric of the day, chose to attempt a nursing shared governance model. Some of this enticing verbiage promised to

Solve personnel shortages, boost staff morale, slash costs, enhance multi disciplinary collaboration, improve clinical outcomes, etc.

But despite the fact that nursing publications have been besieged with articles about models that empower nurses, nursing administrators still are hard-pressed to differentiate one nursing governance innovation from another—beyond rearranged organizational charts and structures, that is.

The waters become that much murkier given the fact that nurse researchers have failed to empirically link any change noted after implementing a governance model to patient or staff outcomes, or to provide hard evidence that successful programs can produce similar results from one setting to another.

It gets worse; there is little agreement on some very key issues: What is shared governance? What exactly is altered by it? And how do we measure the change? This ambiguity contributes little persuasion—beyond a leap of faith—to enlist support from hospital CEOs and to fuel staff enthusiasm for new programs.[2]

Shared governance is an excellent example of what should have been a local performance improvement attempt that instead became a national band wagon. It seemed that every nursing leader in America was caught up in the concept of empowerment for *nurses* and clamoring for permission to jump on the rolling wagon. In response to their nurse leaders, the more astute CEOs called other organizations to check out the nurses' word-of-mouth glowing reports. They spoke with similar nurse leaders who bubbled with enthusiastic proclamations of decreasing costs, improving processes, and improved patient care.

In truth, the original concept of shared governance was narrow and myopic. It revolved around registered nurses organizing themselves into councils in order to assume the responsibilities of nursing leadership along with control of their practice—including electing one RN to sit on the board of directors. It was a beautiful, but brief, nursing dream.

Shared governance was not based on scientific research, and there were no identified outcomes for which data was systematically being gathered to confirm or disprove the validity of the shared governance concept. This is how rituals and myths find their way into nursing folklore and, unfortunately, myths get perpetuated as truths. Shared governance was a "quick fix" effectively used to silence the nurse faction of the health care industry by seeming to give nurses the thing they wanted most—complete, autonomous, independent control of their practice. Morale of the nurses improved as they dreamed of empowerment. They quickly got back in line—many voting against unionization because shared governance was becoming a reality—and scurried about creating councils and jockeying for positions of perceived authority within the councils!

It was our opinion during this tumultuous period in nursing's history that the concept of shared governance was destined to fail. It was, we reasoned, impossible to empower one segment of health care workers over others without imposing controls. It is still impossible. Shared governance did not meet the test of time because it was not directed by the CEO and it did not meet organization-wide needs of all workers.

Robert Hess states,

Nurse administrators have used labels, such as shared, collaborative, professional, and participatory governance to describe, what are in fact, dissimilar programs that share just one common thread—an intention to augment nurses' sphere of influence within the organization. However, these models typically emphasize clinical practice...and limited management functions, such as scheduling, patient care assignments, and quality assurance monitoring—problematic areas that managers would just as soon delegate.[2]

We believe that "governance permeates so many facets of an organization that it cannot be viewed unidimensionally. Governance is a fused phenomena, a multidisciplinary concept that portrays the distribution of control, influence, power, and authority in an organization."[2] Therefore, any framework or model, strictly designed to empower nurses or to direct their practice, is destined to fail. There is no such thing as an independent practice for any segment of worker in the health care industry. All employees within a health care organization, including physicians, are interdependent. Not one group of health care employees can do their assigned jobs without all other workers of the organization also performing their jobs.

Barrier #2: If It Costs Money, Forget It!

A second monumental barrier to restructuring lies in the philosophy of the organization's governing board of directors. Many have a fixation on what we call the "VNO Requirement." *VNO* stands for "visible numbers only," and it describes those governing boards that demand only one thing from their CEO: a positive quarterly profit report. These governing boards, at the peak of the hierarchical pecking order, are little concerned with processes, systems, employees, customer complaints, services delivered, work redesign, or the real performance capabilities of the organization. Their eye is fixed on what they deem to be a profit margin this quarter. This leads them to set an arbitrary numerical target profit each quarter that the CEO must meet. Because there is often an underlying, unspoken threat that profits are synonymous with job security, the CEO passes on the numerical target, right on down the line, until every employee also feels the pressure.

Although Peter Scholtes[6] calls this management style "Management by Results" and we call it "VNO Management," it is the same style with slight variations. Scholtes notes that when profit is the primary

motivating factor in an organization's existence, it fosters a host of organizational problems. Here are six problems of this management style identified by Scholtes that will block a restructuring initiative by the CEO.

Short-term thinking. In a system of numerical objectives, standards, and quotas, rewarded efforts are measurable and of short duration. The near horizon gets attention and countable results receive priority even though the organization's survival may depend on unmeasurable activities undertaken to reach long-term goals. This attitude wreaks havoc with all performance improvement initiatives as well as worker morale along the way.

Misguided focus. If managers and workers do not understand the system's capabilities, a numerical goal is nothing more than guesswork. Decisions will be made by "gut feeling," "the seat of their pants," "hunches," or "knee-jerk reactions." Deming addressed this phenomenon in his famous red bead experiment that is discussed in Chapter 11. In any event, a misguided focus does nothing to help the workers, the organization, or the customer.

Internal conflict. Heeding the numbers instead of the processes and workers causes internal conflict. Controls that affect one department will likely affect several other departments and this leads to conflict. The conflicts between departments lead to finger pointing, the blame game, and an endless series of excuses for why their department's numbers are not as good as the other departments. Everyone is trying to look good to the top management and turf wars flourish.

Fudging the figures. Frequently, imposed measurable goals are unattainable; they lie beyond a system's capability. Workers are forced by the system to fudge figures, alter records, or just "play the game" to work around the system, because they understand that the organizational hierarchy will not permit them to utilize the organization's resources to improve it. For the sake of job security, this charade fosters guarded communication and minor, sometimes major, dishonesty.

Greater fear. The worst shortcoming of the hierarchical, VNO management style is fear—fear of what will happen if quotas are not met, being out of favor, not getting the promotion, or even losing the job. Fear is the prime motivator in this type of system. The more rigid and unrealistic the controls are, the deeper the fear is.

One story that exemplifies the fear principle among employees involves a midnight buffet on a cruise. While standing and chatting with a guest, an employee in charge of the beverage bar suddenly glanced up at the deck above him. The captain of the ship was standing a bit to the left of center on the upper deck. Without noticeably moving a muscle, he said softly to his fellow worker, "Enemy at 11 o'clock." Without looking up, that worker softly said, "Thanks." He took four steps and said to the next worker, "Enemy at 11 o'clock." The word spread around the deck—even onto the dance floor where employees were dancing with guests! This was accomplished by one employee jumping onto the dance floor, laughing and gyrating as he made the rounds to each employee engaged in the dance.

Blindness to customer concerns. A hierarchical management style with emphasis on the bottom line quarterly profit report encourages a company to look inward, rather than outward, at the world in which the customer operates. The emphasis will be greater on profits than on customer satisfaction. Customers no longer need to come to our health care organization for service. There are a plethora of health care organizations ready and waiting for their business. Today there are many options in a variety of settings for people who need health care services.

Peter Scholtes ends by saying, "When people finally realize that the indicators of control may be focused on the wrong measurements, it's too late. The ship is going down and 'Nearer My God To Thee' is heard from the afterdeck."[6]

Scholtes was correct in stating that the VNO Management system is fraught with problems. One of the greatest problems lies in the fact that quotas or bottom line profits may be impossible to achieve, because each part of a health care organization is totally dependent on all others doing their jobs well.

Since employees in departments have little or no control over their colleagues from other departments, when a service crosses several departments, such as environmental services, housekeeping, lab, radiology and surgical services, interdisciplinary problems are bound to arise. Services that require cooperation and coordination from several different departments often are a source of trouble unsolved by the traditional chain-of-command approach. And there is universal agreement that the team approach is the ideal performance improvement mechanism. However, under the hierarchical management style of governance, when a performance improvement opportunity arises, it is virtually impossible to initiate and maintain the momentum of a team of interdisciplinary employees working through the improvement process until improvement is actually achieved.

When a team is suggested in response to the performance improvement opportunity, questions immediately arise. Which department will call the meeting? Whose department budget will support meeting attendance? Which manager will conduct the meeting? Whose job is it to implement a solution? What if one

manager refuses to implement the solution the team agrees would be the best? May that manager overrule the team's decision? Whose department budget will pay for the solution? The idea of an organized response to a performance improvement opportunity flounders and dies for lack of a system to initiate change.

If an organization-wide performance management system is to be successful, it will have to start at the very top of the organization. Empowerment for restructuring will be given to the CEO, who in turn will create a system that fosters a continuum of service between departments to eliminate turf battles, interdepartmental bickering, and hierarchical chains-of-command. No longer may limited resources such as time, money, personnel, equipment, and supplies be devoted to nonproductive squabbles, while performance improvement opportunities within the health care organization go unresolved. Although everyone agrees that teams closest to the performance improvement opportunity should seek solutions, teams cannot function without the empowerment of top management. Paradigms that provide every employee with a stake in conserving resources and controlling outcomes will be actively pursued by those who wish to succeed. CEOs who now bear the responsibility and accountability for organizing and directing the organization-wide performance management system will discover that they like the new role.

THE DRIVING FORCE BEHIND CHANGE

A French author once described heaven and hell in a way that brings home the deepest meaning of cooperation. He described hell as the most exquisite and inviting dining room imaginable. But when new residents of hell sat down to eat, they made a shocking discovery: their elbows did not bend. And so they spent eternity the way they spent their time on earth: futilely trying to stuff themselves.

An adjoining banquet hall, which was heaven, was just like hell in every respect. And when new residents of heaven sat down to eat, they also found out that their elbows did not bend. The people in heaven also spent eternity the way they spent their lives on earth: feeding the person across from them.[3]

A health care organization can be either heaven or hell for internal or external customers. It all depends on the degree to which the health care organization is willing to serve the needs of others and satisfy customers.

The increasing necessity for cooperation instead of competition in the workplace is another driving force behind restructuring the health care organization.

The key to making this happen lies within the power of the CEO. Senge states that "the definition of leadership refers to 'one person' as the leader."[7] This would seem to contradict the shared leadership concept. It does not. One-person leadership enhances the shared leadership concept and makes CEOs comfortable implementing it, because while governance is shared, authority is retained. (See Chapter 18, Empowering the Workforce.)

Behind every profitable health care organization lies a CEO—the "one person" leader—with a vision! He or she most likely has abandoned the traditional hierarchical management style in favor of a "flatter," more interdisciplinary organizational management approach. As one CEO put it, "Our management team is newer and fewer but every single man and woman knows his importance to our success."

Many CEOs are already involved in designing and experimenting with systems of governance in which performance management plays the most significant role. They are already convinced that they must restructure their organizations so that every employee participates in an integrated and continuous performance management system. Furthermore, CEOs of shared leadership organizations will not be the traditional autocratic rulers but will display an ability to work with others and be collaborators and negotiators. "They will blend individual creativity and energy with a value of team effort."[4] In the health care industry, what the CEO buys into, works!

One early outcome of change that is fostering the advancement of the shared leadership concept is the positive performance improvements created and inspired by employees who have been permitted to work on CEO-driven teams. A bevy of benefits have emerged:

- Employees often have a better feel than managers for how processes could be improved; shared leadership breeds creativity ("How would I do this if it were up to me? How could I make my job easier?") Hands-on experience creates an awareness of performance improvement opportunities unknown by many managers.
- Employees may have more diverse backgrounds than managers; they are probably more transient than managers and therefore have picked up many ideas from other jobs ("Where I used to work we solved this problem by . . ."). Management may pick up some great ideas.
- Employees can experiment without upsetting the apple cart; employees can tinker with a new idea and generate little attention, whereas managers investigating the same process would create major concerns among employees.
- Employee-based ideas fare better in the unfair game of politics. Which ideas get a better reception from the work force: proposals from peers or management-mandated manifestos? You got it!

- Employee suggestion programs strengthen important organizational dynamics. You cannot do all the work yourself. You have to delegate. A sound, structured program involving all employees will facilitate your efforts.[8]

With all of the positive benefits of utilizing a shared leadership model driven by the CEO and utilizing every employee's input, are there any negatives? The greatest drawback to implementing a shared leadership model lies in the necessity for organization-wide education to the new leadership style—which means an upfront investment of the organization's resources.

A FRAMEWORK FOR CHANGE

The performance management system of shared leadership displayed in Figure 5-1 is an integral part of THE BLUEPRINT—the synergistic model described in Chapter 3. The evaluation portion of THE BLUEPRINT model is given "life" through the *Shared Leadership* framework. (For 10 characteristics of shared leadership see Appendix 5-2 at the end of this chapter.) By using the principles of this framework, CEOs swiftly and simply are able to restructure a health care organization.

This successful Shared Leadership framework proposed by Katz and Green portrays four councils and two boards that are necessary to organize and manage an organization-wide performance management system. Four groups of interdisciplinary leaders are called *councils*, because a council is "an executive body whose members are equal in power and authority."[3a] There are also two boards. One is the governing board of directors. The governing board of directors exercises a continuous sovereign authority over the entire organization, especially to control and direct the making and administration of policy. The second is the quality management board (QMB). This group has been given the title of "board" because it maintains sovereign authority over the performance management system of the entire health care organization, and the four councils are subject to it. The authority and responsibility for all performance improvement activities lie with the QMB. The QMB, chaired by the organization's CEO, serves as the pivotal point where the performance improvement "buck" stops.

Shared Leadership implemented throughout the health care organization by the CEO provides a method for maintaining control, responsibility, and accountability of the key functions and their processes of service, practice, and governance. Furthermore, the responsibility and accountability of assessing the 11 functions of JCAHO (see box on p. 49) or the 6 areas of accreditation of the NCQA (see box in Chapter 7 on

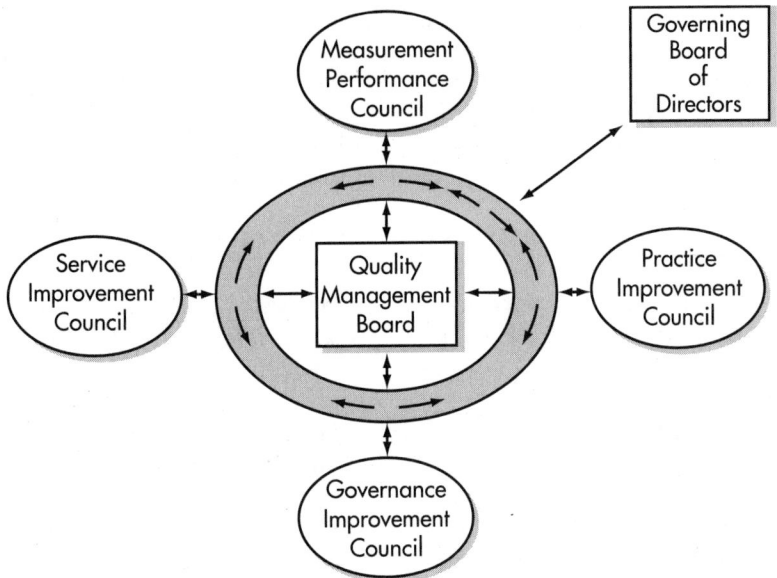

Figure 5-1   The shared leadership framework.

JCAHO'S MANDATED FUNCTIONS FOR 1996

Patient-focused Functions

1. Patient Rights and Organizational Ethics
2. Patient Assessment
3. Care of Patients
4. Education
5. Continuum of Care

Organizational Functions

6. Performance Improvement
7. Leadership
8. Management of the Environment of Care
9. Management of Human Resources
10. Management of Management
11. Surveillance, Prevention, and Control of Infection

Structures with Functions

(These must be in place but are not formally assessed as are the first 11 functions.)

12. Governance
13. Management
14. Medical Staff
15. Nursing

Modified from the 1995 Comprehensive Accreditation Manual for Hospitals by The Joint Commission for the Accreditation of Healthcare Organizations.

p. 77) may be distributed among the councils to share the work of preparation for accreditation.

The councils are named according to how they function within the organization. They are

- the governing board of directors (BOD)
- the quality management board (QMB)
- the performance measurement council (PMC)
- the service improvement council (SIC)
- the practice improvement council (PIC)
- the governance improvement council (GIC)

The four councils and the BOD orbiting the QMB in Figure 5-1 feed into a circle of conductivity. This circle is like a steering wheel of an automobile—driving, directing, and maintaining control by steering the organization via its four council arms. The wheel enables interaction among all councils as well as with the hub or central board, the QMB. The QMB is placed in the center of the wheel as the "horn," or alarm device, ready to sound at the first hint of trouble.

Overview of the Work of Councils and Boards

Governing Board of Directors (BOD). This board retains overall responsibility and accountability for the successful operation of the entire organization.

Suggested BOD members
- Board chairperson
- Chief executive officer
- Chief financial officer
- Vice president for patient services
- Chief of staff
- Community members as consumer representatives
- Corporation representatives
- Philanthropic representatives
- Representatives of managed care contracts/alliances
- Community spiritual leaders

Suggested BOD responsibilities

1. Establish corporate mission
2. Appoint the chief executive officer
3. Establish long-range strategic plan for the organization
4. Establish the annual organizational budget
5. Appoint members of the medical staff
6. Oversee interdisciplinary shared leadership framework
7. Assess and measure organizational performance against plans, budgets, national databases, and measurements of performance

Suggested BOD meetings. Meetings are held either monthly or quarterly.

Suggested BOD term of office. Members of this board serve as long as bylaws permit.

Quality Management Board (QMB). This board retains the responsibility and accountability for the organization-wide performance management program. The CEO is chairperson of this board and members serve at his or her discretion.

Suggested QMB members

- Chief executive officer (Chair)
- Chief financial officer
- Chief operating officer
- Vice president for patient services
- Chief of medical staff
- Risk manager
- Utilization management manager
- Director of market/public relations
- Chairperson of the four other councils
- Any other employees deemed appropriate by the CEO

Suggested QMB responsibilities

1. Implement the corporate mission, philosophy, and goals
2. Actualize strategic planning
3. Implement policy development as well as resource utilization
4. Management planning
5. Performance management organization-wide
   - create councils
   - create job descriptions for all councils
   - implement team worksheet guidelines
   - oversee education for performance management
   - appoint all team leaders, team members, cost out teams, etc.
   - create reporting flow chart
   - review all data
   - prepare facility for accreditation survey
6. Determine delivery of care methodology, acuity, and staffing mix

7. Manage budget and allocation of resources
8. Oversee all risk and utilization management variances
9. Determine contract employment
10. Oversee all marketing, media/public relations, community interface
11. Appoint all council chairs and council members
12. Any other duties as described by the CEO

Suggested QMB meetings. Meetings are held monthly or at the discretion of the CEO.

Suggested QMB term of office. Members of this council serve by virtue of their position within the organization or by the discretion of the CEO.

Service Improvement Council (SIC). This council maintains responsibility and accountability for all clinical patient services within the organization. The chairperson and members of this council are appointed by the QMB. Any staff member with a strong clinical background and education as well as people skills is qualified to chair this council. The chairperson of this council becomes an automatic member of the QMB.

Suggested SIC membership

- chairperson appointed by the QMB
- medical staff
- nursing staff (one from each unit)
- discharge planning staff
- home care services staff
- outpatient services staff
- laboratory staff
- pharmacy staff
- radiology staff
- housekeeping staff
- dietary/nutritional services staff
- materials management staff
- medical records staff
- bio-medical/environmental services staff
- any other staff members deemed necessary/appropriate by the QMB

Suggested SIC responsibilities

1. Support the corporate mission, philosophy, and goals
2. Oversee the development of all patient care standards, including those related to case/outcomes management
3. Approve all patient care standards
4. Oversee the development of patient's rights and organizational ethics standards
5. Oversee the integrity of all clinical documentation of the organization
6. Interact and cooperate with infection control requests and recommendations

7. Participate in clinical research and communicate relevant data to other councils
8. Oversee the organization's patient profile tools, matrices of scope of service, practice and governance and prioritizing matrices from all departments; keep each current for the QMB
9. Follow communication channels as designated by QMB
10. Create, distribute, analyze, and act on the information derived from patient satisfaction surveys
11. Other duties deemed appropriate and assigned by the QMB

Suggested SIC meetings. Meetings are held monthly.
Suggested SIC term of office. A minimum of 2 years' commitment is necessary for members of the SIC. Terms of service should be staggered so that there is never a complete turnover of council membership. Bringing new people onto the council as terms of service end provides a constantly renewed pool of tested talent for the organization.

Practice Improvement Council (PIC). This council retains the responsibility and accountability for the practice of all employees. This permits staff members to govern themselves and to determine issues of competency, dress, behavior, and collaborative practice. Council members are appointed by the QMB.

Suggested PIC membership
- chairperson appointed by the QMB
- medical staff
- nursing staff (one from each unit)
- education staff
- human resources staff
- bio-medical/environmental services staff
- housekeeping staff
- dietary/nutritional services staff
- laboratory staff
- pharmacy staff
- physical therapy staff
- cardiopulmonary staff
- library staff
- materials management staff
- home care services staff
- outpatient services staff
- medical records staff
- discharge planning staff
- any other staff members deemed appropriate by the QMB

Suggested PIC responsibilities
1. Support the corporate mission, philosophy, and goals
2. Oversee the development of all professional practice standards, including those related to competency, dress, behavior, collaborative practice, floating, patient assignments, work duties, conflicts, interdepartmental conflicts, cross-training, all staff member education, patient and family education, etc.
3. Approve all professional practice standards
4. Oversee development of staff rights including distribution of written document
5. Oversee professional ethics issues
6. Participate in professional research and communicate relevant data to other councils
7. Follow communication channels as designated by the QMB
8. Plan and oversee the implementation of professional recognition strategies
9. Resolve competency issues (e.g., professional credentialing and/or certification)
10. Create, distribute, analyze, and act on the information from staff and physician satisfaction surveys
11. Other duties deemed appropriate and assigned by the QMB

Suggested PIC meetings. Meetings are held monthly.
Suggested term of office. A minimum of 2 years' commitment is necessary for members of the PIC. It is suggested that terms of service be staggered so that there is never a complete turnover of council membership. Bringing new people onto the council as terms of service end maintains a constant pool of tested talent for the organization.

Governance Improvement Council (GIC). This council retains the responsibility and accountability for the day-to-day governance of the organization. This council provides managers with a forum for interaction on the day-to-day problems of the organization.

Suggested GIC membership
- chairperson appointed by the QMB
- managers of every department (and unit) of the organization

Suggested GIC responsibilities
1. Support the corporate mission, philosophy, and goals
2. Oversee the development of all administrative standards, including those related to administrative policies, procedures, and practice guidelines
3. Approve all administrative standards
4. Participates in administrative research and communicates the relevant data to other councils
5. Oversee new product evaluation, equipment function, adequacy of supplies, and technology measurement including feedback of all faulty equipment; new equipment requests
6. Resolve day-to-day operational/system difficulties

7. Follow communication channels as designated by QMB
8. Oversee the fire and safety committee
9. Create, distribute, analyze, and act on the information derived from manager satisfaction surveys
10. Other duties deemed appropriate and assigned by the QMB

Suggested GIC meetings. Meetings are held monthly and may also be called into emergency session by the chairperson to handle an immediate system crisis situation.

Suggested GIC term of office. The members of this council serve by virtue of their position within the organization. As long as a member is a manager within the organization, he or she is a member of this council.

Performance Measurement Council (PMC). This council retains the responsibility for receiving, aggregating, and packaging all data of the organization; participation in national data banks, and for overseeing all mandated performance measures. This council is responsible for the routine collection of all quality control information from units/departments. Furthermore, the PMC serves as a resource center for the education and execution of accurate and appropriate performance measurement processes within the organization, such as current methods for conducting teams, use of statistical process control tools, development of story boards, etc.

Suggested PMC membership
- chairperson appointed by the QMB
- medical staff
- nursing staff
- infection control staff
- administration staff
- discharge planning staff
- outpatient services staff
- home care services staff
- laboratory staff
- pharmacy staff
- radiology staff
- housekeeping staff
- dietary/nutritional services staff
- materials management staff
- medical records staff
- bio-medical/environmental services staff
- any other staff member deemed necessary/appropriate by the QMB

Suggested PMC responsibilities
1. Support the corporate mission, philosophy, and goals
2. Oversee organization-wide quality control data

3. Collect, send, receive, and report data to and from national data banks designated by the QMB
4. Oversee the integrity of incoming QC data (from other councils and departments)
5. Participate in quality improvement research and communicate relevant data to other councils
6. Follow quality communication channels as designated by the QMB
7. Determine performance measurement policies and procedures, including the type of assessment tools, sample size, determining data collection methodologies, determining by whom and how data will be tabulated
8. Design appropriate action plans to correct quality problems
9. Spearhead organization-wide preparation for accreditation surveys
10. Any other duties deemed appropriate and assigned by the QMB

Suggested PMC meetings. Meetings are held monthly.

Suggested PMC term of office. A minimum of 3 years' commitment is suggested for members of the PMC. It is suggested that terms of service be staggered so that there is never a complete turnover of council membership. Bringing new people onto the council as terms of service end provides a constantly renewed pool of tested talent for the organization.

REFERENCES

1. Anderson R: Atlas of the American economy: an illustrated guide to industries and trends, *The congressional quarterly,* Washington, D.C., 1994, Elliott & Clark Publishing.
2. Hess Jr, RG: Shared governance: nursing's 20th-century Tower of Babel, *J Nur Adm,* 25(5): 14-17, 1995.
3. Mannello T: *A CQI system for healthcare: how the Williamsport Hospital brings quality to life,* New York, 1995, Quality Resources.
3a. *Merriam-Webster's collegiate dictionary,* ed 10, Springfield, Mass, 1993, Merriam-Webster.
4. Merry MD: Shared leadership in health care organizations. *Topics in health care financing,* 20(4): 26-38, 1994.
5. Roberts M: *Your money or your life: the health care crisis explained,* New York, 1993, Doubleday.
6. Scholtes PR: *The team handbook,* Madison, Wis, 1990, Joiner Associates, Inc.
7. Senge P et al: *The fifth discipline fieldbook: strategies and tools for building a learning organization,* New York, 1994, Doubleday.
8. Tylczak L: *Increasing employee productivity: an introduction to value management,* Menlo Park, Cal, 1990, Crisp Publications.

Appendix 5-1   10 Reasons Why Nursing's Shared Governance Phenomenon Didn't Work

1. Nurses are not independent, autonomous practitioners subcontracting their services to a health care organization. They are an integral part of a health care *team*.
2. Nurses receive their power from management. To unite could cost their jobs. Empowered *nursing* councils that control management decisions were a myth.
3. Society and therefore hospital management undervalues care, particularly that given by nurses. There is a strong belief that family members or servants or other personnel can substitute for nurses.
4. Nurses have failed to document that their services make any difference to patient outcomes. Why should a profession portrayed as making no appreciable difference to outcomes be granted empowerment?
5. The division of nursing does not generate a revenue. People value what they pay for.
6. Nurses do not mandate nor control the labor hours per patient day. The organization's acuity system and staffing mix are determined by management based on a budget that is not shared with the workers.
7. Nurses have no power to admit, discharge, or prescribe. They function on the orders of physicians and by the policies of management. Nurses have systematically given away pieces of their profession (respiratory care, nutritional care, discharge planning, spiritual care, etc.) and, in doing so, have failed to create an area of expertise critical to positive patient outcomes.
8. Nurses have no formal control over the organization's resources.
9. Conflicts and divisions within the nursing profession are legendary. A group that cannot control itself is seen as powerless to control others or areas outside the profession.
10. Most registered nurses lack knowledge of health care finances as well as statistical knowledge necessary to plan and analyze resource utilization. Lacking knowledge of the business environment of mergers, managed care, corporations, health care reform, and the nuances of Medicare and Medicaid, RNs are crippled in their efforts to effect change.

Appendix 5-2   Characteristics of Shared Leadership

1. Shared leadership provides a shared, understandable, visual framework for organization-wide performance management.
2. All councils are interdisciplinary, made up of workers from both within and without the health care organization, which fosters collaboration across the continuum of health care.
3. Resource conservation and utilization become the responsibility of each council and all team leaders by virtue of the organized methodology to construct and manage team projects.
4. The QMB, chaired by the CEO, serves as the pivotal quality focus of the organization.
5. All duties and responsibilities of each council are delineated in writing.
6. There is no attempt by workers to wrest control of the organization from management, nor is there an attempt by management to sabotage staff members' assumption of their responsibilities, since all councils are interdisciplinary and all council members work toward meeting the interdisciplinary outcomes of the organization.
7. The work of measuring the required functions of health care organizations in anticipation of an accreditation survey by JCAHO or NCQA may be divided among the councils for a more even distribution of responsibility and accountability as well as a more equitable method of meeting accreditation requirements.
8. Councils are designed so that problems are addressed by staff members closest to the problems, since council positions are appointed based on expertise within the organization.
9. Teams are empowered to act within the guidelines of the organization.
10. This framework fosters cooperation rather than competition.

Part Three

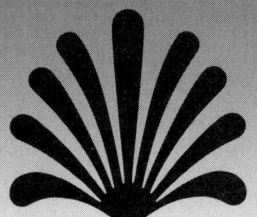

CREATING AN ORGANIZATION-WIDE PERFORMANCE AWARENESS PROGRAM

Chapter 6

Identifying Customers and Delineating the Scope of Business

If you don't know where you are going, when you get there, you don't even know you're there.

Herb Cohen

Perhaps you have read the poem about the five wise men who wanted to learn about elephants, so they observed one. But because they were all blind, they could not see the elephant. Each wise man touched a different part of the elephant to determine what the animal felt like; each man drew a different conclusion:

- The first stumbled into the elephant's side and decided that an elephant is like a wall.
- The second touched the elephant's tusk. He compared the elephant to a spear.
- The third held the elephant's trunk and concluded that elephants are similar to snakes.
- The fourth felt the elephant's leg and decided that elephants are very much like fans.
- The fifth, who grasped the elephant's tail, claimed that all elephants are like ropes.

The poem concludes . . .

And so these men of Indostan,
Disputed loud and long.
Each in his own opinion,
Exceeding stiff and strong.
Though each was partly in the right,
And all were in the wrong!*

---

*John Godfrey Saxe's well-known fable appears in many collections, including *100 More Story Poems*, selected by Elinor Parker, New York, 1960, Thomas Y. Crowell Company.

A similar behavior is sometimes manifested by those seeking to identify customers and delineate the scope of service, practice, and governance in today's health care organizations. Many organizations are so large and complex it is difficult to see the entire picture. If a CEO, for example, tries to understand each manager's service, practice, and governance problems, the information received will be biased. Each manager will relate the complexities of his or her particular department because that is his or her frame of reference.

As illustrated in the elephant story, when the whole is seen from a biased perspective, there is a tendency toward fragmentation of information. Fragmentation of information is the death knoll of a performance management system. If fragmentation is permitted, critical facets of health care organization's delivery of service, practice, and governance may be overlooked and opportunities to improve missed. A three-domain, or tri-focus, approach, i.e., identifying customers and delineating the scope of service, practice, and governance in a health care organization, is a key concept for successfully implementing an organization-wide performance management system. Using this approach provides top management leaders with a global view of an organization's customers and scope of services, practices, and governance issues. This view is essential to the proper distribution of resources as well as to the prioritization of key processes of an organization's functions for assessment and improvement. The organization that uses the tri-focus *team* approach to service, practice, and governance in considering each facet of its processes will quickly see the benefits. Customers fall into three domains and in identifying those of a service delivery business we look at end service users, company employees, and company managers (Figure 6-1). Problems are more easily pinpointed and solved when this organized approach is used.

However, this approach is not a quick fix for CEOs so that some quality busy work is underway to satisfy accreditation requirements. There is an old adage that says, "There is a big difference between motion and direction." CEOs cannot distribute forms, demand that management staff complete them, and when the forms are completed, ignore them. Delineating the scope of service, practice, and governance is not a new trick that will quickly boost the quarterly profits. But in the long term, rational predictions about trends and resource expenditures will be made from data rather than gut feelings and hunches.

This chapter describes a new thinking process and some associated tools to implement the technique. In fact, a CEO may find that this chapter forms the basis for reinventing the health care organization. To reinvent the organization, it may be necessary to completely abandon the traditional operational policies and procedures as well as the "chain of command" philosophy and create an entirely new set of rules and methods. Old ideas about how health care organizations should be managed and problems should be solved will be abandoned and the new organizational structures will look entirely different. Health care organizations, regardless of how small and isolated, will be designed specifically to operate in a complex global market with shared information, responsibility, and accountability. Customers, degreed professionals, and health care workers will design processes to collaborate across a broad continuum of care network that begins in the community and reaches both into and beyond the walls of an acute care facility. Organizational patterns will shift from bureaucratic to interdependent frameworks, such as the one described in Chapter 5.

Hammer and Champy refer to this shift as *reengineering*. [5] They say that

> *Business reengineering means putting aside much of the received wisdom of two hundred years of industrial management. It means forgetting how work was done in the age of the mass market and deciding how it can best be done now. In business reengineering, old job titles and old organizational arrangements—departments, divisions, groups, and so on—cease to matter. They are artifacts of another age. What matters in reengineering is how we want to organize work today, given the demands of today's markets and the power of today's technologies. How people and companies did things yesterday doesn't matter to the business reengineer."* [5]

Health care organizations are service delivery businesses, and as stated in Chapter 3, every service delivery business requires (a) someone to receive the service, (b) someone to deliver the service, and (c) someone to govern the service. Therefore, we can assume that there are three critical facets to every

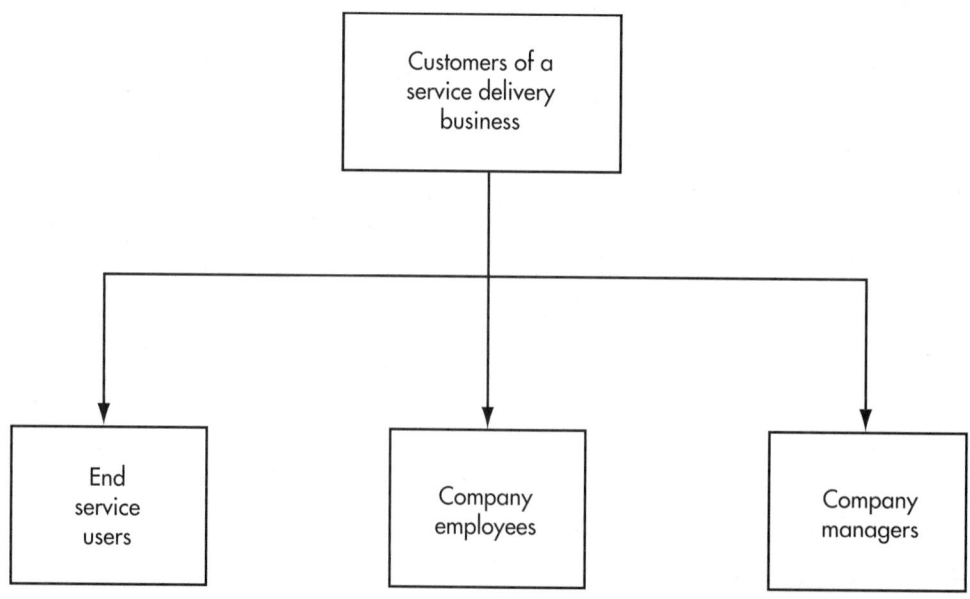

Figure 6-1   Tri-focus/three-domain approach to customers of a service delivery business.

health care organization: service, practice, and governance. Assuming the CEO has reorganized responsibility and accountability via a model such as the one described in Chapter 5, and councils are organized to govern the three domains of a service delivery business, where does the organization go from here?

KNOW THE CUSTOMER

If we are going to reengineer a health care organization, we must begin by answering the question, *Who is my customer?* If performance improvement is truly to occur in health care organizations, then performance *efforts* require a new way of thinking about the *customer.* Why focus on the customer? Because, as quoted in Zemke's *The Service Edge,* John Guerra, an AT&T branch manager, states, "Quality is not measured by me. It's not even measured by you. Quality is in the eyes of your customer."[14] Furthermore, "Businesses succeed or fail one customer at a time."[1]

Who is the customer of a health care organization? The typical answer, "the patient," is only partly true. The patient is not the *only* customer.

Many customers exist within the organization. A system for identifying them is desirable, because the delineation process looks at each domain for a comprehensive listing of all customers receiving the services, the practices, and the governance of the health care organization.

Before delineating the scope of service, practice, and governance of a health care organization, it is important to understand *who customers are.* You are then able to understand to whom or to what end the service, practice, or governance is directed. When a problem occurs, it then becomes easy for staff members to identify the domain(s) in which the problem occurs and direct the complaint to the relevant council(s). The council(s) overseeing the involved domain(s) may create a team to brainstorm the problem, find a solution by consensus, and then carry out the planned steps to resolution.

The 1990s are the decade of rediscovering the customer. This rise of customer information is the result of Japan's example of building economic strength based on customer satisfaction. Indeed, knowing the customer has become the driving force behind America's quality revolution. Here is one example of the Japanese view of customers. "On a train ride back to Tokyo from Japan's northern regions, a long-time Japanese friend explained to us the Japanese approach to business, 'In the United States,' he observed 'you say the customer is always right. In Japan, we say, *"okyakasuma wa kamisama desu"*—the customer is God. There is a big difference.'"[9]

Many trace the increased emphasis on customers in the American business world to the 1980 NBC program "If Japan Can...Why Can't We."[12] However, long before the program, "Walt Disney Productions, a current world-wide model for quality and customer service, practiced the principles of knowing its customers. Like Japan, in a Walt Disney theme park, the customer is god—and this idea was not dependent on the Japanese. In fact, the 'Disney Way' has been in effect since Steamboat Willie changed his name to Mickey Mouse."[10]

However, Disney did not limit his customer concept to those who walked through the gates of his theme parks. His concept of customer involved each domain or area of his service delivery business: customer service, staff practices, and management processes. The idea that each domain—service, practice, and governance—was equally important and required equally as much attention was revolutionary at the time. Disney had the odd notion that if he placed prime importance on (a) pleasing and meeting the needs of the paying customers who came to his theme park, (b) pleasing his employees in their daily on-the-job practices by providing them with all the necessary equipment and supplies to do their jobs well, and (c) creating planned, organized governance systems and processes as well as an intense educational program to teach these functions and processes to every employee, profits would follow like sunshine after rain.

The enormous financial success of Walt Disney Productions sometimes clouds the simplicity of Disney's business philosophy. Seven decades ago, Disney said that his customers are the people who come through his gates, the staff members that work for him, and his management team. This tri-focus, three-domain approach to customer identification and service is still viable today. It continues to catapult the Disney business, which began in 1928, into a global empire.[10]

Today's health care organizations would do well to emulate some of the Disney philosophy and reengineer its organizations with a tri-focus, three-domain focus on customers. Disney proved the accuracy of the philosophy that says, "when all customers are happy, profits and productivity soar." Identifying customers and delineating scope of service, practice, and governance provide the solid foundation upon which the rest of the performance management system is built.

For ease of explanation this concept is divided into two parts: A and B (Figure 6-2). Part A identifies customers in the service, practice, and governance domains. Part B identifies the scope of services routinely rendered by health care organizations, by request or as needed, and in an emergency. Tools have been devised to assist a health care organization in obtaining this necessary information.

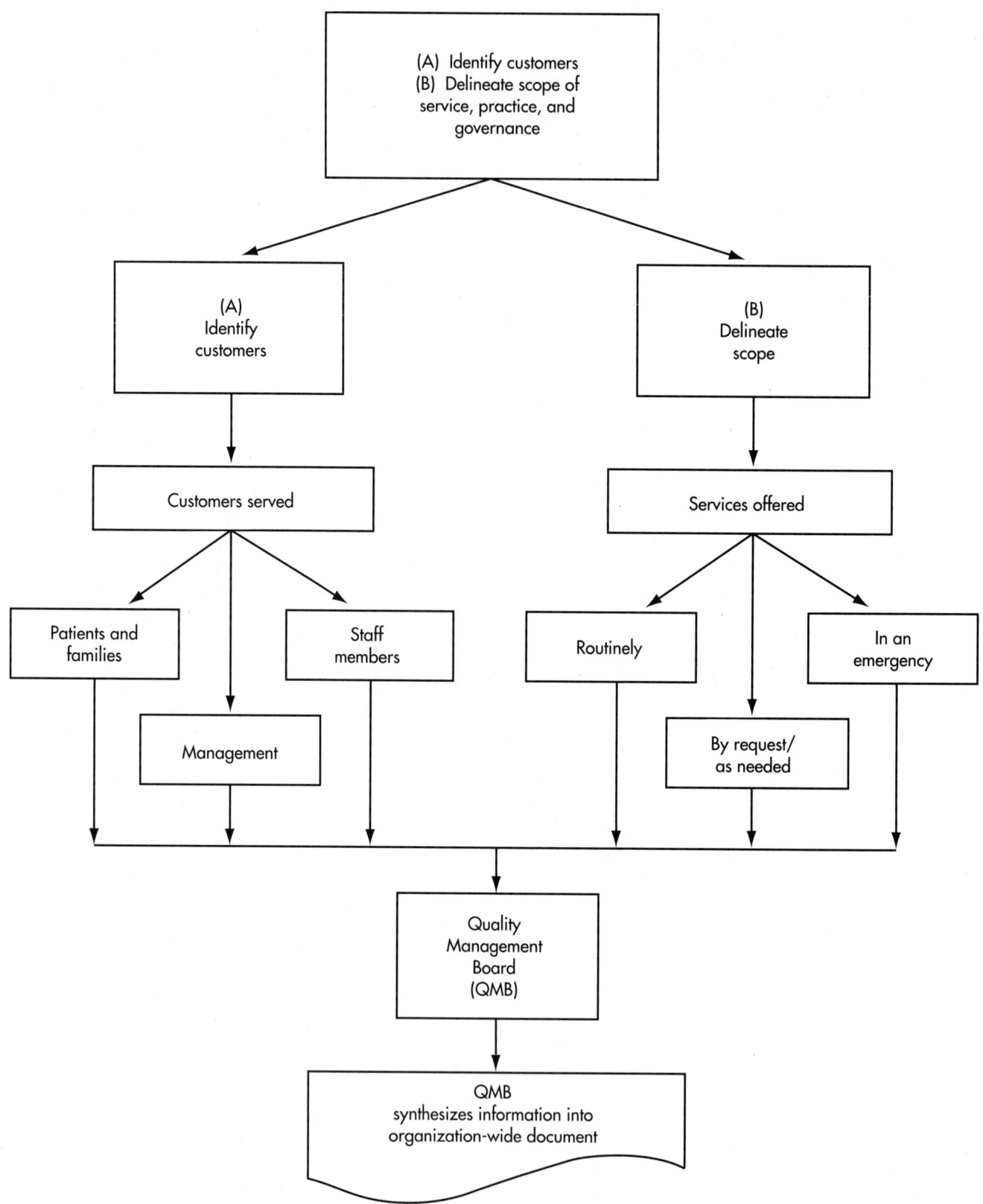

Figure 6-2   Identifying customers and delineating scope of service, practice, and governance.

PART A: IDENTIFYING CUSTOMERS WITHIN EACH DOMAIN

Part A involves answering the question, *Who are our organization's customers, both internal and external?* You may create an understanding of the organization-wide customers by first identifying each department's customers. This departmental identification of customers then may be sent to the QMB. The QMB then pools the data from each department and uses it to create an accurate, organization-wide profile of customers.

The tools that have been devised to assist with identification of customers in each domain are referred to as a profile. Profile tools have been developed to assist health care organizations to identify customers in each domain. These tools serve to organize your thoughts and may be modified to suit your organization.

"Who is the customer?" is the first and the crucial question in defining business purpose and business mission. It is not an easy question nor an obvious one. How it is being answered determines, in large measure, how the business defines itself."

L.L. Bean, the legendary catalog retail giant, puts it this way:

A customer is the most important person ever in this organization . . . in person, on the telephone, or by mail.

A customer is not an interruption of our work, he is the purpose of it.

A customer is not dependent on us, we are dependent on him.

We are not doing a favor by serving him, he is doing us a favor by giving us the opportunity to do so.

A customer is not someone to argue or match wits with. Nobody ever won an argument with a customer.

A customer is a person who brings us his wants. It is our job to handle them profitably to him and to others.[1]

The importance of understanding your customer and the impact of a thoughtful answer is shown by the carpet industry in the United States since World War II.

The carpet industry is an old one, with little glamour and little sophisticated technology . . . For thirty years, and until well into the early fifties, the industry had been in a steady, long-term and apparently irreversible decline. Then, within a few years, the industry completely reversed the trend . . . traditionally the rug and carpet manufacturer had defined his customer as the homeowner, and especially as the family buying its first home. But . . . the young couples had no money so they postponed buying rugs—and this meant they were not likely to buy them at all.[4]

It wasn't until the carpet industry saw the home *builders* as its customer that the industry began to turn around. The industry convinced the builders that wall-to-wall carpeting can be put over cheap unfinished flooring—resulting in a better house at lower cost to the builder.

Viewing the homeowner as the only customer for carpet sales was a marketing mistake of the carpet industry, just as viewing the patient as the only customer of a health care organization is a mistake. Viewing the patient as the only customer indicates that the organization has addressed only the service domain. The customers in the practice and governance domains have been ignored. A complete, total performance management system with a tri-focus approach will be successful in a health care organization long after competitors have fled the playing field. In other words, many errors are made and many resources wasted when organizations fail to identify their internal *and* external customers.

The idea of identifying customers and treating them nicely began in the health care industry in the early 1980s. Many hospitals, following the lead of Memorial Hospital of South Bend, Indiana, assumed that the patient was everyone's customer and insisted upon "guest relations" training for all employees.[13] It soon became clear, however, that simply renaming patients "guests," and conducting "Smile, staff, smile!" courses had little effect on the organization. Why? Only the customer in the service domain was being addressed in this popular program; no mention was made of the customers in the practice and governance domains. It is a business error in today's environment to believe that the health care organization's only customer is external and consists solely of the patient. There are far more internal customers than external in health care organizations.

From a business perspective, it is imperative that health care organizations delineate clearly who the customers are—internally and externally—in all three domains: service, practice, and governance. How can an organization improve customer service, stay competitive, and retain long-term business goals if the customer is unknown?

In one study, Russell C. Coile, Jr., and Randolph M. Grossman asked *Health Care Forum's* "Panel of 300" to anticipate what's new and what's next "in the coming 1,000 days" for American health care. Overwhelmingly, the Delphi panel's answers revolved around quality—both quality of care and quality of caring. *The Service Edge* by Zemke, Coile, and Grossman concluded that measurement and the ability to "prove" customer satisfaction will be increasingly important.[13]

Companies such as Disney, Frito-Lay, and IBM have identified the importance of both external and internal customers and have used this knowledge to their advantage in becoming service leaders.[8] Remember, quality is in the eyes of the customer, whether the customer be the patient, family, or significant others in the service domain, or staff members, physicians, and ancillary service workers in the practice domain, or managers, supervisors, vendors, contractors, or other health care alliances in the governance domain.

But what does delineating the customers in three domains have to do with quality? Consider this fundamental rule: *with the customer as the reference point, priorities for action in each domain are easy.*

In other words, irrespective of domain, all performance management activities revolve around a customer. This means that all employees of the organization have an understanding of their customers in order to identify their scope of service, practice, and governance. Furthermore, the customers within each domain are clearly identified in writing on a profile such as the one shown in Figure 6-3. There are four advantages of identifying customers in each domain: (1) it permits delineation of a particular target audience for program development, (2) areas of difficulty may be more closely identified, (3) it facilitates problem solving when customer complaints arise, and (4) it permits interdepartmental teams to flowchart processes to identify weaknesses and determine where breakdowns occur.

Here is an example of an organization that did not utilize the concept of customer identification in the service, practice, and governance domain:

Work that requires the cooperation and coordination of several different departments within a company is often a source of trouble. When retailers return unsold goods for credit to a consumer products manufacturer we know, thirteen separate departments are involved. Receiving accepts the goods, the warehouse returns them to stock, inventory management updates records to reflect their return, promotions determines at what price the goods were actually sold, sales accounting adjusts commissions, general accounting updates the financial records, and so on. Yet no single department or individual is in charge of handling returns. For each of the departments involved, returns are a low-priority distraction. Not surprisingly, mistakes often occur. Returned goods end up "lost" in the warehouse. The company pays sales commissions on unsold goods. Worse, customers do not get the credit that they expect, and they become angry, which effectively undoes all of sales and marketing's efforts. Unhappy retailers are less likely to promote the manufacturer's new products. They also delay paying their bills, and often pay only what they think they owe after deducting the value of the returns. This throws the manufacturer's accounts receivable department into turmoil, since the customer's check doesn't match the manufacturer's invoice. Eventually, the manufacturer simply gives up, unable to trace what really happened. Its own estimate of the annual cost and lost revenues from returns and related problems runs to nine figures. From time to time, the company's management has attempted to tighten up the disjointed returns process, but it no sooner gets some departments working well than new problems crop up in others.[5]

If a health care organization fails to delineate the customers in each of the three domains of its service delivery business, the organization, like the manufacturer in this example, will wind up with performance problems. Can one department solve the interdepartmental puzzle of this example? It is doubtful. The solution lies in an interdepartmental team, under the direction of the QMB tackling the problem of service, practice, and governance issues that have a bearing on the returned, unsold goods of this manufacturer.

This example illustrates the fallacy of customers being addressed only in the service domain. They are *external* to the organization. What of those customers that are *internal* and lie within the practice and governance domain?

Traditionally, customer complaints in any domain other than clinical have been ignored because they were not viewed as customer complaints but, rather, as unavoidable staff disgruntlement, more to be accepted and tolerated than given serious consideration. Often staff complaints were not given serious consideration, because health care organizations had abundant resources of time, money, personnel, and patients at their disposal. This abundance gave rise to the cavalier attitude that health care workers were "a dime a dozen" and that there would always be sickness, trauma, death, and a surplus of physicians and ancillary staff members. Few observers could have predicted the national economic chaos in the health care industry today. After decades of this "take it or leave it" approach, many health care organizations find that their survival today depends on adopting different tactics. They are faced with limited budgets, controlled reimbursements from managed care, and contracts with large companies to provide all health care services for thousands of employees. Today, keeping patients *out* of their facilities is profitable, hiring lesser levels of workers is profitable, and hiring physicians as staff employees is profitable. Who could have predicted that registered nurses would be out of work with few jobs available and physicians would accept a paycheck and practice controls?

In the face of these tremendous health care changes, both internal and external customers play a vital role in the prosperity and longevity of a health care organization. If they go unrecognized, the organization will suffer both financially and productively. Financially, because there will be a lack of organization and continuity of interdepartmental performance and productivity because employees, because of a lack of clear, understandable processes, simply will fail to perform. Morale will be low and turnover of employees

CUSTOMER PROFILE: PATIENT

Date of survey: from _____ to _____   DRG: _____
Average length of stay: _____   Admitted from: _____

Average age: _____   Sex: _____   Marital status: _____   Education: _____

Personal habits affecting recovery or employment:

Substance abuse: _____ %   Type of abuse: _____
Smoking: _____ %   Obese: _____ %   Undernourished: _____ %

Socioeconomic status:

Employed: _____ %   Own telephone: _____ %   Automobile: _____ %
Lives approximately _____ miles from health care organization
Primary language of this patient population group: _____

Common medical/nursing/ancillary interventions/processes delivered to this patient group:

Diagnostic: _____
Therapeutic: _____
Medications: _____

Co-morbidity/coexisting conditions:

1. _____   2. _____
3. _____   4. _____

Common complications seen in this patient group:

1. _____   2. _____
3. _____   4. _____

Possible emergencies that could occur in this patient population group:

1. _____   2. _____
3. _____   4. _____

Specific in-house planning needs of this patient population group:

1. _____   2. _____
3. _____   4. _____

Specific discharge planning needs of this patient population group:

1. _____   2. _____
3. _____   4. _____

A

Figure 6-3   Example of customer profile for a patient. **A,** Blank form. **B,** Form filled out using survey results.

Continued.

CUSTOMER PROFILE: PATIENT

Date of survey: from _1/15/91_ to _1/15/92_   DRG: _#88 C.O.P.D._

Average length of stay: _21.2 days_   Admitted from: _Emergency Dept._

Average age: _66_   Sex: _Male_   Marital status: _89% S_   Education: _5th Grade_

Personal habits affecting recovery or employment:

Substance abuse: _66_ %   Type of abuse: _Alcohol_

Smoking: _88_ %   Obese: _22_ %   Undernourished: _62_ %

Socioeconomic status:

Employed: _24_ %   Own telephone: _31_ %   Automobile: _20_ %

Lives approximately _5-15_ miles from health care organization

Primary language of this patient population group: _English_

Common medical/nursing/ancillary interventions/processes delivered to this patient group:

B

Diagnostic: _A.B.G.'s, Chest x-rays_

Therapeutic: _Chest PT, inhaler, postural drainage, oxygen_

Medications: _Steroids, antibiotics_

Co-morbidity/coexisting conditions:

1. _Liver dysfunction_   2. _Diabetes_
3. _Dyspnea_   4. _____

Common complications seen in this patient group:

1. _Altered skin integrity_   2. _Respiratory infections_
3. _Pneumonia_   4. _Depression_
5. _Self-care deficit_   6. _Role dysfunction_

Possible emergencies that could occur in this patient population group:

1. _Respiratory arrest_   2. _Pneumonia_
3. _Skin breakdown (infection)_   4. _____

Specific in-house planning needs of this patient population group:

1. _Education on pursed-lip/diaphragmatic breathing_   2. _Schedule tests to conserve energy_
3. _Nutrition consultation_   4. _Substance Abuse Education_

Specific discharge planning needs of this patient population group:

1. _Extra pillows or foam wedge_   2. _Bedside telephone_
3. _Oxygen vendor_   4. _Humidifier_

Figure 6-3, cont'd.

likely will be high and costly. In organizations that have shifted their focus from quality management to performance management, the meaning of the term *customer* has been broadened to include all who are users or providers of the organization's services, practices, or governance processes.

Performance-managed health care organizations understand that internal customers are just as necessary for the perpetuation of the business as external customers. Today, the combination of managed care and capitated reimbursement, information management and national data bank comparisons of outcomes, alliances with other health care organizations, too few dollars, too few workers and too few patients—who have ever increasing expectations and demands—is shaking health care organizations to the core.[13] In this environment, *all* customers of the organization become vitally important. Recognizing customers in all three domains is critical to a transformation from the traditional quality programs to new performance management programs as well as a complete reengineering within the health care organization.

Identifying Customers: Service Domain

Before delineating scope of care and service in any health care organization, there must be an understanding of who receives most of the care or service in each department. Knowing the intended recipient in the service domain controls or dictates how the care or service will be delivered. For example, if the patient profile reveals that the most frequently admitted patients have the diagnosis of chronic obstructive pulmonary disease, are male and homeless, and are primarily alcoholics with less than a third-grade education, this will influence how care and teaching must be carried out in this setting. There must be a plan of care that is tailored to this patient population. Furthermore, handing the patient a pamphlet on chronic obstructive pulmonary disease and returning 30 minutes later for a "discussion" would be inappropriate. In this setting, specific, simple teaching plans should be developed using numerous illustrations and few, simple words.

Understanding the customer in the service domain also enables the organization to channel resources appropriately. For example, if a majority of customers seeking the services of the radiology department is poorly educated and does not speak English, resources expended to create departmental signs for client directions or to create a sophisticated patient satisfaction questionnaire written in English would be wasted— even if it were an award-winning project—because it would be inappropriate for the radiology department's typical customer. Instead, such an organization should create signs in two languages and a simple sat-

isfaction questionnaire in two languages to record patients' responses about their treatment in this department. Likewise, designing a follow-up telephone call of discharged radiology customers may be inappropriate if the patient population is largely indigent and has no telephones.

In addition, knowledge of the intended customer assists health care organizations to predict outcomes of care and establish target parameters for performance improvement of their services. For example, consider a free-standing clinic participating in an alliance with an acute care health system that treats a very high number of IV drug abusers. In this instance an organization-wide intravenous therapy (IV) standard that specifies that all intravenous procedures be inserted with one stick would be inappropriate, because in these types of customers it may be virtually impossible to insert a needle into a vein in one stick. Furthermore, a target outcome such as, "no infections resulting from IV therapy," could prove unachievable for the staff of this clinic. Who can determine the cause of infection in a vein of a drug-addicted client who has abused every accessible vein? Without knowing the primary customers in the clinic, data would be skewed.

Ideally a customer profile will be completed for all departments within the organization. Each clinical department may create a profile for the top three DRGs, medical diagnoses, or services that are provided. All other departments also need to create customer profiles. For example, customer profiles may be completed for each housekeeping department by identifying the various internal customers served. For example, housekeeping services are extended to patients' rooms, the labor and delivery department, surgical services, administrative staff offices, dining rooms, and so on. The housekeeping profile should include each customer and the specific facets of cleaning service required. In this way, each department may provide a useful picture of the majority of its services. This, in turn, enables the organization through its QMB to create a composite organization-wide profile of primary customers served, as well as the specific services rendered. Figure 6-3 presents an example of a customer profile related to a patient. However, this tool may be modified by an organization to capture desired information about each department's customers who are not patients, such as the housekeeping department, the cafeteria employees, the bookkeeping department, medical records, and so on.

Identifying Customers: Practice Domain

Customers in the practice domain consist of every worker in the health care organization, including physicians. Every worker has a "practice." There is a laundry practice, a housekeeping practice, a dietary practice, a radiology practice, a laboratory practice, an admitting practice, a bookkeeping practice, and so on. *Practice* implies the "use of one's knowledge, or a person who practices a profession."[12]

One health care consultant during a recent visit to a large midwestern hospital presented the idea that each department in the hospital hired workers into a *practice*. The response from one nurse was, "Absolutely not! I am educated and *I* have a practice! If the kitchen help wants to obtain an education then they also may have a practice! But I, for one, refuse to share the word *practice* with them." This is a divisive attitude that impedes the interdisciplinary performance improvement process and perpetuates the myth of one worker group being superior to other groups.

Every employee is significant! Every worker makes an invaluable contribution to the organization and deserves to feel a pride of workmanship. Employees who are taught the value of their worth and their importance to the overall operation of the organization will, in return, feel a commitment and loyalty to the people who hired them.

In *Mickey Mouse Marketing*, N.W. Pope explains the Disney concept of employee importance. He relates a personal event that involved his two children working for Walt Disney World in Orlando, Florida:

> *My two kids, ages 18 and 16, average intelligence, reasonably quick, are accepted to be Casual Temporaries—summer, Christmas, Easter, etc., employment.*
>
> *They are to take tickets. That's it. How tough can that be?*
>
> *Four eight-hour days of instructions are required before they can go "on stage"! They are paid to learn, but before a Disney cast member (CM) interfaces with a Guest, the management must be absolutely certain that the CM can, and will, perform properly. After all, we are dealing with Customer Satisfaction, they say. Nothing is spared to assure customer satisfaction.*
>
> *"Why," I inquired, "does it take four days to lean how to take tickets?" Waste of time I thought.*
>
> *My two **Traditions I** graduates, with his new haircut and her "a-little-lipstick-only" makeup, jump to the defense of 32 hours of education in the fine art of taking tickets.*
>
> *I was informed there are x varieties of tickets, each having special meaning. What happens if someone wants to know where the restrooms are, where do we eat inside, and what happens if I lose my child, how many bricks in the castle? Questions ad infinitum.*
>
> *"We need to know the answers or where to get the answers quickly," I am advised. "After all, Dad, we're on stage and must produce the show for our Guests. Our job, every minute, is to help the Guest enjoy the park."*
>
> *After the first day on the job Pope said to his children, "How does it feel to be ticket takers?"*
>
> *Again he was berated.*
>
> *"Ticket takers? Dad, we're WDW Hosts." (Walt Disney World Hosts.)*

> *Walt Disney was a marketing magician, no doubt. But his keen insight into personnel and customer relations, separately and collectively, enabled him to create the world's most successful entertainment conglomerate by starting with a mouse he drew and named Steamboat Willie in 1928.*[10]

There are no "little people" employed at Walt Disney Productions. This concept is also true in a health care organization. Every job is critical for overall success. At one hospital a health care consultant posed the question, "Who is the most important employee in the surgical services department?"

One of the surgical scrub technicians answered, "The Surgical Chief of Staff."

Again the health care consultant posed a question. "If the surgical services department personnel were to vote on who may come to work next week, the professional housekeeping staff or the chief of surgery, for whom would the employees vote?"

Without hesitation the technician answered, "The professional housekeeping staff! Without them not one surgical case could begin." So, which worker is the most critical to the smooth operation of the surgical services department? The answer, of course, is *every employee* who works there!

Although most health care organizations have little trouble identifying the customers in the service domain, they often have trouble identifying other *employees* as customers. Furthermore, although many have programs that emphasize treating patients as valuable customers, some might question the need for treating staff from the housekeeping, kitchen, laundry, and the environmental control departments as valuable customers. As one vice president for nursing stated, "It's never occurred to me that the kitchen staff and laundry staff are also customers. The idea of catering to these workers as though they are valuable customers is a brand new thought. I'll have to think it through." It will be a *giant* step forward toward performance improvement when *all* employees of health care organizations are viewed as an indispensable resource and treated accordingly. The survival of many health care organizations may depend on it! Megatrend tracker John Naisbitt has predicted that by the turn of the century, as many as 2,000 hospitals will have either closed their doors or been absorbed into other hospital systems.[13]

A staff profile is a composite tool used to assist in recognizing the needs of the customer receiving direct assistance or interdependent cooperation assistance from staff in the practice domain. This profile, which averages staff data, is used for the following:

- The values of the organization can be matched with those of the staff members.

- The values of the staff members can be matched with those of their customers.
- The experience and qualifications of the staff members can be matched with their expected role or job description.
- This profile may be used to predict future staffing patterns and trends.
- Employee development opportunities can be planned in accordance with needs of the staff members.
- The continuum of care function can be broken into relevant processes permitting staff members to apply, modify, or discard an action based on patient population needs.

The staff profile from each unit and department should be sent to the QMB. The QMB processes these profiles to create an organization-wide staff profile. This global, composite profile then becomes the basis for organizational staffing, acuity mix, hiring decisions, and future staff educational plans. These staff profiles should be updated every 3 years to enable the health care organization to track and trend staffing mix and patterns.

Identifying Customers: Governance Domain

If health care organizations are to be successfully reengineered into stable, profitable businesses, the philosophy of customer satisfaction should extend not only to those external customers, which include patients, but also to internal customers, which include all management staff.

Customers in the governance domain consist of every manager, supervisor, director, "head," chief, or any of a myriad of other creative title designations that indicate a rank or title of leadership in a health care organization. These employees in health care organizations often are perceived as "one of us" and are therefore completely overlooked by the CEO as his or her prime customer. Yet managers are one of the most valuable customers and resources of the organization. To overlook this can result in a vicious circle of non-productivity and corporate negativity that pervades the organization. Management morale affects the overall perception of the organization by the customers it is designated to serve. Managers are the oil that makes the organizational engine run smoothly.

The concept of the manager as the customer of the administration of the health care organization is critical to corporate success in today's competitive environment. Yet there is little documented evidence that managers are cultivated as valued customers of the administration.

The philosophy of managers as valued customers lies in the fact that each manager represents a sizable investment by the organization. As Betty Holcomb points out in *Nurses Fight Back*, the cost of hiring and orienting a professional nurse for an organization has been estimated at $20,000.[6] Curran states that the cost of turnover in the U.S. hospital industry in 1988 was *$3.2 billion.*[2] These costs do not include the time that colleagues spend helping to orient and socialize the newcomer to the organization, and all the other resources expended in helping the newcomer gain proficiency. Over time, the total investment in a manager, in formal and informal training, is very great. Despite this, traditional CEOs often allowed these vital participants in the organization's well-being to run down, become technically obsolete, or burn out because they failed to recognize and treat managers as valuable customers.

In today's health care environment this nonchalance toward the treatment of valuable customers may prove to be the missing competitive edge that would have ensured a long future for the organization. One common element in today's successful health care organizations is the practice of placing both external and internal customers as a top priority for special attention. Like other businesses, health care's CEOs are learning that "if they're going to be in the business of providing satisfied customers, they must first be in the business of providing satisfied employees."[3]

Health care organizations often expend much effort on personnel or human resources. Practically all of them have active recruitment and retention programs. However, they expend only limited efforts on the *maintenance* of managers. Rarely do CEOs poll their managers on a regular basis to solicit their opinions and assess their job satisfaction, nor do they gather statistics for a manager profile that identifies the characteristics of the majority of its managers. Many organizations operate without a fundamental knowledge of the primary customers in the governance domain, despite the fact that managers vary in experience, longevity, academic preparation, and style. Not knowing management's needs, CEOs blunder in dictating assignments and performance measures for this level of worker.

A manager profile can assist the organization to identify this important customer. Organizations that know their management team profile can match potential managers with organizational values, discern compatibility with staff members' values, and estimate this employee's potential productivity based on home environment and other commitments, as well as the person's interest in personal and professional growth.

Manager profiles should be obtained and utilized by the QMB in its decision-making processes. They should be reviewed and updated every 3 years.

These management profiles enable the QMB to track and trend management patterns of employment and productivity.

Creating Profiles

The work of creating profiles begins in each department of the organization. Start by having each department manager appoint a team of three to five people to (a) identify the customers of the department, (b) identify the customers' expectations of the department, and (c) identify major inputs and vendors of the department. Table 6-1 will guide the team's thinking. The team may then use Figure 6-4 to answer the questions from the outline. After these forms are completed, the team may use the answers to construct a customer profile in each domain of their department: service, practice, and governance. This is an informational guideline from which the team may brainstorm. However, each team should add its own external and internal customers to the brief list that appears in the box on p. 70.

Before beginning data collection for the profiles about patients, employees, or managers, seek the services of the organization's legal department. Ask, "If the profile is anonymous, with no place for the employee or manager's name, is it an invasion of the privacy laws in this state?" Gathering the data is important; however, refraining from invading the privacy of our fellow workers is also important. Ideally, all data from each department of the health care organization would be computerized and updated each year. The data processing department then would have the capability of providing employees with composite information whenever needed to assist in organization-wide decision-making.

Additional data can be collected about employers and managers. For example, one organization is using the Meyers-Briggs tool to ensure a good fit between staff and managerial styles.

PART B: DELINEATING SCOPE OF SERVICE, PRACTICE, AND GOVERNANCE

Once Part A is completed, the team is ready to begin Part B: delineating the scope of service, practice, and governance within the team's department. As with Part A, this information, when completed, is channeled to QMB. It is the job of the QMB to analyze the data from each department and create a composite, organization-wide master matrix of the scope of service, practice, and governance of the organization.

Part B answers the question, *What services, practices, and governance do we provide for our customers and under what situation?* This is an extremely important process, because it serves as the cornerstone on which the prioritizing information in Chapter 7 is built. A matrix tool is used to help delineate the scope of service, practice, and governance (Tables 6-2 through 6-4, pp. 71-74).

TABLE 6-1   Identify customers: team brainstorming outline

Steps	Questions to consider	Tools to use
IDENTIFY CUSTOMERS	Who are our customers? Do we have different types of customers? Who are our external and internal customers?	Identify customers worksheet
IDENTIFY CUSTOMER EXPECTATIONS	Do we really know what the customer wants? Are there other needs that the customer has not stated? Have we negotiated the requirements with the customer? Do all our customers have the same needs?	Surveys Focus groups Face-to-face meetings Research
IDENTIFY MAJOR INPUTS AND VENDORS	What materials/information do we use routinely? Who supplies it to us? What services do we provide? Do our vendors know exactly what we want from them?	Flow chart Fishbone diagram Brainstorming Storyboard

IDENTIFY CUSTOMERS: TEAM WORKSHEET

1. With the team, identify the customers in our department. Label each of them as external or internal.*

External	Internal
_____	_____
_____	_____
_____	_____
_____	_____
_____	_____
_____	_____
_____	_____
_____	_____
_____	_____
_____	_____

2. What are our external and internal customers' expectations of our department?

External	Internal
_____	_____
_____	_____
_____	_____
_____	_____
_____	_____
_____	_____
_____	_____
_____	_____
_____	_____
_____	_____

3. What are the major inputs and who are the major vendors for this unit? In other words, who or what is critical to the functioning of this department?

External	Internal
_____	_____
_____	_____
_____	_____
_____	_____
_____	_____
_____	_____
_____	_____
_____	_____
_____	_____
_____	_____

*Use another sheet of paper if necessary.

Figure 6-4   Team brainstorming outline for identifying customers.

INTERNAL AND EXTERNAL CUSTOMERS

Internal

- All employees of the health care organization
- Physicians
- All other departments in the organization
- The entire administrative staff: bookkeepers, secretaries, and resource personnel, such as librarians and house supervisors

External

- Patients
- Patients' families
- The community
- Other health care institutions that transport or receive our patients
- People who require medical records of our patients (physicians, lawyers, etc.)
- Vendors and suppliers of the products with which we work
- Ambulance services
- Funeral companies
- Florists
- Fire companies
- Police
- Accrediting agencies, including the state and federal government
- Third party payers, such as insurance companies and the federal government

The matrix tool is organized vertically into these three domains. It is organized horizontally into three divisions: (a) the service, practice, or governance routinely offered by this department, (b) the service, practice, or governance offered by this department by request or as a need arises, and (c) the service, practice, or governance offered by this department in an emergency. These three divisions horizontally provide space for listing all possible services, practices, and governance delivered by the department.

To delineate the scope of service, practice, and governance in a department, the appointed team simply fills in the name of the department at the top of the page and then brainstorms about three questions:

1. What services does this department offer/provide/ contribute to its internal and external customers
   a. routinely?
   b. by request or as need arises?
   c. in an emergency?
2. What practices does this department offer/ provide/contribute to its own staff members
   a. routinely?
   b. by request or as need arises?
   c. in an emergency?

3. What governance does this department offer/ provide/contribute to the administration of the organization
   a. routinely?
   b. by request or as need arises?
   c. in an emergency?

The matrix permits each department to provide a thorough inventory of its service, practice, and governance processes. Identifying all of the processes in each domain that are offered, provided, or contributed to by each department allows the QMB to look at the multiple, interacting processes that are carried out between departments and identify problem areas. Most processes in a health care organization involve several departments and multiple workers. The matrix will help organize them into manageable groups for discussion of methods for performance management.

There is a widely held belief that an organization would have few, if any, problems, if workers would do their jobs correctly. As Dr. Joseph M. Juran pointed out years ago, this belief is incorrect.[1]

In fact, the potential to eliminate mistakes and errors lies mostly in improving the *systems* through which work is done, not in changing the *workers*. This observation has evolved into the rule of thumb that at least 85% of problems can be corrected only by changing systems (which are largely determined by management), and less than 15% are under a worker's control—and the split may lean even more towards the system.

For example, a production line worker cannot do a top-quality job when working with faulty tools or parts; a surgical technician cannot do a good job with gloves that do not fit. The environmental control department cannot carry out the organization's safety plan without fire alarms that function properly and doors that are not jammed, and hallways, stairways, storage areas, and patient rooms free from clutter.

Even when it does seem that an individual is doing something wrong, often the trouble lies in how that worker was trained, which is a system problem. Once people recognize that systems create the majority of problems, they will stop blaming individual workers. They will instead ask which system needs improvement and will be more likely to seek out and find the true source of a problem.[11]

The matrix provides a worksheet to be used by each department's team. Further, it serves as a worksheet to organize and capture the processes of each department that are performed routinely, as the need arises, and in an emergency. This visible representation of processes within each of the health care organization's departments should prove invaluable to the planning of the organization's performance management plan. Once the processes are identified in each department and sent to the QMB, a comparison may be made between

TABLE 6-2   Scope of service, practice, and governance matrix

Dept: CCU	Service domain	Practice domain	Governance domain
SERVICES ROUTINELY OFFERED BY THIS DEPARTMENT	1. Medication administration (all routes) 2. Skin care 3. ECG monitoring 4. Use of nursing process 5. Documentation 6. 1:2 ratio nursing care 7. Infection prevention 8. Falls prevention 9. ACLS-prepared staff 10. Cardiac education	1. Staff safety 2. Orientation 3. Preceptorship 4. Certifications: Basic ECG, ACLS, IABP, IV therapy 5. Written standards for CCU 6. Employee development plans 7. Employee evaluation every 6 months 8. Cross-training to incoming float staff	1. Participation in organization-wide teams 2. Peer review 3. Unit quality control 4. Participation in organization-wide data collection 5. Carrying out the mission, philosophy, and goals of the organization 6. Adherence to organization-wide policies 7. Scheduling of staff
SERVICES OFFERED BY THIS DEPARTMENT BY REQUEST OR AS NEED ARISES	1. Ratio of 1:1 nursing care 2. Hemodynamic monitoring 3. Pain control 4. Arrhythmia control 5. Ventilator care 6. Intraaortic balloon pump monitoring 7. Arterial line monitoring 8. Acid-base monitoring 9. Visitor control	1. Performance counseling 2. Cross-training 3. Time off 4. Education time 5. Maternity leave 6. Ethics counseling	1. Intensive review of sentinel events 2. Floating to other units 3. Transportation of patients 4. Drawing blood samples 5. Participate in special team research projects 6. Cleaning and reorganizing unit work space, closets, drawers
SERVICES OFFERED BY THIS DEPARTMENT IN AN EMERGENCY	1. Bolus therapy 2. Thrombolytic therapy 3. Advanced cardiac life support	1. Sick leave 2. Ethics counseling	1. Emergency staffing 2. Triage in-house patients with chest pain on 11-7 shift 3. Perform ECGs in-house on 11-7 shift 4. Start IVs in-house if other staff unable to gain access

TABLE 6-3   Scope of service, practice, and governance matrix

Dept: Homecare	Service domain	Practice domain	Governance domain
SERVICES ROUTINELY OFFERED BY THIS AGENCY	1. Patient plan of care 2. Patient assessment 3. Patient teaching 4. Case coordination with physician 5. Documentation 6. Infection control/prevention 7. Medication administration 8. Skin care including wound/ulcers 9. Respiratory care including oxygen 10. Intravenous care (peripheral and central lines) 11. Gastrointestinal care including feeding/meal preparation 12. Genitourinary care/catheters 13. Rehabilitation services	1. Staff safety 2. Orientation 3. Preceptorship 4. Regular staff meetings 5. Paid travel time 6. Employee development plans 7. Employee evaluation every 6 months 8. Defense training/emergency whistle, spray, etc. 9. Cellular telephone 10. Cast load of 5 to 8 visits/day 11. Written standards for Home Care	1. Participation in organization-wide quality improvement teams 2. Peer review 3. Agency quality control 4. Participation in agency-wide data collection 5. Carrying out the mission, philosophy, and goals of the home care agency 6. Adherence to agency-wide policies 7. Scheduling of staff 8. Ordering of equipment and supplies 9. Budget management 10. Case management of top three populations
SERVICES OFFERED BY THIS AGENCY BY REQUEST OR AS NEED ARISES	1. Epidemiology screening 2. Hospice care 3. Arrange transportation to acute care facility when necessary 4. Ventilator care 5. Pronounce death	1. Performance counseling 2. Detailed road maps 3. Time off 4. Education time 5. Maternity leave 6. A "partner" to visit question-able behavior-problem patients 7. Inservices 8. Ethics counseling 9. On-site ECGs 10. On-site blood samples drawn	1. Intensive review of sentinel events 2. Meeting with parent organization's discharge planning team 3. Referrals to other health care providers 4. Maintaining equipment/supplies 5. Participate in special team research projects 6. Cleaning and reorganizing agency work space 7. Communication with other branches of agency: QA data, etc. 8. Meeting JCAHO standards for accreditation
SERVICES OFFERED BY THIS AGENCY IN AN EMERGENCY	1. Oversee calling of ambulance when necessary 2. CPR	1. Sick leave 2. Emergency leave 3. Ethics counseling	1. Emergency staffing 2. Participate with American Red Cross disaster relief plan

TABLE 6-4 Scope of service, practice, and governance matrix

Dept: Dietary	Service domain	Practice domain	Governance domain
SERVICES ROUTINELY OFFERED BY THIS DEPARTMENT	1. Patient meals 2. Employee meals 3. Visitor meals 4. Free meals to rescue squad 5. Documentation 6. 24-hour vending machines 7. Sanitized utensils, plates, etc. 8. Infection prevention (staff with colds, etc. wear masks, all food techs wear gloves) 9. Hot food in appropriate containers 10. Printed menus to each in-house patient	1. Staff safety 2. Orientation 3. Preceptorship 4. Regular staff meetings 5. Written standards for dietary dept. 6. Employee development plans 7. Employee evaluation every 6 months 8. Free meals 9. Cross training between dietary, housekeeping, and nursing assistants	1. Participation in organization-wide teams 2. Peer review 3. Unit quality control 4. Participation in organization-wide data collection 5. Carrying out the mission, philosophy, and goals of the organization 6. Adherence to organization-wide policies 7. Scheduling of staff 8. Ordering of food and supplies 9. Budget management 10. Menu planning 11. Delivery of meals to patients
SERVICES OFFERED BY THIS DEPARTMENT BY REQUEST OR AS NEED ARISES	1. Cater special patient functions 2. Prepare and deliver late trays 3. Special patient food requests including kosher, vegetarian 4. Patient dietary education 5. Distribution of literature on special diets	1. Performance counseling 2. Cross training 3. Time off 4. Education time 5. Maternity leave 6. Cater special employee functions 7. Inservices 8. Free diet advice and menus	1. Intensive review of sentinel events 2. Floating to other units 3. Delivery of meals to patients 4. Maintaining equipment/supplies 5. Participate in special team research projects 6. Cleaning and reorganizing work space 7. Tours of kitchen to special interest groups 8. Meeting JCAHO standards for accreditation
SERVICES OFFERED BY THIS DEPARTMENT IN AN EMERGENCY	1. Disaster plan	1. Sick leave 2. Emergency leave	1. Emergency staffing 2. Participate in preparing food and feeding disaster victims

73

departments to discover the interrelated processes and the impact they are having on the primary functions of the organization. The processes causing problems for the organization may then be prioritized and targeted for performance management. In this way, health care organizations may fix their systems by fine-tuning departmental processes for, as Dr. Juran pointed out, at least 85% of an organization's problems lies within its *systems.*

Using the profiles and the matrix provides a systematic, planned approach for health care organizations that are contemplating reengineering their systems. It assists in laying the groundwork upon which a health care organization can build a stable, understandable, and measurable performance management system in which processes within each key function are analyzed and improved.

Dr. Arthur Kaplan, Director of the Center for Medical Ethics at the University of Minnesota, states in *The Service Edge,* "We have expectations of health care providers that have never existed before. We have yet to come to grips with the difficult choices that go with those demands."[13] Before health care organizations can "come to grips with the difficult choices," spoken of by Dr. Kaplan, an understanding of customers and their expectations is essential. A thorough understanding of the service, practice, and governance of each department also is essential. Before we can confront the choices that go with the customers' rising expectations and demands, some strategic planning by each department followed by the QMB is of paramount importance. Without this information, health care organizations cannot plan for the future.

CONCLUSION

The ideas and tools presented in this chapter will assist you to organize and focus each department's work team on a common goal and will provide the foundation for creating an organization-wide performance management system. When finished, that foundation will consist of a shared leadership framework such as the one described in Chapter 5; an understanding of both internal and external customers; an understanding of the scope of each department's processes within the service, practice, and governance domains; and an understanding of the prioritizing process that will be discussed in the next chapter. This foundation will provide the structure for a stable, well-constructed performance management system that will endure well into the future.

REFERENCES

1. Bowles J, Hammond J: *Beyond quality: how 50 winning companies use continuous improvement,* New York, 1991, G.P. Putnam's Sons.
2. Curran C: Critical care update, issues, trends, and opportunities. Keynote address at the National Conference Resource Applications, Inc, October 18, 1990.
3. Dobyns L, Crawford-Mason C: *Quality or else: the revolution in world business,* Boston, 1991, Houghton Mifflin Co.
4. Drucker PE: *Management: tasks, responsibilities, practices,* New York, 1985, Harper & Row.
5. Hammer M, Champy J: *Reengineering the corporation; a manifesto for business revolution,* New York, 1993, Harper Business.
6. Holcomb B: *Nurses fight back.* In Lindeman CA, McAthie M, editors: *Readings in nursing issues and trends,* Springhouse, Penn, 1990, Springhouse Publishing Co.
7. Neuhauser D, McEachern JE, Headrick L: *Clinical CQI: a book of readings,* Chicago, 1995, Joint Commission.
8. Peters T, Waterman R: *In search of excellence,* New York, 1982, Harper & Row.
9. Peters T: *The pursuit of WOW: every person's guide to topsy-turvy times,* New York, 1994, Random House.
10. Pope NW: Mickey Mouse marketing. *American Banker,* July 25, 1979, pp 5-21.
11. Schultz P: *The team handbook,* Madison, Wis, 1990, Joiner Associates, Inc.
12. Walton M: *The Deming management method,* New York, 1986, Putnam.
13. Zemke R: *The service edge,* New York, 1989, Penguin Books.

Chapter 7

Prioritizing Organization-Wide Performance Improvement Processes

Our systems invariably measure "the wrong stuff."
Tom Peters

Imagine a fantastic smorgasbord. The tables are overflowing with scrumptious food. You are famished, and the mere sight of all that good food starts your salivary glands working overtime. This food fantasy, however, could be a nightmare if you are not careful. Falling prey to one of the following food traps could result in a gastronomic disaster.

The first trap is bingeing. With reckless abandon, you attack the tables, overloading your plate. You eat until you can eat no more. The error here is overindulgence, and the lack of self-control results in a tight waistband and the burning desire for an antacid. You forgot that "all you can eat" does not mean "eat it all." What should have been a satisfying experience has deteriorated to an unpleasant feeling of discomfort.

This also occurs when you try to overload your performance management system. This "binge" assessment style represents an "eat it all" mentality. The misconception is that you have to assess everything you do multiple times every year. The result is an awareness, measurement, and improvement plan that is unmanageable. "More" is not necessarily "better."

Every time a problem arises, regardless of its importance, it is integrated into the performance management system's programs. Staff members become frustrated with the volume of measurement data to be collected. In an attempt to streamline the process and appease staff members, you reduce the number of measurement activities. This binge-purge cycle creates an unstable performance management system. Staff members begin to question the value of assessment activities when they are important one day and are discontinued the next. Like overeating, overmeasurement can transform what should be a positive, validating activity into an unpleasant experience.

The second food trap is grazing. Everything looks great. You want it all but do not want to overeat, so you taste a little bit of everything. Your plate overflows with bits and pieces of many different foods. Soon you are full, but you have not had your fill of any one food. You want to go back to the table for more of something that you enjoyed, but your stomach is too full.

In performance measurement there also are grazers. This school of thought suggests that you collect a little bit of data about a lot of things in an attempt to obtain a full picture of your services. There are two key problems with this approach. First, you may sacrifice measuring something essential to assess an activity of lesser importance. Second, you scatter your measurement resources with little gain. The misconception is that everything you do must be assessed every year—and once you begin, you may not discontinue it. Many believe that no matter what is examined, some measurement activity such as data collection should have taken place. Dividing the measurement time over so many issues usually means that all issues are treated the same. However, some parts of your service, practice, and governance require more frequent and intense measurement.

Indecisiveness is the root of this trap. The result is a measurement program that does not provide enough data to identify problems and initiate change. This indecision often stems from not knowing who the major customer of the service is and what key processes are critical to achieving desired outcomes.

In the final food trap, you indulge your "sweet tooth." You skip the meal and head right for the dessert table, discovering the strawberry shortcake and cherries jubilee. You fill up on empty calories and sacrifice good nutrition for palate pleasure.

Similarly, measuring superficial processes is a common performance measurement trap. It usually results from a misunderstanding of which processes of your service are most critical to the outcomes you need to accomplish. It is an attempt to keep data collection easy. The activities measured may have little impact on the quality of your service. Staff members become frustrated with the data collection, perceiving it as busywork, instead of the basis for problem-solving analysis.

Just as your body requires a nutritionally sound diet to ensure effective functioning, your department requires a sound performance management system to ensure its effectiveness. Eating a balanced diet is a means to good personal health, and a well-balanced diet is based on the four basic food groups. Similarly, a well-balanced performance management system is based on four basic analysis groups or criteria of your service. These four criteria are the test of whether or not to add a process to your performance management system and start the ball rolling toward improvement. The four analysis criteria include the *high-risk, high-volume, problem-prone,* and *high-cost processes* that are most critical to the service, practice, and governance offered by your organization.

The Joint Commission defines a process as: "A goal-directed, interrelated series of actions, events, mechanisms, or steps."[5] This broad definition encompasses all processes performed in all types of situations and all types of institutions providing health care services—from acute care to walk-in clinics. The key concept of measuring processes lies in prioritizing and measuring only those of greatest significance to the situation under review. Although health care workers believe that everything they do is important, only those activities that are appropriate and essential to achieving the desired outcomes are of greatest importance. Choosing to measure only the important processes streamlines the appraisal process and makes the best use of resources.

PROCESS CONCEPTS REPLACING ASPECTS OF CARE

The focus on aspects of care, which has been popular for the past several years, has been replaced by a new accreditation concept. Aspects of care briefly advocated by the Joint Commission for the Accreditation of Health Care Organizations (JCAHO) proved of little value in affecting outcomes. Because the scope of its influence was department-based, little information was shared organization-wide. As a result of this narrow focus, many health care workers were poorly prepared for the organization-wide scope of the accreditation survey. Even *without* a survey these organizations were unprepared for all departments and employees to cooperate instead of compete. Many health care providers thought "aspects of care" were synonymous with quality control and therefore set up "checksheets" with criteria to check off when certain processes were completed. For example, patients' skin integrity was frequently listed as an important aspect of care and a checksheet listing routine skin care became the quality assessment tool. When it was checked every shift, providers thought they had "done" QA!

Even more distressing was the notion that quality was an activity of *only* the nursing department. Many health care providers did not understand that "important aspects of care" applied to *all* departments of a health care organization. As far back as 1994, the *JCAHO Accreditation Manual for Hospitals* stated, "The important functions . . . include both direct patient care activities . . . and management and support processes and functions. . . . Reframing the standards in terms of these organization-wide, multidisciplinary functions emphasizes the interdependent nature of all the activities of a health care organization."[4] (See the box on p. 49 in Chapter 5 for a list of JCAHO's functions; for an explanation of the 11 functions see Appendix 7-1.)

Even though the American business world was exhorting all industries to concentrate on *improving* the processes involved in delivering services, carrying out practices of workers, and managing governance systems, health care organizations kept on doing what they'd always done, which was, essentially, quality control. Quality control was simplistic, understandable, and produced information that was manageable. Never mind that it did not change outcomes.

As the complexity of health care organizations increased and technology became more and more sophisticated, interdisciplinary performance measurement seemed a far-off dream. Peters and Waterman state that "along with bigness comes complexity, unfortunately. And most big companies respond to complexity in kind, by designing complex systems and structures. They then hire more staff to keep track of all this complexity, and that's where the mistake begins."[9]

NATIONAL COMMITTEE FOR QUALITY ASSURANCE (NCQA): SIX AREAS REVIEWED DURING AN NCQA SURVEY

1. Quality improvement
2. Utilization management
3. Credentialing
4. Members' rights and responsibilities
5. Health services
6. Medical records

EXERCISE: KEY FUNCTIONS OF THE DEPARTMENT

Identify the key functions within the department. Create a pie chart to carve up the resource allocations according to key functions. Indicate the percentage of time, dollars and staff spent for each function. Use a second pie chart to segment the resource allocation by department service, practice, and governance. Have the staff complete the same exercise. Compare their results with those of the department's leaders to identify discrepancies. Use the results as a springboard for discussion of priority functions. Ask questions such as the following:

- Is the distribution of time and dollars in line with the priorities of the organization?
- Is the inordinate amount of time, energy, and dollars being spent on one function at the expense of another function?
- If so, what would be a more equitable distribution of resources?

It may prove to be an enlightening exercise to ask administration to predict how much of the department's resources are being spent for each function for comparison with actuals.

Modified from Katz J: *Designing a quality management program in educational services.* In Rodriguez L: *Manual of staff development,* St. Louis, 1995, Mosby.

Given all the multitude of problems facing health care organizations today, it is little wonder that restructuring the organization to measure performance outcomes takes a low priority.

There was a decided lack of organization-wide implementation of a systematic, planned, organized performance management system driven by top management based on a model or framework. There was also a lack of understanding of the performance measures that were decreasing costs and improving performance in the business world. It gradually became apparent to health care organizations that improved fiscal outcomes occurred when processes within the health care organization were controlled—not when checksheets were filled in.

Both the National Committee for Quality Assurance (NCQA) and JCAHO, along with other organizations, invested time, money, personnel, and research searching for an ideal method to move health care organizations from the traditional QA to a more sophisticated system of statistical process control that would yield data upon which rational predictions of resource utilization could be based.[8]

It became apparent that a focus on primary functions that existed within the health care organization provided performance improvement as well as control of resource utilization. Therefore, a functional approach to the accreditation process was devised by both JCAHO and NCQA.

This means that health care organizations must examine each of their key functions and consider the processes that lie within each function. The exercise in the box in the above right corner will assist in identifying each department's key functions. Then, using tools of statistical process control, they must decide which processes are "in control" or "out of control" and how best to improve the key function by capitalizing on small, incremental improvements of processes. (For a discussion on statistical control see Chapter 12.)

This results in organizations being able to demonstrate that positive service, practice, and governance outcomes are the direct result of a smoothly functioning organization-wide performance management system.

Both patient outcomes and resource use are directly influenced by the performance of the organization: doing the right thing (the extent to which service is efficacious and appropriate), and doing these right things well (the extent to which service is available, timely, continuous, safe, efficient, respectful).[4]

The design and operation of many important functions strongly influence whether the organization's services exhibit these qualities, or dimensions of performance. The effect of an organization's performance on its important functions and on the processes that lie within functions is reflected in its patient outcomes, the cost of its services, and the judgments made by patients, staff, purchasers, and others about the quality and value of the care provided.[4]

This multidisciplinary functional approach is far more valuable to a health care organization than the former "aspects of care" approach. This approach emphasized a method for meeting requirements of JCAHO, whereas the functional approach emphasizes an organization's outcomes more than the methods used to achieve it. "This approach is valuable because it is anchored in the real work of health care professionals and in the real improvements that can be achieved to benefit patients and others."[4] Furthermore, this perspective is based on the understanding that "organizational performance is the key determinant of four important results—that is, patient outcomes, costs, quality, and value."[4]

The new accreditation system works like this: functions are inherent in every health care organization as are the many processes that make up a function. In the JCAHO's accrediting format, five functions are patient focused, six are organizational focused, and four are structure functions. With the exception of the four structure functions, the accreditation process mandates that each health care facility *assess* and *improve* processes under each of the 11 functions (Appendix 7-1). Here it is in simple language: "Performance is made up of functions, which are composed of processes which, when performed, lead to outcomes."[7]

The nine dimensions of performance are the yardstick by which you measure the efficacy of the performance management system. Furthermore, consider David Garvin's eight characteristics of quality when an organization-wide performance management system is devised (see Chapter 1).

DIFFERENCE BETWEEN PROCESSES AND FUNCTIONS

Important processes are those activities that are central to your service. Each process performed falls directly under one of the 11 functions outlined in Appendix 7-1. Processes are the service, practice, and governance activities that add value to your performance and for which your performance is valued.

Consider a typical American family. Regardless of the members of the family, there are certain functions necessary to maintain its operation. Some of these functions include providing (a) nutrition/food, (b) transportation, (c) clothing, (d) cleaning/maintenance, (e) health care, and (f) fiscal management.

For example, consider the processes under function *a*, nutrition/food. These processes might include menu planning, purchasing groceries, storing groceries properly in the home, preparing meals, serving meals, and cleaning up after meals. To improve the function of nutrition/food, it would be necessary for the members of the family to sit down and discuss each of the important processes. Improving the processes would ensure improvement of the function.

Similarly, improving processes within a health care organization improves key functions. For example, under the function "management of the environment of care," one important process involves hazardous waste disposal. Likewise, in a hospice department, pain management is a multidisciplinary process vital to the function "care of patients." In the lab, blood usage is an important process under the function "patient's rights and organizational ethics." In the kitchen, proper cooking temperatures for meats and refrigerator temperatures for storage are important processes under the function "surveillance, prevention, and control of infection."

You may have noticed that each process may fall under several functions, depending upon the problem and the focus of the study for improvement.[2] Each process also may involve a variety of health care providers from several different departments. Competence, and therefore the practice or performance, of each health care worker involved in an identified process is a critical component in delivering quality service: "the ability of a health care professional to perform or support a patient care activity in the correct manner (i.e., without fault or error) and to perform or support the *correct* patient care activity (i.e., conform with or adhere to pre-established guidelines) often has a direct bearing on quality of patient care."[6]

DEFINING THE FOUR CRITERIA USED TO PRIORITIZE PROCESSES

Not all processes are of equal importance. Some are critical, and a health care organization might want to give them immediate attention by appointing a process improvement team. How does an organization decide which processes receive top-priority action from a team, which may be handled by one employee, and which are of lesser importance and may be left with no direct improvement action until weeks or perhaps months later? To assist an organization in developing a performance management system, predetermined criteria against which to measure and/or prioritize each process has been identified. Percentages of delivered services have been added to further refine and separate critical processes from those that are simply important. The predetermined criteria against which to measure and/or prioritize processes include deciding which are high-volume, high-risk, problem-prone, and high-cost. Once measured, a strategy to categorize each process is carried out.

The following is an explanation of each criterion against which to measure processes as well as our recommended percentages of services involved. Using these percentages as a guide helps to further refine the work of prioritizing processes.

High-Risk Processes

High-risk processes include those in which harm or lack of significant benefit may occur if the activity is either performed or not performed, i.e., acts of commission and acts of omission. A process is high risk if its performance or omission could result in trauma, death, litigation, or loss of accreditation or license.

Taking a routine blood pressure using a sphygmomanometer and stethoscope usually is not considered high risk, because it is not invasive in nature and its omission usually does not *directly* result in adverse outcomes. However, monitoring a critically ill patient's arterial line blood pressure on a monitor may be considered high risk because the blood pressure may be fluctuating and dangerously low. Add to that the invasive nature of arterial lines and the potential for infectious and bleeding complications, and what is normally a routine procedure that nursing assistants perform becomes a high-risk activity that only a licensed professional may perform. Other examples of high-risk patient processes that may fall into both service and practice domains include administration of potentially lethal medications and subduing a violent psychiatric patient. High-risk governance processes would include failure to ensure licensure and credentialing of medical staff and lack of properly maintained disposable containers for used sharps, laboratory errors, lack of a system for blood usage, and unsanitary kitchen conditions. Furthermore, governance processes that may be considered high risk include a performance management system, staffing, annual licensure validation, and product evaluation. In each domain there are processes that can be categorized as high risk.

High-Volume Processes

High-volume processes are those that occur frequently or involve a large number of customers, employees, or organizational systems. However, high volume does not always indicate a critical process. We may give numerous bed baths, but their significance to the patient's recovery depends on the diagnosis of the patient and his or her level of acuity. A bed bath may not be a critical process for a patient with an acute, evolving, myocardial infarction, but it may be of great significance to a patient with a large draining wound.

If more than 50% of any of the top three customers of a department (or, in a clinical unit or department, use the top three DRG or patient diagnoses) receive a particular process, that process should be considered high volume. For example, in the dietary department, if more than 50% of the patient meals prepared are 1800-calorie diabetic diets, this process is considered high volume. Likewise, if more than 50% of the repairs performed by the maintenance department involve repairing broken beds, this process is high volume.

If 25% to 50% of a department's customers receive a process, it is of medium volume, and if less than 25% receive a process, it is considered low volume. Likewise, if the top three customers of a department receive a process once per day or more often, it is high volume. More than once a week but less often than once per day is medium volume, and once a week or less is low volume. Examples of clinical high-volume processes include receiving mouth care, meal service, and routine vital sign checks.

Here is a practice example of high volume. Chest auscultation and arterial blood gas analysis may be identified as a priority diagnostic process for patients with chronic obstructive pulmonary disease (COPD). In this department, chest auscultation is performed at least once per shift on all patients with COPD as part of the practice guidelines for managing the patient with impaired gas exchange. Improvement in the patient's oxygenation is monitored using this technique. The process is provided frequently to a large number of patients in a high-volume DRG, and because it is appropriate to their condition and essential to track improvement; therefore, it is a high-volume practice activity.

On the other hand, arterial blood gas analysis is performed only if the patient's condition deteriorates. It is not performed routinely and is not performed on more than 50% of the COPD patients. Although critical to positive outcomes, arterial blood gas analysis cannot be considered a high-volume practice activity in this department. It may, however, be classified as another type of important process.

Other examples of high-volume practice processes might include completing time cards correctly, fire and safety preparedness, and documentation. Again, regardless of frequency, processes are considered "important" only if they will directly affect outcomes if they are not carried out properly.

Employee payroll is an example of a high-volume governance process. A governance process should be considered high volume if it affects more than 50% of employees in any given position or if the process occurs frequently. "Frequently" is defined as once a week or more. If a process occurs less than once a week but at least once a month, it is of medium volume. Those activities occurring on a quarterly basis or less are low volume.

High-volume governance processes, such as the process for preparing the payroll every other week, also will affect outcomes; the outcome is that staff members will terminate employment if they fail to be reimbursed for their service. Scheduling, maintaining the patient classification system, capital expenditures, marketing, hiring, and firing are all examples of high-volume governance processes.

Problem-Prone Processes

Problem-prone processes in the service domain include those processes that produce problems for the customer. In the practice domain, these include processes that produce problems for the employees, and in the governance domain, those processes that produce problems for the system.

Some of these problem-prone processes in the service domain might include failure to receive correct instructions on admission, failure to understand the physician's explanations about treatment and medication options, and strict visiting hours that preclude a loved one's presence at the bedside. They might also include broken call bells, cold meals, infrequent physician rounds, uncomfortable room temperatures, repeated drawings of blood that require multiple sticks each time, missed pulmonary treatments, or waiting hours on a stretcher for a radiology test.

Examples of problem-prone customer populations might include geriatrics, immunosuppressed patients, chemically dependent patients, as well as neonates and women in labor.

Some problem-prone processes in the practice domain might include adhering to the fire and safety code, filling in time cards correctly, and credentialing surgeons in new procedures.

Other problem-prone practice processes might include adherence to the dress code, professional conduct, and absenteeism. Examples of problem-prone staff populations might include graduates from other countries, new graduates, or chemically impaired workers.

Problem-prone processes in the governance domain might be meeting the continual requirements of regulating and accrediting agencies, maintaining a balanced budget, and ensuring vendor response to the organization. Additionally, governance problem-prone processes might include patient classification systems or capital expenditures greater than the budget, frequent sick calls of employees, high turnover of staff, or lack of an organization-wide performance management system.

Unionized employees or physically challenged employees might be an example of a problem-prone group from the governance perspective.

High-Cost Processes

Health care costs in the United States have risen to more than 13% of the gross national product (GNP). Some estimates suggest that medical expenses would escalate to more than 15% of the US GNP by the year 2000.[1] High-cost processes of health care delivery systems are not always obvious. It is easy to identify the very expensive items, such as the use of specialized beds for skin care; however, small costs, if amassed in high volume, also can significantly deplete resources.

High-cost service processes might include those processes or items not covered by insurance, such as invasive procedures (e.g., pacemaker insertion and hemodynamic monitoring), the cost of consultants, out-of-pocket expenses for family travel to and from the hospital or the customer to and from the clinic. It might also include no third-party payer at all, indicating that all hospital and physician expenses are the responsibility of the individual patient.

High-cost processes in the practice domain include such processes as basic life support certification and the mandatory inservices. High-cost governance processes are those that result in large expenditures for the organization. They may include maintaining the organization's information database, the patient classification system, and even the performance management system.

Additionally in the governance domain, absenteeism, use of agency personnel, continuous purchases of scrubs for employees, and unwarranted use of overtime by employees are all examples of high-cost governance processes.

A METHOD TO PRIORITIZE KEY FUNCTIONS AND PROCESSES

As stated, all processes that lie within the functions of a health care organization are not equally important. Some are more critical than others. How, then, will we decide which to assess first and which to assess second? Perhaps there are some processes that are being performed with excellence and there is no need to attempt to improve them at the present time. The department team members will categorize each process and then prioritize it. They will then send the completed project to the QMB. The QMB will use the information from each department to create a master list of prioritized processes and select the ones with highest priority to be improved this year.

CATEGORIZING AND PRIORITIZING PROCESSES

Three tools have been devised to simplify this necessary preliminary work of categorizing and prioritizing processes in each department. Each tool falls under one of three steps. It is important to read the entire chapter before attempting to use these tools. With a clear understanding of the reasons for performing each step and using each tool, the team will be highly productive.

The three tools designed to assist you to categorize and prioritize processes in your department are shown in Figures 7-1, 7-2, and 7-3. This three-step method will lay the foundation for departmental and organization-wide performance management. Each of the three steps is progressive in that the first tool (Figure 7-1)

IDENTIFY KEY FUNCTIONS AND PROCESSES WORKSHEET

DEPARTMENT: _____   DATE: _____

TEAM: _____   TEAM LEADER: _____

FUNCTION: _____

PROCESS: 1. _____

2. _____

3. _____

4. _____

5. _____

FUNCTION: _____

PROCESS: 1. _____

2. _____

3. _____

4. _____

5. _____

FUNCTION: _____

PROCESS: 1. _____

2. _____

3. _____

4. _____

5. _____

FUNCTION: _____

PROCESS: 1. _____

2. _____

3. _____

4. _____

5. _____

FUNCTION: _____

PROCESS: 1. _____

2. _____

3. _____

4. _____

5. _____

Are there duplicate processes under the functions? If yes, combine them here.

Duplicate processes:

_____

_____

_____

_____

_____

_____

Figure 7-1   Worksheet for identifying key functions and processes.

must be completed before beginning the second tool (Figure 7-2), and the second tool must be completed before beginning the final prioritizing tool (Figure 7-3). This three-step method using the three tools provides the "how to" of prioritizing processes.

Step I

The tool presented in Figure 7-1, Identify Key Functions and Processes Worksheet, will help the team members to organize their thoughts. Notice that the

DATE: _____   **MATRIX FOR PRIORITIZING PROCESSES**

DEPT.

	SERVICE	PRACTICE	GOVERNANCE
HIGH RISK	1.	5.	9.
HIGH VOLUME	2.	6.	10.
PROBLEM PRONE	3.	7.	11.
HIGH COST	4.	8.	12.

A

Figure 7-2   Matrix for prioritizing processes. **A,** Blank form. **B,** Completed matrix.

Continued.

MATRIX FOR PRIORITIZING PROCESSES

DEPT.

Dietary

	SERVICE	PRACTICE	GOVERNANCE
HIGH RISK	1. Sanitized utensils, plates, etc. 2. Infection prevention 3. Cross training/floating	1. Infection prevention 2. Staff safety 3. Written standards for dietary dept. 4. Cross training/floating	1. Scheduling of staff 2. Ordering food/supplies 3. Unit quality control 4. Sanitized utensils, plates, etc. 5. Infection prevention 6. Written standards for dietary dept. 7. Cross training/floating 8. Intensive review of sentinel events 9. Maintaining equipment and supplies
HIGH VOLUME	1. Hot food in appropriate containers 2. Sanitized utensils, plates, etc. 3. Infection prevention 4. Patient dietary education 5. Distribution of literature on special diets 6. Cross training/floating	1. Hot food in appropriate containers 2. Infection prevention 3. Patient dietary education 4. Distribution of literature on special diets 5. Staff safety 6. Cross training/floating 7. Education time	1. Hot foods in appropriate containers 2. Sanitized utensils, plates, etc. 3. Infection prevention 4. Scheduling of staff 5. Ordering food/supplies 6. Unit quality control 7. Written standards for dietary dept. 8. Cross training/floating 9. Maintaining equipment and supplies
PROBLEM PRONE	1. Hot food in appropriate containers 2. Sanitized utensils, plates, etc. 3. Infection prevention 4. Patient dietary education 5. Distribution of literature on special diets 6. Cross training/floating	1. Hot food in appropriate containers 2. Infection prevention 3. Patient dietary education 4. Distribution of literature on special diets 5. Staff safety 6. Cross training/floating 7. Education time 8. Written standards for dietary dept. 9. Staff schedule	1. Meeting JCAHO standards for accreditation 2. Maintaining equipment and supplies 3. Cross training/floating 4. Written standards for dietary dept. 5. Unit quality control 6. Ordering food/supplies 7. Scheduling of staff 8. Infection prevention 9. Sanitized utensils, plates, etc. 10. Hot food in appropriate containers
HIGH COST	1. Sanitized utensils, plates, etc. 2. Infection prevention 3. Hot food in appropriate containers 4. Distribution of literature on special diets 5. Cross training/floating	1. Education time (not paid by hospital) 2. Cross training/floating (Have to carry personal insurance)	1. Meeting JCAHO standards for accreditation 2. Maintaining equipment/supplies 3. Ordering food/supplies 4. Cross training/floating 5. Scheduling of staff 6. Hot food in appropriate containers

B

Figure 7-2, cont'd.

FINAL PRIORITIZING WORKSHEET

DATE: _____ DEPT: _____ TEAM LEADER: _____ SENT TO QMB; DATE: _____

CRITICAL PROCESSES	EXTREMELY IMPORTANT PROCESSES	VERY IMPORTANT PROCESSES	IMPORTANT PROCESSES

Figure 7-3 Final prioritizing worksheet.

tool (Figure 7-1) has a space for the name of the department, the date, the team name, and the team leader's signature. This is followed by an organized brainstorming outline. There is then space for listing five key functions of the department and the most critical processes that lie within each function.

The team conducts a brainstorming session to list the major functions of the department. You may choose to use the 11 key functions (Appendix 7-1) identified by the JCAHO or to develop your own list. Some departments may decide that they have more than five key functions that are critical to their service, practice, and governance. In that case, use the same format on a sheet of blank paper and continue brainstorming until all of the key functions of your department have been listed.

The departmental team is now ready to conduct a second brainstorming session to decide which processes under each key function should be placed on the worksheet. These are the processes that are the "driving force" within each key function. For example, under the function Patient Rights and Organizational Ethics some processes might include (a) the patient process for notifying the health care organization of the patient's decision to exercise the "right to die" policy, (b) the process to carry out abortion decisions, (c) the process for conflict resolution with staff members' cultural, religious, or ethical values, and (d) the process for maintaining medical record confidentiality.

There will be numerous processes under each function. The team must choose the *most* critical of these for priority performance improvement. Once key functions of the department are listed and processes under each function have been selected, the team should review each process looking for duplicate processes. Combine duplicates and place them in the box provided for this purpose in the lower righthand corner of the worksheet. Then mark through the duplicate process under the function. By doing this, processes will not appear multiple times in each box of the next tool. There should be no process listed more than once on the Identify Key Functions and Processes Worksheet. Once this worksheet is completed, your team is ready for the next step.

Now the team is ready to use the tool shown in Figure 7-2.

Step II

Figure 7-2 is divided vertically into the three domains of a service delivery business: service, practice, and governance. It is divided horizontally into the four prioritizing headings previously discussed: high risk, high volume, problem prone, and high cost.

Here is how to use the matrix: First, place the name of the department in the top lefthand corner of the matrix. Then, using the first tool, Figure 7-1, as the reference point, categorize each listed process under the vertical criteria of high risk, high volume, problem prone, and high cost and the horizontal column, service, practice, and governance. A process may fall into one or more of the categories of criteria: high volume, high risk, problem prone, and high cost. For example, if a process includes oncology patients, administration of chemotherapeutic agents may be high volume because of the number of patients receiving it, high risk because of the toxicity of the agents, and problem prone because of their numerous side effects. It may also be high cost because of the cost of the drugs themselves, the equipment used, and the fact that the nurses administering them must be credentialed.

As you look at each process that was listed under a function on the Step I worksheet, ask yourself, "Is this process high risk to those who *receive the service* of this department? Is it high risk to the practitioners who *deliver the service* of this department? Is it high risk to those who *govern the service* of this department?" If the answer is yes, then write the process in boxes 1, 5, and 9. Then ask, "Is this process high volume to those who *receive the service* of this department? Is it high volume to the practitioners who *deliver the service* of this department? Is it high volume to those who *govern the service* of this department?" If the answer is yes to each of these questions, write the process in boxes 2, 6, and 10. Ask, "Is this process problem prone to those who *receive the service* of this department?" If the answer is no, leave box 3 empty.

Continue until you have analyzed each process and have made the decision to either place it or not place it in a box on the prioritizing matrix tool. When the exercise is finished and all processes of the Matrix for Prioritizing Processes have been listed, count the number of times each process appears in the boxes on the matrix. Weight should be given to the processes that appear the most times, in all domains, on the matrix. The maximum number of times a process may appear on the matrix is 12. A process would occur in each box of the matrix if it met the four prioritizing criteria in each domain. Rank each process by the number of times it appeared in a box and list the rank order on the back of the form in Figure 7-2.

Step III

Now the team is ready for the final step of the prioritizing process. Look at Figure 7-3. There is a space at the top of the tool to enter the date, the department name, the team leader's name, and the date that this final tool is sent to the QMB. There are four columns with four headings. The headings are critical processes, extremely important processes, very important processes, and important processes. How do we know which processes go into each of the columns? Here are criteria for proper column selection:

Processes that fall into four categories of any domain are **critical processes.** They are the first level of priority in the performance management system. Processes that fall into three of the four categories in any domain are **extremely important processes** and should be measured at least three times each year. They are prioritized as follows:

1. *High risk, problem prone, high volume.* Examples typically include medication administration, ventilator care in ICU, handling of hazardous wastes, patient and staff safety, equipment checks, proper collimation and radiation doses, proper food storage and handling, and checking for electrical hazards. These are the assessments that the organization must do frequently and continuously.
2. *High risk, problem prone, high cost.* Examples typically include care of the patient who is ventilator-dependent or on hemodialysis, bypass surgery, running a code, caring for the indigent or high Medicare or Medicaid population, laundry, employee needle sticks, patient falls, patient's skin integrity, use of agency personnel, and turnover.
3. *High risk, high volume, high cost.* Examples typically include purchasing food, supplies, capital equipment, and laundry; piping oxygen into the walls, purchasing and maintaining safety equipment such as crash carts and fire alarms, orientation of new employees, and continuing education.
4. *Problem prone, high volume, high cost.* Examples typically include skin care, blood administration, medication errors, shift reports, cafeteria service, absenteeism, invasive procedures, housekeeping, and nosocomial infections.

Processes that fall into two of the four categories in any domain are *very important processes* and require measurement at least twice each year.

Next list those processes that fall into two of the four categories according to the following priority order:

1. High risk, problem prone
2. High volume, problem prone
3. High cost, problem prone
4. High risk, high volume
5. High risk, high cost
6. High volume, high cost

Finally, list the processes that fall into only one of the categories. These are *important processes* and may or may not require measurement.

Now it is time for the final tally of all boxes. Until this point we have been addressing each domain singularly under Step III. We have been looking at how many times processes fall into the boxes of one domain. Now it is time to use the final tally numbers by counting how many times processes fell into any box in any domain. List the processes that were placed in 10 to 12 boxes on the Matrix for Prioritizing Processes under the *critical processes* heading. These represent the processes that deserve the performance management system's highest priority. List those processes that were placed in seven to nine boxes of the matrix under the *extremely important processes* heading. These represent the processes that deserve the organization's second highest priority.

List those processes that were placed in four to six boxes of the matrix under the *very important processes* heading of this final prioritizing tool. These are the processes that deserve your third highest measurement priority.

Finally, list those processes that were placed in one to three boxes under the *important processes* heading. These represent the processes that are the last priority in the 5-year plan. This tool is now ready to be sent to the QMB for comparative analysis with other departments.

It will be virtually impossible for the QMB to assign a performance improvement team to every process listed from each department of the organization. To do so would require two staff members for every process, one to perform the process and the other to measure your technique and outcomes. Remember, the purpose of the performance improvement process is to spot-check those processes that are *most* critical in defining performance of your service. The cost of administering your performance management system is, of course, an important concern. Therefore, it may take 3 to 5 years to incorporate into the system all of the various categories of processes that you provide in your department as part of your delivery of service, practice, and governance.

Because it is impossible to measure everything in a busy department, prioritization of the department's critical processes to be measured is vital to the organization-wide performance management system. This worksheet, when completed in every department, is sent to the QMB. The QMB will review each department's Final Prioritizing Worksheet and create a master composite list of top-priority processes that need to be improved over the next 5 years.

This presents the QMB with necessary data from each department to create an organizational master performance management priority plan. The QMB may then decide upon process improvement team leaders and team members to address the top-priority processes of the organization.

When there is a systematic method for identifying functions and processes in each department, and that information is "fed" into a central clearinghouse for performance management such as the QMB, important information is communicated about each department's functions and processes and purposeful inter-departmental performance improvement may be planned.

The smooth, multidisciplinary performance of processes in all domains is necessary to successful outcomes of the health care organization. These outcomes include costs, performance improvement, value, and customer satisfaction. Ignoring a process that has a direct impact on positive outcomes of service, practice, or governance of a health care organization jeopardizes its reputation and future economic prosperity.

NARROWING OPTIONS

Narrowing options begins with a plan. Many health care organizations have adopted a 5-year performance management calendar. This is reasonable, given the plethora of processes involved under each function. Once the QMB's list of organization-wide priorities is completed, the 5-year performance management strategic plan may be created by deciding which of the processes will be assessed for each year of the 5-year period.

The organization may target one fourth to one third of the processes to be part of the performance management plan. Of the processes targeted for improvement, we suggest you select these percentages for balance: 60% of the processes to be addressed pertain directly to service delivery; 20% of the processes to be addressed pertain directly to staff performance; and 20% of the processes to be addressed pertain to governance performance. These will be the processes for which standards will be developed and indicators will be chosen.

Each year QMB reviews all departments' scope of service, practice, and governance and the important processes relevant to each domain. They then validate and/or amend the 5-year plan by reviewing each process targeted for performance improvement during the next year. Changes in the 5-year plan will be based on any changes that have occurred in customer services, staff practices, or governance systems.

By completing the critical work in each department outlined in Steps I through III, you will construct the foundation for a sound 5-year performance management strategy. Additionally, the content presented in Chapters 4, 5, 6, and 7 will create a sound structure for turning the performance management philosophy into a "how-to, hands-on" methodology for getting a job done! Taking the time to plan and organize the system as described in these chapters is very time-consuming, and annoying to some busy employees who cannot see the big picture. But once completed by each department, the methodology serves to streamline the rest of the performance management system. Well-defined responsibilities, well-delineated customers, differentiated scope of service, practice, and governance, and prioritization of critical processes are the keys to developing a performance management program that continually measures and improves the essence of the organization's overall performance.

This careful planning eliminates the haphazard, "knee-jerk" busywork that can occur when measurement becomes a response to isolated instances or specific situations. You will be assured that your performance management system is on target with the priority processes of your organization and that those priority processes are consistent with your mission.

REFERENCES

1. Anderson R: Atlas of the American economy: an illustrated guide to industries and trends, *Congressional Quarterly*, Washington, D.C., 1994, Elliott & Clark Publishing.
2. Green E: Eleven functions for '95, *Quality connection*, vol 4, no 4, January/February 1995.
3. Joint Commission on Accreditation of Healthcare Organizations: *The measurement mandate*, Chicago, 1993, The Commission.
4. Joint Commission on Accreditation of Healthcare Organizations: *1994 accreditation manual for hospitals*, vol 1, Chicago, 1994, The Commission.
5. Joint Commission on Accreditation of Healthcare Organizations: *1995 accreditation manual for hospitals*, Chicago, 1995, The Commission.
6. Joint Commission on Accreditation of Healthcare Organizations: *Quality review bulletin*, Chicago, 1989, The Commission.
7. Katz JM: Defining excellent performance, *Nursing quality connection*, vol 4, no 1, March/April 1994.
8. National Committee for Quality Assurance: *Reviewer guidelines: standards for accreditation*, Washington, D.C., 1995, The Committee.
9. Peters T, Waterman R: *In search of excellence*, New York, 1982, Harper & Row.

Appendix 7-1   Explanation of JCAHO's 15 Functions; 11 Are Mandated for Performance Improvement

Hospitals seeking accreditation will be required to measure, assess, and improve critical processes of their choice under each of the 12 JCAHO-mandated functions for performance improvement. The 15 functions are divided into 3 sections: patient-focused functions, organizational functions, and structures with functions. (The structures with functions must be in place but are not formally assessed as are the first 11 functions.)[5]

Patient-focused Functions

1. **Patient's rights and organizational ethics.** *Patient's rights* includes access to care, treatment that includes advanced directives, active participation in care, conflict resolution, and care at end of life. *Organizational ethics* includes networking with prior and post health care givers beyond the walls of the organization, disclosure of ownership of referred services, organ donation, medication or clinical trials and patient involvement in research. Furthermore, *organizational ethics* includes establishment of policies and mechanisms to address any request by a staff member not to participate in an aspect of patient care. This function also includes billing and marketing practices of the organization.

2. **Patient assessment.** Institutions must now address how assessments and reassessments in each department that deals directly with patients will be conducted. This includes radiology, laboratory, admitting, all nursing units, and emergency triage. Physical, psychologic, and social assessment by nursing and medical staff must occur within 24 hours of admission. Patient-specific populations drive the timeliness and extent of the assessment and reassessment process. This function further delineates structures supporting assessment and care decisions.

3. **Care of patients.** Multidisciplinary, patient-focused teamwork emphasizing collaboration, communication, coordination, and integration of care is the focus of this function. These areas should be specifically addressed:
   - Planning and providing care
   - Anesthesia care in all settings
   - Medication administration in all settings by all caregivers
   - Nutritional care
   - Operative and other invasive procedures
   - Rehabilitation care and services
   - Special treatment procedures

4. **Education.** Evidence that each of seven educational areas has been addressed as appropriate is required. Education should
   - facilitate patient's and family's understanding of the patient's health status, options, and consequences of options selected
   - encourage patient and family participation in the decision-making process about health care options
   - increase the patient's and family's potential to follow the therapeutic health care plan
   - maximize patient and family care skills
   - increase the patient's and family's ability to cope with the patient's health status/prognosis/outcome
   - enhance the patient's and/or family's role in continuing care
   - promote a healthy patient lifestyle

   There must be a systematic approach to education throughout the organization.

5. **Continuum of care.** Each health care organization also must view the care it provides as part of a continuum that over time enables patients to have access to an integrated system of settings, services, and care levels. This includes the patient's pre-entry phase; the entry phase; the coordination of care among practitioners while within the organization; pre-exit phase, which includes discharge planning; and exit phase, which includes provision of information or data to help others meet the patient's continuing care needs.

Organizational Functions

6. **Performance improvement.**   This function shifts the primary focus from the performance of individuals to the performance of the organization's systems and processes, while continuing to recognize the importance of the individual competence of medical staff members and other staff. The goal of this function is that the organization designs processes well and systematically measures, assesses, and improves its performance to improve patient health outcomes. Performance is what is done and how well it is done to provide health care.

7. **Leadership.**   Effective leadership (a) defines a strategic plan that is consistent with the organization's mission, vision, and values, (b) clearly communicates the organization's mission and vision and strategic plan throughout the organization, and (c) fulfills the organization's vision by providing the framework to accomplish the goals of the strategic plan. (THE BLUEPRINT is such a framework.)

8. **Management of the environment of care.**   This function requires seven environmental control plans: (1) safety management, (2) security, (3) hazardous materials/waste management, (4) emergency preparedness, (5) life safety, (6) medical equipment, and (7) utility systems. There is particular emphasis on smoking policies, construction and renovation, fire doors and fire extinguishers, fire drills, security incidents, high-risk equipment, and performance criteria for employees that work in this department.

9. **Management of human resources.**   The Joint Commission has combined requirements from orientation, competency assessment, training, and education. The human resource department must demonstrate a written plan for ensuring organization-wide orientation and competency assessment for all employees—this requirement is no longer "just for nurses." All education now falls under this function. There is no longer a requirement for a nursing education department.

10. **Management of information.**   This function includes information about the science of care, the individual patient, the care provided, the results of care, and the performance of the organization itself. Furthermore, because many individuals and departments within the organization provide care, their work must be coordinated and integrated. Because of this dependence on information and the need to coordinate and integrate services, health care organizations must treat information as an important resource to be managed effectively and efficiently. JCAHO recognizes that this function may take up to 5 years to complete and the scoring guidelines will accommodate the time needed for this transition. Emphasis will be placed on greater collaboration and information-sharing to enhance patient care.

11. **Surveillance, prevention, and control of infection.**   The goal of the surveillance, prevention, and control of infection function is for the health care organization to identify and reduce risks of endemic and epidemic nosocomial infections in patients and health care workers. The scope of this function is broad. It includes activities at the direct patient care level and at the patient care support level to reduce risks for nosocomial infections. The function also links with the support systems to reduce the risks of infection from the environment, including food and water sources. There must be a written, organization-wide plan to carry out this function.

Structures with Functions

12. **Governance.**   This function deals with approval of budget and capital expenditure plans, bylaws, organizational structure, relation to medical staff, executive committee role, rules and regulations, avoidance of conflict of interest, hospital ownership/control disclosure, level of patient care, self-evaluation, selection of volunteers, etc.

13. **Management and administration.**   Contract services performance evaluation, employee health service, internal controls, legal compliance, medical record review, organ and tissue donors, patient complaints, personnel policies, smoking policy, etc.

14. **Medical staff.**   This includes appointments, reappointments, and terminations actions by MD applicants, peer review and recommendations, approval of outside patient care services, bylaws, clinical privileges, continuing education of MD staff, quality monitoring activities, peer review of individual MD performance problems, role of departmental chairperson, overseeing selection of appropriate surgical procedures, etc.

15. **Nursing.**   This includes assignment of responsibilities, education, competence, evaluation of nursing staff members, standards development, competencies, collaboration with other disciplines, committee assignments, data collection, decision making, diagnoses, delegation of responsibilities, documentation of licensure, etc.

Chapter 8

Developing and Disseminating Standards

No amount of travel on the wrong road
will bring you to the right destination.
Ben Gaye III

In 1898 a struggling author named Morgan Robertson wrote a novel, *Futility,* about an oceanliner. The oceanliner was far larger than any other ship and was labeled "unsinkable." One cold night in April, laden with passengers, it wrecked on an iceberg with enough lifeboats for only a fraction of its 3,000 passengers. Robertson called his ship *Titan.*[10]

Fourteen years later, a real ship left Southampton on its maiden voyage to New York. It too was a mammoth vessel: eleven stories high and four city blocks long. It was the world's largest and most glamorous ship, and it was "unsinkable." Its name was the *Titanic.*

When one of the passengers, Mrs. Albert Caldwell, asked a deck hand who was carrying luggage if the ship was really unsinkable, he answered, "Yes lady, God himself could not sink this ship."

Perhaps the most convincing feature of the *Titanic* was its watertight construction. It had a double bottom and was divided into 16 watertight compartments formed by 15 watertight bulkheads running across the ship. It could float with any two compartments flooded and thus was labeled "unsinkable."

But sink it did. At 11:40 P.M. on April 14, 1912, the Titanic hit an iceberg, which ripped a gash in 6 of the 16 compartments. The ship sank in 2 hours and 40 minutes.

Because no one could imagine a situation where a watertight ship would ever need to evacuate all of its passengers before help could arrive, the Titanic carried only 16 lifeboats. Each of the 16 state-of-the-art Welin davits was designed to carry 4 lifeboats, a total of 64 lifeboats in all.

The British Board of Trade regulations for vessels weighing more than 10,000 tons required a minimum of 16 lifeboats with a capacity of 5,500 cubic feet and rafts and floats equal to 75% of the lifeboat's capacity. The Titanic weighed 46,328 tons and was required to carry boats for only 962 people. The White Star Line, who built the ship, exceeded the requirements by adding the four canvas collapsible boats stowed on deck. In all, the boats could carry 1,178 people. On this fateful night, the Titanic carried 2,207 passengers on board.[11]

The passengers that night were calm but confused as they stood on the boat deck. There had been no lifeboat drill. The passengers had no boat assignments. The crew had assignments, but hardly anybody bothered to look at the list. Not all the lifeboats being lowered were filled to capacity and the collapsible ones were virtually useless. Boat number 1, built to hold 40 passengers, contained only 12.

Only 651 passengers survived. Had the Titanic been fully equipped with lifeboats and had the correct emergency procedures been communicated and practiced, all on board could have been saved. Even with only 16 lifeboats and 4 collapsibles, had the proper procedures been followed, more than half of the passengers could have been saved. Only about 25% of the passengers of the Titanic survived. It remains history's greatest sea disaster.

Standards as well as fate played a key role in what happened on the Titanic. The lack of adequate equipment, the lack of proper procedures, and the lack of communication about those procedures contributed to the loss of life. Standards are the bulkheads of a truly "watertight" organization.

"If standards are to carry any weight, they are not merely set down and communicated in writing. They are lived out in daily practice."[12]

PERFORMANCE MANAGEMENT STANDARDS

To be truly effective, standards must be well-developed and communicated to every individual within the organization. A culture of commitment to the standards must permeate the organization if excellent performance is to be achieved. A performance management system is built upon clearly defined standards. A standard is a written statement that specifies expectations. Donabedian suggests that a standard serves as a precise quantitative or qualitative specification of a structural component of the health care system or an aspect of care based on process or outcome expectations. A standard is a written value consisting of the rules that apply to key processes, the processes themselves, and the results that can be expected when those processes are enacted. A standards-based performance management system defines the specifications of performance.

Standards must be

- specific
- measurable
- appropriate
- reliable
- timely

Well-developed standards provide a qualitive measure of the fit between what we say and what we do. "Well-organized standards translate the abstract nature of corporate values into actions at even the most basic level of detail."[8]

Each domain has its own specialized standards: standards of service, standards of practice, and standards of governance. Within each standards domain, three types of standards are written: structure, process, and outcomes (see box above).

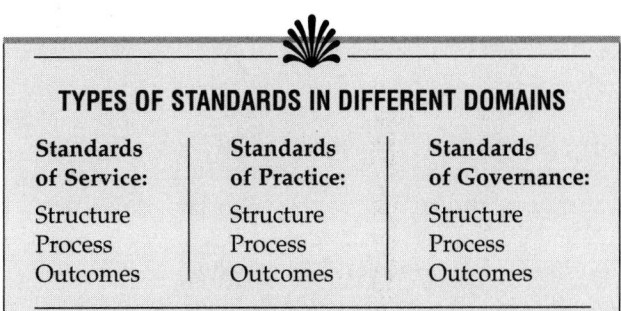

TYPES OF STANDARDS IN DIFFERENT DOMAINS

Standards of Service:	Standards of Practice:	Standards of Governance:
Structure	Structure	Structure
Process	Process	Process
Outcomes	Outcomes	Outcomes

Standards help the individuals working within the organization to adhere to generally accepted contemporary practices in service delivery. Clearly defined standards eliminate the element of connotation. Crosby states, "'Quality of life' is a cliché because each listener assumes that the speaker means exactly what he or she, the listener, means by the phrase."[3] In health care, many individuals are professing quality of life as an indicator of quality health care. Crosby believes this is precisely why we must define quality as conformance to requirements if we are to manage it. "Thus those who want to talk about quality of life must define that life in specific terms, such as desirable income, health, solution control, political programs, and other items that can be measured. When all criteria are defined and explained, then the measurement of quality of life is possible and practical."[3] Likewise, defining quality of life as health requires specific, measurable terms.

Crosby also believes standards eliminate the norm references by setting up objective criterion benchmarks. Thus a Taurus is not compared with a Mercedes, but rather each is compared with the specifications for that car. If the Taurus conforms to all the specifications for a Taurus, then it is a quality car, regardless of the fact that it may not have all of the features of a Mercedes. Likewise in health care if a traditional procedure meets all of the requirements and achieves the desired outcomes, it is a quality procedure, whether or not it uses the latest technology.[3]

The values of the organization as expressed by its standards provide a source of stability for organizations. Those standards are virtually worthless unless they are shared with the members of the organization and the customers it serves. These shared values represent what the organization stands for.

Standardization brings predictability, and it is that predictability that is critical to improving process capability. It is because of standards that we have a degree of comfort and stability in both our personal and professional lives. Standardization allows us to move within the environment with ease. Lack of it causes discomfort. You can travel throughout the U.S. and in any hotel room feel fairly confident that you will be able to blow dry your hair, because the plug will fit into the socket and the current flowing through the walls will match that required by the blow dryer. It has been standardized. However, if you travel to Europe without some type of adaptor, you will be air drying your tresses.

The same predictability that frees you from traveling with your current adaptor in the U.S. can be useful professionally, too. Predictability within the organization is essential to performance management. Everyone in the organization needs to sing not only from the same hymnal but also from the same page. Once the choir is singing the same tune, modifications can be made to enhance the beauty of the performance. Once standardization has been achieved, performance measurement and improvement efforts can begin.

STRUCTURE STANDARDS

Structure standards outline the legal parameters that govern performance expectations. They include the mission, philosophy, goals, policies, and job descriptions of the organization/department. They are nonnegotiable and cannot be situationally modified. That means that the individual employee cannot choose to ignore or modify the rules at will. For example, a policy outlines which employees may perform venipuncture. Regardless of individuals' prior training or experience, if their position title is not on that policy, they may not under any circumstances perform venipuncture within that organization. Structure standards represent the absolutes of behavior that cannot be changed at will.

Structure standards are those that if ignored or modified would put the customer, the staff, or the organization at risk. Structure defines the scope of authority within which the individual or group representing the organization may function. When confronted with a situation contrary to the "rules," an individual or group must seek additional counsel from someone in a higher position of authority or within the legal department before pursuing the matter.

Any time there is a variance from structure standards, it should be documented and reported to the risk management department. These are the standards to which 100% compliance is essential. Noncompliance cannot be tolerated.

Noncompliance indicates actions that are out of sync with the mission, philosophy, goals, policies, or position requirements of the organization. To achieve peak performance requires that all individuals within the organization are working together to achieve the organization's goals. This cannot occur when various individuals or groups within the organization are working at odds with each other.

In defining structure standards it is important to identify any exceptions. If so, the issue probably is process and not structure.

Because structure standards represent the absolutes of the organization, a thorough scrutiny of all existing policies is needed to separate the policies that are nonnegotiable under any circumstances from those that, conceivably, can be negotiated. Those issues to which adherence is expected less than 100% of the time are not structure and should not be labeled as such. In most cases, misuse of structure standards has occurred most frequently in the arena of policy. Organizations have had a tendency to react to negative situations by creating new policy and drafting a memo for immediate distribution. "Policy by memo" is a favorite form of management in many health care organizations. The policy manual grows with each memo and the policy is in effect until the next knee-jerk reaction. Policy manuals become unwieldy and are not read. A thorough scrutiny of existing policies would enable the organization to significantly reduce the number of policies. In one organization, a review of policies related to staff leave resulted in a reduction of policies from five pages to two. The remainder of the information about applying for the various types of leave was reformatted into a process standard.

Mission

The mission statement addresses the overall business in which the organization is engaged. The organization's mission identifies what it is about. It is shaped by the relationship between the present or potential needs and desires of the community. "Some organizations falter or fail because they attempt to produce a service that lies outside their capabilities, others because the demand fails to materialize or declines."[17]

To formulate a sound mission, answer these questions:

1. What services are we providing? What are we really about?
2. For what purpose are we in this activity?
3. What tasks must be carried out to meet community needs, provide services, and survive?[17]

The mission defines the primary interests of the organization, including the organization's inherent values and what it intends to accomplish. The mission clarifies what the organization does and who it tries to serve.[5]

Mission statements also help confirm an organization's identity. From the mission statement can be derived the typical deliverables expected by its customers. These deliverables include the following:

1. the level of customer satisfaction expected
2. the inventory level to be maintained or turns to be attained
3. the unit cost or cost level to be achieved

Philosophy and Goals

Philosophy is a written statement of an organization's beliefs regarding the three domains, i.e., what is believed about customer service (patient care), what is believed about staff practice, and what is believed about governance.

Philosophy is converted to goals that demonstrate how the organization operationalizes its philosophy. For example, the philosophy of the equality of man can be enacted in this goal: to be an equal opportunity employer. The accompanying box shows a philosophy written in all three domains.

Goals define measurable end results that individuals, groups, or organizations attempt to achieve by expending resources. Until the long-term goals of the

organization have been identified, it is difficult if not impossible to write yearly objectives.

Schulz suggests a contingency approach to goal formulation because of rapidly changing environments. The contingency approach varies based on where power is concentrated and includes problem solving, when power is concentrated among policy makers; coalition formation, when power is dispersed or parties are in conflict and bargaining; conflicting objectives, occurs when power is balanced between policy makers and other active parties and there are conflicting goals among parties to the goal formulation process.

"The reason that goals go undefined, are unused in guiding the evaluation of performance, or are seen merely as a process to undergo before getting back to

PHILOSOPHY WRITTEN IN THREE DOMAINS

Excellence in Service

We believe . . .

- that each of our patients, regardless of circumstances, possesses intrinsic value from God and should be treated with dignity and respect.
- that each encounter with patients and families should portray compassion and concern.
- that each patient should receive quality care that is cost-effective, competitive, and based on the latest technology.
- that patient confidentiality and privacy should be preserved.
- that meeting the needs of patients and other customers should always be our number one priority.

Excellence in Practice

We believe . . .

- that the primary duty of health care professionals is to restore and maintain the health of patients in a spirit of compassion and concern.
- that the scientific process is an integral part of practice as health care professionals.
- that collaboration within the health care team is essential to meet the holistic needs of patients, which include physical, psychosocial, and spiritual aspects of care.
- that we should aggressively promote patient and family education to allow each individual the opportunity to prevent illness and/or achieve optimal health.
- that we are accountable to patients, patients' families, and to each other for our professional practice.
- that monitoring and evaluating health care services is our responsibility and is necessary to continuously improve care.
- that we should pursue professional growth and development through education, participation in professional organizations, and support of research.

Excellence in Leadership

We believe . . .

- that we should provide a progressive environment, utilizing current technology, guided by responsible stewardship to promote the highest quality patient care and employee satisfaction.
- that we should encourage and support collaborative decision making by those who are closest to the situation, even at the risk of failure.
- that compassion should be characterized in our day-to-day personal interactions as well as being a motivating factor in management decisions.
- that we should be sensitive to individual needs and give support, praise, and recognition to encourage professional and personal development.
- that we should possess an energy level and personal style that empowers and inspires enthusiasm in others.
- that we should consider suggestions and criticisms as challenges for improvement and innovation.
- that justice should be applied equitably in all employment practices and personnel policies.

what the group considers are the real issues is a lack of incentives for using the goals."[17]

Goals are also written in three domains. Goals are written about customer service, practice, and governance and are derived directly from the philosophy.

For example, if the philosophy states

We believe that each patient should receive quality care that is cost effective, competitive, and based on the latest technology,

then a goal statement might be written as follows:

To provide quality patient care that is cost effective, competitive, and based on the latest technology.

Annual objectives are then derived from each goal statement and are increasingly specific. For example, an annual objective based on the above goal might read as follows:

To design quality care for the patient undergoing coronary artery bypass surgery that is competitively cost effective, and based on the latest technology.

Specific outcomes for this service objective can then be designed and indicators of success developed to chart progress toward this annual objective.

In the practice arena, the philosophy statement might read:

We believe that we should pursue professional growth and development through education, participation in professional organizations, and support of research.

A goal statement might read:

To pursue professional growth and development through education.

The annual objective might relate to the educational opportunities for a specific staff population or a specific type of educational opportunity.

In relation to the governance domain, a philosophy statement might read:

We believe that we should encourage and support collaborative decision making by those who are closest to the situation, even at the risk of failure.

A goal might be to develop a risk-accepting environment for collaborative decision making. An objective may outline the desire to develop a system of self-directed performance improvement teams.

Policy

Policy defines the organization's "laws"—those tenets that when not adhered to, create a legal or physical threat to the customer, employee, or organization. Policies are in concert with the mission, philosophy, and goals of the organization. There cannot be a policy that does not support the basic beliefs and goals of the organization. Policy can be altered only by a recognized authority within the organization, although state and federal law changes may dictate to that authorizing board changes that must be made. Typically any policy changes should be reviewed by the organization's legal department.

Policy is a guide to action. The purpose of policy is to explain who will take action, what action is required, and when action will be taken. For example, there may be an organizational goal related to being an equal opportunity employer and policy related to the diversity ratio.

Policies are significant because they permit a rational and/or realistic approach to controversial situations. A controversial situation is one in which an individual or group is unsure which course of action to pursue. This indicates a disruption in the relationship between a person or organization and the environment. Policies guide behavior.

"However, because a policy is in written format does not mean that it will be read, understood and accepted."[17]

Many organizations confuse structure with process. This leads to bulky policy manuals and confusing procedure manuals. Staff members become frustrated because they are unclear about which pieces of information in the policy and/or procedure manual are required and which permit modification. Policies may not be situationally modified because they function as a framework for decision making by defining desirable and undesirable behavior. Policies are structure standards.

Carlson and Ranney believe the policies are "usually indicative of an organization's value system, its assumptions about people and human behavior, and its understanding of and beliefs about what makes organizations effective."[2] They assert that in the absence of formal policies, de facto policies spring up. De facto policies represent what really happens in practice (repeatedly). These policies are embedded in everyday work and are less visible. They might be completely contradictory to the formal policies and totally inconsistent with the mission, thus undermining the organization's efforts toward its goals.

Policies should be periodically reviewed to

- consider whether the policy supports the mission and goals of the organization.
- consider whether it is consistent with the major philosophical concepts/contracts adopted by the organization.
- examine whether the policy is needed.
- examine its clarity and effectiveness.

"Policies that react to problems are wasteful." Emphasis should be on removing the causes of the problems. Punitive policies such as those related to medication errors should be eliminated. It is not often that the people making the errors are bad. More likely they were busy and short-staffed.

Carlson and Ranney suggest asking the following questions about policies:

1. How complex is the policy?
2. Will it be easy to administer?
3. Will it be readily understood by the people it affects?
4. Is it brief, concise, unambiguous, complete?
5. Will it address the issues it is intended to address?
6. Is it presented in a language and form appropriate for the situation?
7. How do you know?
8. Will it produce the desired results?
9. Is it stated positively or negatively (should vs. should not)?
10. Does it clearly explain why this rule or policy is necessary?
11. What is the plan to determine whether it is producing the desired results and whether it needs improvement?
12. Is it possible to test the policy or rule before applying it to the whole organization? Such a trial might permit some needed modifications before company wide implementation.
13. How is it (or will it be) communicated to the organization?
14. Who will communicate the policy or rule?
15. How, when, and where will it be announced?
16. Will it need to be communicated periodically for new employees or to keep it fresh in people's minds?[2]

Job Descriptions

Job descriptions are structure standards because they outline the requisite knowledge, skills, attitudes, responsibilities, and scope of authority of a specific position within an organization for the organization to function at maximum performance.

By ignoring the job description in hiring practices, the organization may end up with unqualified staff or individuals without the necessary experience to fulfill the specifications of the job. Organizational performance is compromised. Valuable resources are consumed in training the individual to perform at the required level, and millions of dollars are lost in opportunity costs while the individual is underperforming. Some individuals never achieve the level of performance expected and problems arise from the constant lack of skills.

Hiring someone whose qualifications vary from the defined job description is outside the scope of authority of the hiring manager and requires additional administrative approval. This is a change in thinking for many organizations that have treated job descriptions as "wish lists" rather than absolutes. However, as the job market becomes more competitive and the stakes for survival become higher, staff members are a critical weapon not to be taken lightly. Hiring is a critical administrative process demanding organizational attention. Human resources are pivotal to peak performance. For job descriptions to be structure standards and ergo absolutes, it is essential that they be purged of all but the most vital requirements and responsibilities that are directly linked to the achievement of the organization's goals.

PROCESS STANDARDS

Process standards are as important as structure standards, but they do not carry the same degree of weight in the organization. As the old adage goes, there is more than one way to skin a cat. Whether skinning cats is allowed in this organization and who has the authority to do so are considered *structure,* how to do it, if it is allowed, is *process.* The organization's decision to skin cats requires a policy—a structure standard. Knowing how to skin a cat requires a procedure, a process standard.

With process standards, there is not an expectation of 100% compliance; some variation is expected. Some of that variation is justifiable and acceptable and some is not. Unlike altering structure, changing process does not require approval by a higher authority. A qualified individual can change process with sound justification and documentation of that rationale. For example, CDC guidelines recommend that peripheral IV sites be rotated every 72 hours. In this particular situation, Mrs. Jones is an emaciated, terminally ill patient. This peripheral IV was started with much difficulty, and after 72 hours the nurse observes that the IV is dripping well with no signs of inflammation or pain at the insertion site. The nurse may choose to leave the IV in place rather than changing the site. However, once the decision not to replace the IV has been made, the nurse is responsible for observing the IV site and documenting its condition closely and more frequently than usual and documenting the rationale for the decision not to rotate the site.

Process outlines how the knowledge, skills, and attitudes of the organization are operationalized. Process is how we get from here to there. Clearly defining the types of process and the actions involved in each is the first step in eliminating process variation. The written process standards define operational norms. Process standards can be modified, based on the situation and the judgment of the individual or work group responsible for making decisions within the context of that situation. Process is situationally negotiable. Situational modification occurs when the practitioner determines that a presenting circumstance does not fit the norm, and therefore a modification of the operational norm is required to achieve the desired outcomes.

Process takes many formats. These include procedures, practice guidelines, plans, and documentation. Process standards translate the organization's values into actions and define in writing those processes for which the organization will be held accountable.

Peters states that because process is negotiable, it must also be flexible. This flexibility is important because there currently exists little information regarding the enigma of client care and which interventions yield the best outcomes under which circumstances. Therefore, the ability to adjust care in accordance with the amount of progress toward the client's expected outcome is significant. Also, the individuality of client/family response to care is great and has many intervening variables, so it is impossible to predict all the potential events during an episode of care.[15]

Process standards include procedures, practice guidelines, plans and documentation.

Procedures

Procedures are psychomotor tasks. They are the step-by-step analysis of a specific task. In procedures, one step is dependent upon another, and the steps are best performed sequentially for optimum results.

Procedures require skill acquired through muscle memory. The practitioner is required only to follow the steps to achieve the outcome. Procedures may be written in narrative form or they may be written as an algorithm or flow chart. Information on constructing a flow chart can be found in Chapter 12.

Practice Guidelines

Practice guidelines outline the ongoing management of conditions or situations. These can be service related, practice related, or governance related. In the service arena, a clinical condition would include symptom management. Clinical practice guidelines are written to outline the management of specific clinical symptoms/conditions, e.g., fever, hypovolemic shock, decreased cardiac output, nausea, and vomiting. Examples of clinical practice guidelines can be found in the appendices of Chapters 9 and 13.

In the practice arena, conditions would include the management of such issues as the credentialing process. Administrative practice guidelines would address such operations as staffing, opening and closing units, and budgeting. Although both procedures and practice guidelines consist of a series of actions, the actions in practice guidelines are not organized into steps and may occur concurrently as opposed to the sequential requirements of procedures.

Grimshaw and Russell's comprehensive review of the literature found that all but 4 of 59 studies detected improvements in the process of care following guideline use. They noted that studies reporting large improvements suggest the potential impact of guidelines when development, dissemination, and implementation are all appropriate.[7]

There are both external and internal practice guidelines. External practice guidelines are those written by an organization other than the institution itself. The Agency for Health Care Policy and Research has generated many practice guidelines as have numerous professional associations. These guidelines tend to present a broad brushstroke of accepted treatment. Internal guidelines are those developed by the institution and are based on patient demographics and institutional-specific resources. They should be in concert with external guidelines; however, they reflect the institution's current state of health care practices for specific conditions.

We have identified four key paradoxes associated with the development of practice guidelines:

1. internal versus external control
2. individualization versus standardization
3. centralization versus decentralization of decision making
4. multidisciplinary collaboration versus discipline-specific development[6]

"These paradoxes represent extremes on a continuum. Each extreme represents a 'black or white' organizational approach. As we all know, we live in a grey world where the subtle shadings of balanced approaches yield more positive results than the absolutism of extremes. The key to survival in weathering the changes that are necessary to eliminate variations in practice patterns is found in a combination approach to each of these major issues."[6]

Plans

A plan is a tool that outlines an intent to act. Plans can exist in the service, practice, or governance domain. A clinical path is a service plan and is probably the type of plan most easily identified in health care. However, practice paths/plans are also used to foster employee growth and development, and certainly the budget represents the fiscal plan used in the governance of the organization.

Plans plot the critical course for outcomes achievement and performance improvement. "Critical paths comprise the predetermined . . . activities involved in a specific project . . . from start to finish and the time to complete each of the activities. They are interdisciplinary guides to the usual treatment patterns for a group of clients with similar needs."[15] Although Peters was referring to a clinical path, the same applies for employee development plans and administrative plans.

Documentation

If you didn't chart it, you didn't do it. In this era of litigation, documentation is one of the most important activities performed within an organization. There are three types of documentation: (a) data collection, (b) planning, and (c) evaluation.

Data collection is defined as the information collected as the result of measurement. This can include clinical data such as vital signs, hemodynamic values, or lab results. However, it also can include data such as the number of staff members attending a fire safety class or the average length of stay for mothers after a normal vaginal delivery. Data collection is best handled on charts and graphs where it easily can be tracked over time. Data are typically recorded on some type of flowsheet.

Planning involves a written record of the intent to act and directs the actions to be taken. Documentation of evaluation is accomplished by keeping progress records, and it is required in each of the three programs and for each of the domains. Documentation of the performance awareness program is in the form of the written standards, their development and approval mechanism, and records of the educational activities undertaken to disseminate the standards to staff. In performance measurement, documentation of the performance studies and their analysis is required. In the performance improvement program, documentation of the action planning process, the implementation of the improvement plan, and the results obtained is imperative. Although documentation can take many forms, the most common formats used are flowcharts for data collection, plans for the planning process, and progress records for recording progress toward outcomes.

OUTCOME STANDARDS

Outcomes are the payoff. Although in health care, as in many other businesses, the payoff may not always be what was desired or expected. Well-defined structure and process standards, however, greatly increase the likelihood of achieving desired outcomes.

Outcomes are the results obtained through enactment and completion of a process. They can be divided into expected (desired) outcomes and unexpected (undesired) outcomes. Expected outcomes are usually achieved when a process is carried out as specified. Unexpected outcomes usually result from nonconformance with specifications or when an uncontrollable force affects the process.

Outcomes never stand alone. It helps to think of outcomes as "piggyback" standards, because outcomes are attached to all process standards. The old song about love and marriage applies to process and outcomes: you cannot have one without the other. Although most practitioners are accustomed to patient outcomes, outcomes relate to practice processes and governance processes as well. For example, an outcome of a credentialing process in advanced life support may be that an individual fulfills the course requirements and passes the test and is able to demonstrate the skill appropriately. An outcome of the staffing process is that there is adequate staff to care for the number of patients on any given unit during any given shift.

Outcomes are written for every procedure, practice, guideline, and plan. An example of an outcome for the venipuncture procedure might be venous access in one stick while maintaining sterile technique. Examples of outcomes for practice guidelines can be found in Appendices 9-1 and 13-1. In order to develop reliable, valid outcomes, the process of benchmarking is extremely helpful.

BENCHMARKING: A CRITICAL TOOL FOR STANDARDS DEVELOPMENT

Benchmarking is the search for industry best practices, which lead to superior performance. It is based on the premise that internal operations cannot always have the best answers for every problem. It is the continuous process of measuring against the best.

Benchmarking is a tool that assists in developing more realistic goals and objectives. Benchmarking is a goal-setting process; it is a means by which the practices needed to attain new goals are identified. "Benchmarking legitimizes goals and targets by basing them on an external orientation . . . It challenges, in a productive, planned fashion, those individuals and organizations to concentrate on what will make operations more successful in the market place and eventually attain superior performance."[1]

The chief benefits of benchmarking are as follows:

- more adequately meeting end user customer requirements
- establishing goals based on a concerted view of external conditions
- determining true measures of productivity

- attaining a competitive position
- becoming aware of and searching for industry best practices

"The bench marks may most importantly indicate the direction that must be pursued rather than specific operationally quantifiable metrics that are immediately achievable."[1] The conversion of benchmarks to operational targets translates the long-term actions into specifics.

Targets are more precise and incorporate what realistically can be accomplished within a given time period.

There are four types of benchmarking:

1. internal: a comparison of internal processes
2. competitive: competitor to competitor comparisons of a specific process
3. functional: comparisons of processes to similar processes within same industry
4. generic: comparison of processes regardless of industry

Once standards have been established, the job is half done. Equally important is the development of, understanding of, and commitment to performance excellence through standards implementation.

ESTABLISHING COMMITMENT

Clarifying values and breathing life into them through written standards is the cornerstone of performance awareness. However, those written standards are not worth the paper on which they are written, unless they have been disseminated throughout the organization and those staff members affected by them have committed to adherence.

Crosby believes that "quality is an achievable, measurable, profitable entity that can be installed once you have commitment and understanding, and are prepared for hard work."[3]

Getting staff to "buy in" to the standards begins when they are being developed. Those individuals involved in implementing the standards must play a major role in their development. The individual is the basic building block of a team and an organization. Achieving the individual's support results in a commitment to improved performance and productivity. "When employees have a sense of purpose that what they are doing makes a difference, phenomenal energies get released. When those energies get channeled into work, the result is outstanding performance and productivity."[18]

Ulschak suggests that high performance and productivity result from the following:

1. Individuals who have a strong commitment and a clear sense of purpose and role

2. Feedback systems that provide individuals with good data

He suggests that the corporate culture needs to clearly define its purpose and communicate it not only during orientation of new employees but also during the recruitment and selection process and throughout the employee's tenure. "There can never be too much communication about purpose."[18] Also, the organization needs to focus on how its purpose fits with that of the individual. If the purposes are at odds, commitment is unlikely and the individual's performance may in fact hamper performance and productivity. This concept applies to the teams and committees as well.[18]

To accomplish this with teams, Ulschak recommends three steps:

1. The corporate culture needs to identify norms among individuals that endorse and support teams and clarify the individuals' commitment and purpose.
2. The corporate culture needs to encourage problem-solving, conflict management, and decision-making skills as they apply to teams.
3. The corporate culture needs to have structures in place for rewarding team accomplishment.[18]

Congruity must exist between the individual, the team, and the organization.

Numerous authors have discussed the relationship of corporate culture and performance and productivity. Standards are a critical part of corporate culture, because they help define how the organization copes with its problems of external adaptation and internal integration. Standards define "how we do it here."

Corporate culture is defined as a pattern of basic assumptions that have worked well enough to be considered valid and therefore to be taught to new members as the correct way to perceive, think, and fall in relation to coping with its problems of external adaptation and internal integration. Standards form the basis of a strong corporate culture. It is through the corporate culture that the performance management system gains its support.

A successful performance management system depends on communication with and commitment of everyone affected. Kern suggests building that commitment through the use of cascading teams. The cascading teams approach starts with the initiation of a small group of vested individuals. This group then involves additional people in the planning process and an even bigger group in the implementation phase. The ultimate objective is commitment through the involvement of all affected individuals.[9]

Creating a Culture of Performance Excellence

According to Deal and Kennedy, a culture is a "system of informal rules that spells out how people are to behave most of the time."[4] Employees should know exactly what is expected of them and should be able to comply without wasted time and effort.

Deal and Kennedy describe five key elements that make up a strong culture:

1. business environment
2. values
3. heroes
4. rites and rituals
5. cultural network

These elements apply directly to the continual enculturalization of performance excellence.

The business environment is the single greatest influence in shaping a corporate culture. The environment in which a company operates determines what it must do to be successful.

Values are the beliefs of the organization made explicit in their written standards. These standards must be well defined and disseminated throughout the organization. Chapter 16 discusses the development of standards for the performance management system.

Rites and rituals are the systematic routines of day-to-day life in the organization. They exemplify the behavior that is expected of employees, and they tangibly demonstrate what the company stands for. In terms of performance, these rites include the measurement activities that are a critical part of each individual's job. These rites and rituals may also be evidenced in the recognition systems that have been established to reward excellence.

Finally, the cultural network serves as the primary (but informal) means of communication within the organization. It is through the network that the true values are passed along from employee to employee and department to department. For example, Mary Jane Moon, RN, may have resigned with official notification of a new job offer. However, the truth according to the "grapevine" may be that Mary Jane made too many medication errors.

Using this informal network can be a powerful method for communicating the organization's vision. For example, it can be instrumental in changing the perception of measurement as "blame fixing."

"Culture causes organizational-inertia; it's the brake that resists change because this is precisely what culture should do—protect the organization from willy-nilly responses to fads and short term fluctuations."[4] Overcoming this inertia requires continuous effort over time. It cannot be accomplished merely by writing new standards. It has been our experience that in moving to a culture of performance excellence, it takes approximately 2 years of consistent effort before overt signs of the new culture are evident. In the fast-paced world of health care where we are accustomed to seeing immediate results, this process can appear painfully slow. So slow, in fact, and so fraught with resistance and cynicism that many people throw their hands up in desperation and stop trying. There is no substitute for time. Developing a culture of performance excellence is analogous to running in a marathon. Those who persist, pace themselves well, and have a long-range strategy will ultimately succeed.[4]

An effective strategy to develop a strong culture of performance requires three elements:

1. a top-down commitment
2. an environment to succeed
3. quality education

A top-down commitment is essential to the development and growth of a culture of performance excellence. O'Leary states, "Leadership can make or break quality improvement efforts in an organization. These initiatives don't just happen; they do not bubble up from the grass roots; they move from the top down." He believes that continuous performance improvement is an organization-wide way of life which is helpful to the organization and good for the patient whom it serves.[13]

Top-down commitment must be apparent throughout the organization. In other words, management has to "walk like it talks." Without that consistency, staff will mistrust management and not take the performance management initiative seriously. For example, if management extols the virtues of performance improvement, but it balks at spending the money for the needed changes, staff receives conflicting messages. Likewise, the nurse manager who constantly stresses the importance of responding to patient call bells but does not respond to staff "call bells" sends a mixed message about responding to customer requests.

The vision of performance excellence is like a seed. If it falls on barren ground, it will lie there and remain a seed. If it is watered and fertilized, it germinates and becomes a strong seedling. That seedling needs constant nourishment and the proper environment if it is to survive and flourish. So too, the performance management system itself needs a supportive environment for its potential to be fully realized. Performance improvement efforts in the performance management system focus on the development and maintenance of a professional practice environment. This involves participatory decision making through shared leadership that promotes a sense of accountability in individuals for achieving the organization's goals and objectives.

The new performance management environment in organizations must be one of security and not fear and one that promotes communication rather than isolation. Deming insists that it is essential to drive out fear: "People are afraid to point out problems for fear they will start an argument, or worse, be blamed for the problem."[19] An environment that utilizes performance measurement to affix blame cannot support a performance management system. That type of environment only fosters deception and mistrust. Porter-O'Grady states that "workers begin to build trust immediately upon joining an organization, expecting a sharing of information that affects their personal and economic welfare. When the hospital does not honestly and freely supply all of the information workers need to do their jobs and to make judgments about their future there, a feeling of basic mistrust insidiously begins to undermine all other supports."[16] An environment of trust encourages the open exchange of information throughout the organization. This environment enables participatory decision making and provides staff with the information needed to make informed decisions. Although staff members are held accountable for their decisions, the environment is free of reprisal and unwarranted disciplinary action. Risks are managed and there is freedom to fail. Dennis O'Leary believes " . . . there is a lot more to be gained by improving the norm than by punishing all of the outliers."[13]

No one can feel comfortable in an environment that does not provide the material and fiscal support necessary for staff members to act responsibly upon decisions. A fertile environment for performance excellence involves valuing staff's administrative responsibilities for measuring and improving the results of services as much as it values the provision of that care. Staff members should be free from clinical responsibilities when attending to their practice or governance responsibilities without the need for worry about who is caring for their patients while staff members are out of the department. Administration must ensure staff members are able to carry out measurement activities as part of their routine job responsibilities, not as an additional task for them to "fit in" as time permits. Commitment of resources to support the performance management functions of the division enhances staff trust in the rhetoric and translates it to reality. Commitment of resources also involves recognizing and rewarding accomplishments. A strong recognition program is necessary to keep the fires of staff enthusiasm for the performance management system burning brightly, and it motivates staff members to even higher levels of excellence.

To participate in this new environment in a meaningful way, staff members must be fluent in the language and processes of performance management. Learning a foreign culture begins with a familiarization with the language and rituals or customs of the country; so too, in the unfamiliar world of performance management, staff members must have an opportunity to acclimate. A solid educational curriculum for performance management is essential at all levels throughout the organization. Education regarding performance management includes training in terminology, data collection, statistical analysis, decision making, strategic planning, and change. The depth and scope of the training are based on position responsibilities. For example, assistants and technicians may be involved in data collection, whereas the members of the Performance Measurement Council would be responsible for data analysis and interpretation. Both groups, however, would need to know the basic, or core, terminology. The educational process is ongoing; it begins with orientation and continues throughout the staff member's tenure. To be meaningful, the information must be repeated periodically to reinforce the message and update all employees to the latest changes taking place at the national, regional, local, and institutional levels.

The provision of an environment for success and the development of education are closely linked to the introduction of technology that will enable employees to collect, process, analyze, and project trends in large volumes of information quickly and efficiently. Computer technology can greatly facilitate performance management activities and education. Its successful implementation requires that the staff becomes literate in yet another language and culture, that of automated information processing. Unless staff members have the knowledge and skills necessary to use computer technology, its use can waste their time and energy. Used appropriately, however, computer technology is the key to taming the paper tiger of performance management.

REFERENCES

1. Camp RC: Benchmarking applied to health care, *The Joint Commission Journal on Quality Improvement,* 20(5): 229-238, 1994.
2. Carlson B, Ranney GB: Reviewing organizational policies and rules, *Quality Progress,* 25(1): 50-56, 1992.
3. Crosby PB: *Quality is free,* New York, 1979, New American Library.
4. Deal TE, Kennedy AA: *Corporate cultures,* Reading, Mass, 1982, Addison-Wesley.
5. Garner JF, Smith HL, Piland NF: *Strategic nursing management,* Rockville, Md, 1990, Aspen Publishers.
6. Green E, Katz JM: *Clinical practice guidelines for the adult patient,* St. Louis, 1995, Mosby.
7. Grimshaw JM, Russell IT: Effect of clinical guidelines on medical practice: a systematic review of rigorous evaluations, *Lancet,* 342: 1317-1320, 1993.
8. Katz JM, Green E: *The BLUEPRINT for Quality Management: The Agenda for the Future.* In Schroeder P, editor: *The encyclopedia of nursing care quality,* vol 2, Gaithersburg, Md, 1991, Aspen Publishers.

9. Kern JP: The chicken is involved but the pig is committed, *Quality Progress,* vol 28, 10, Oct 1995, 37-42.

10. Lord W: *A night to remember,* Mattituck, NY, 1987, Amereon House.

11. Lynch D: *Titanic—an illustrated history,* Ontario, 1992, Madison Press Books.

12. Mannello T: *A CQI system for healthcare: how the Williamsport Hospital brings quality to life,* New York, 1995, Quality Resources.

13. O'Leary D: Accreditation in the quality improvement mold- a vision for tomorrow, *Qual Rev Bull,* 17(3): 72-77, 1991.

14. O'Leary D: CQI—a step beyond QA, *Qual Rev Bull,* 17(1): 4-5, 1991.

15. Peters DA: Outcomes: the mainstay of a framework for quality care, *Journal of Nursing Care Quality,* 10(1): 61-69, 1995.

16. Porter-O'Grady T: *Creative nursing administration,* Rockville, Md, 1986, Aspen Publishers.

17. Schulz R, Johnson AC: *Management of hospitals and health services,* ed 3, St. Louis, 1990, Mosby.

18. Ulschak FL: *Corporate culture: the impact on productivity and performance.* In *Productivity and performance management in health care institutions,* Chicago, 1989, American Hospital Publishing.

19. Walton M: *The Deming management at work,* New York, 1990, G.P. Putnam's Sons.

Part Four

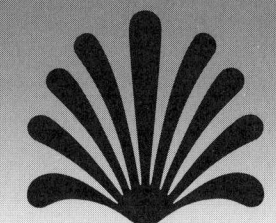

CREATING AN ORGANIZATION-WIDE PERFORMANCE MEASUREMENT PROGRAM

Chapter 9

Developing Performance Measures

Toto, I don't think we're in Kansas anymore!
The Wizard of Oz

In the classic film "The Wizard of Oz," when the farmhouse finally lands and Dorothy steps through the door, you know immediately that something has happened. Up to that point, the film was shot in black and white. As Dorothy opens the door and steps through, the beautiful technicolor world of Munchkinland appears. The director used color as an indicator of a significant change.

Indicators are ubiquitous. They are positive or negative signs of change. Indicators measure various things. On a piece of machinery, an indicator monitors its function. The gas gauge in your car measures how much fuel is in the tank, thereby indicating approximately how many miles you can travel until you must refuel. In meteorology, indicators monitor the weather. A rise or fall in barometric pressure indicates a change in the weather pattern. In chemistry, indicators such as litmus paper measure the presence of a substance such as an acid or a base.

Indicators alert you—they forecast a deviation from the norm and may warn of impending problems. Economists pay special attention to indicators such as interest rates, unemployment rates, and inflation as predictors of an impending recession. Signs of a labor shortage are evidenced by higher vacancy rates, increased help wanted ads, increased retention activities, and higher salaries.

Indicators are a part of daily life. The clock indicates whether we are early, late, or on time. The calendar indicates the month, date, and day of the week. Traffic signals indicate stop, go, or caution, and a growling stomach indicates that it is time for a meal.

Just as "Hail to the Chief" heralds the arrival of the president and the first robin is the harbinger of spring, indicators may represent something else. They may not be a direct representation of measurement. Although "Hail to the Chief" is not the president and the first robin is not spring, when you hear the first notes of that song or see the first robin, you know the president or spring has arrived.

We use indicators in health care, too. There are clinical, practice, and governance indicators. Some are direct measures; others are not. Vital signs generally indicate overall patient status. A thermometer directly measures body temperature, and the presence of a fever, rapid pulse, and increased respirations may signal an infection. A practice indicator might include completed documentation of patient admission and discharge forms. A governance indicator might include the number of shifts on which staffing ratios were met.

INDICATORS

In performance management *indicator* refers to a particular type of measurement. An indicator is a performance measure. It is a valid and reliable quantitative process or outcome measure related to one or more dimensions of performance. These dimensions were described in Chapter 1. Performance is composed of competence and productivity. Competence means that the individual or organization has the ability to provide an identified level of performance. Productivity means that those abilities are translated into appropriate actions that achieve performance outcomes.

Traditionally, accrediting agencies surveyed the capabilities of an organization—its competence. Was the organization able to provide quality care? Today, however, the thrust of accreditation activities has shifted to productivity, or the yielding of favorable results. No longer do accreditation surveys focus on the question, "Is the organization *able* to provide quality services?" but rather, "*Does* the organization provide quality services?" Today, the accreditation process focuses on actual performance rather than simply the capacity to perform well.[6] For example, rather than deciding solely whether an institution follows a program to prevent patient falls, the reviewer will evaluate whether that program has any effect on the number of falls associated with injuries.

Indicators provide a critical method for focusing on the desired outcomes and/or the key processes. To date, the development has focused on indicators related specifically to patients. These are called clinical indicators. A clinical indicator is "a quantitative measure that can be used as a guide to measure and evaluate the quality of important patient care and support services."[2] It is not a direct measure of quality but rather a flag that points to specific issues that require more intensive review. Indicators enable organizations to measure customer outcomes as a function of individual and organizational performance.

Today, however, a much broader approach to indicators is required. As each department within an integrated delivery system provides a service to its customers, each has a need for service-related indicators. Some of the customers of departments will be patients. Others, although not dealing in direct patient care, nonetheless have a specific set of customers and thus need service indicators.

An indicator is an event. It is expressed as the number of events compared with a specified universe of events. The ratio is expressed as:

$$\frac{\text{Number of customers for}}{\text{whom a specified event occurs}}{\text{Number of customers involved in}}$$
$$\text{the event the indicator is measuring}$$

For example:

$$\frac{\text{Number of patients with acquired stage IV pressure ulcers}}{\text{Number of patients with pressure ulcers}}$$

or

$$\frac{\text{Number of urinary tract infections in patients with indwelling urinary catheters}}{\text{Number of patients with indwelling urinary catheters}}$$

Categories of Indicators

An indicator is categorized by the type and seriousness of the event it measures. The type of event measured by an indicator may be structure, outcome, or process and is service, practice, or governance in scope.

Types of measurement. *Structure, process, or outcome.* Measurement may be related to structure, process, or outcome. Structure refers to the rules that govern how the service is provided. Process encompasses all of the activities provided and outcomes are the results of the process. For example, structure defines all the equipment necessary and available to perform surgery, process is how the surgery was performed, and the outcome is the patient's status after the surgery. For the function of patient education, structure relates to the necessary teaching aids, process is the act of patient teaching, and outcome is whether and how much the patient learned.

Another example would relate to the environmental control department. Structure indicators might define the rules related to handling hazardous waste materials. Process indicators relate to the process of disposing of hazardous waste or the process of reporting and cleaning of a waste spill. Outcome indicators measure the number of spills that occur and/or danger or damage to individuals and/or property as the result of a spill.

Structure indicators are derived from the written structure standards. These standards include the mission, philosophy, goals, policies, and job descriptions of the organization. Structure indicators measure whether or not the rules of the organization are being adhered to. For example, if the key process being monitored is safety and the clinical policies state that all patients who are in a wheelchair or on a stretcher must have a seat belt on, a structure indicator might read:

$$\frac{\text{The number of geriatric patients}}{\text{up in a wheelchair with seat belt on}}{\text{Total number of patients up in wheelchairs}}$$

Process indicators measure specific aspects of the service that are critical to outcomes. Examples of process indicators include assessments, routine and emergency treatments, and management of complications.[2]

Process indicators are derived from written process standards. These include the procedures, practice guidelines, plans, and documentation that outline how service in each department is to be delivered and recorded. Process indicators may be used in conjunction with outcome indicators or in situations in which an outcome is not readily achievable in a time frame relevant to the organization. Pain management in terminally ill cancer patients is an example of a process indicator. Eradicating the cause of the pain to alleviate it is not feasible; therefore, pain control becomes the best available indicator of the process of managing the pain. It may be written:

$$\frac{\text{The number of patients with terminal cancer experiencing pain who achieve a 0-2 level of pain control on a 1-10 scale}}{\text{The number of patients surveyed with terminal cancer experiencing pain}}$$

Outcome indicators measure what does or does not happen to the customer, staff, or system after something is or is not done.[2] These results may be desirable or undesirable. Outcome indicators are based on the written outcome standards of service, practice, or governance that have been integrated into the process standards. For example, the outcome standard for the venipuncture procedure might be to establish venous access in one stick. The outcome indicator would read:

$$\frac{\text{The number of one-stick venipunctures achieved}}{\text{The number of venipunctures attempted}}$$

An infection control outcome might read:

$$\frac{\text{The number of ventilated patients who develop pneumonia}}{\text{The number of ventilated patients}}$$

On a safety practice guideline, the outcome standard might be to avoid level IV falls, i.e., unsupported falls resulting in injuries. In this case, the outcome indicator would read:

$$\frac{\text{The number of level IV falls in patients} > 65 \text{ years old within 4 hours of sedative administration}}{\text{The total number of level IV falls}}$$

Service, practice, or governance. The type of event measured by an indicator may also be categorized as service, practice, or governance. A service event relates to the customer. It measures key factors in the care that a patient receives or the outcomes of that care. For example, there is no evidence of physical injury to the patient as a result of application and maintenance of physical restraints. A practice event relates to an aspect of practice affecting customer outcomes. It measures key factors of professional practice that have an impact on the quality of customer results. For example, in the

nursing department there is evidence of the use of the nursing process in each nurse's practice. In the admitting department there is evidence of advanced directives obtained on every admission. In the radiology department there is use of a gonadal shield for every abdominal x-ray. A governance event deals with organizational factors that affect patient outcomes. It measures key aspects of the system that affect the results of service delivery. Examples of governance events include understaffing, bed utilization, and availability of equipment.

Service, practice, or governance indicators can measure structure, process, or outcomes. Examples of service structure, process, and outcome indicators have been stated above. The number of staff members attending CPR classes is a professional process indicator. The number of staff members correctly initiating CPR in a code situation is a professional outcome indicator. An example of an administrative structure indicator is the number of times the crash cart was fully stocked and ready to use.

Service indicators are based on service standards; likewise, practice and governance indicators are based on their respective standards. These indicators are just as important as the service indicators in determining organizational performance. If not enough workers are present in a department on a given shift, the governance standards will not be met, regardless of how well they are written. Similarly, if there are a sufficient number of workers, but an insufficient number of them possess the requisite knowledge or skills, the practice standards are meaningless.

Seriousness of events. Indicators are also classified by the seriousness of the events they measure. A sentinel event measures a serious, undesirable, and often avoidable process or outcome.[7] Although the frequency is low, the event is so severe that individual case review is required. This type of indicator is described in Chapter 6. "Sentinel event indicators are generally viewed as being of limited value because they represent the extremes of performance measurement. In this regard their most practical applications relate to risk management activities. Even then, analysis and investigation of a sentinel event may prove to be inconclusive."[4]

An aggregate data indicator quantifies a process or an outcome related to many cases, as opposed to isolated cases as in a sentinel event. Aggregate data indicators measure both discrete and continuous variables.

A discrete variable is a measurement that is limited to specific options such as "greater than" × amount of time or "less than" × amount of time. It measures whether the event falls in one category or the other. A discrete variable indicator is called a rate-based indicator.[4] Examples might include stat lab results that take more or less than 15 minutes to be reported, and emergency room wait time of more or less than 1 hour.

Both discrete and continuous variable indicators measure an event that requires intensive review only if the rate of occurrence exceeds preset control limits. These are situations for which a variance in care is allowed. For example, the number of patients with acquired stage IV dermal ulcers is a rate-based indicator because of the virtual certainty that among these patients will be an aged diabetic in end-stage renal failure associated with peripheral vascular disease, stroke, hemiplegia, and incontinence. In such a patient, it is impossible to prevent skin breakdown. Moreover, a small number of other patients will acquire dermal ulcers despite optimal nursing. The indicator acknowledges these inevitable occurrences. This type of data is expressed as a ratio or proportion based on the population being measured. A proportion defines the numerator as a subset of the denominator:

$$\frac{\text{The number of emergency room patients waiting more than 1 hour}}{\text{The total number of emergency room patients}}$$

$$\frac{\text{The number of stat lab results taking more than 15 minutes to report}}{\text{The total number of stat lab results reported}}$$

A ratio describes the population being measured in terms other than population itself. For example:

$$\frac{\text{The number of central lines that result in bloodstream infections}}{\text{The number of central line days}}$$

$$\frac{\text{The number of delinquent accounts}}{\text{The number of billable patient care days}}$$

A continuous variable is a measurement that can fall anywhere along a continuous scale, e.g., the amount of time it takes to receive stat lab results, the length of wait time in the emergency department, or the length of time it takes to turn over a patient room. The actual values for each continuous variable are recorded, and the process or outcome is monitored using statistical process control tools such as a run chart, control chart, or histogram. Continuous variable data is usually expressed as a mean or average.[4]

Characteristics of indicators. Olivas and coworkers describe the lack of understanding and the inability to control the care delivery process as major barriers to achieving quality.[13] The result is a failure to select appropriate variables that will forecast change, a failure to measure these variables, and a failure to adjust activities to conform to the standards for the service.

Indicators are those forecasting variables that serve as the barometers of performance in health care service, practice, and governance and are the best predictors of quality or its absence. To provide meaningful information, indicators must possess five key characteristics: they must be reliable, valid, measurable, specific, and relevant.

Indicators must be reliable. Reliability refers to the accuracy of indicators over time, between raters, and across patients; that is, results are consistent regardless of who is collecting the data, when the data are collected, or from which source the data are obtained. To be considered reliable, a thermometer must provide an accurate reading of body temperature regardless of which practitioner is taking the temperature, what time of day the temperature is taken, or which patient's temperature is being taken. In one organization, the reliability of the newer digital thermometers was questioned. Many health care practitioners preferred the glass thermometers; however, there were numerous infection control and cost issues related to the use of glass thermometers. To assure health care practitioners of the accuracy of the digital thermometers, a study was done comparing the results obtained with each type. The findings confirmed the reliability of the digital thermometers in measuring body temperature, and the use of glass thermometers was abandoned.

Indicators need to be reliable. The practitioner using them has to feel confident in their ability to measure the variables that they are designed to measure, regardless of who is collecting the data, when, or from which patient. The indicators that measure the number of dermal ulcers ensure that there is a consistent and accurate means by which dermal ulcers are staged. The use of a standard tool such as the Norton scale provides that assurance.

Indicators must be accurate and valid. Just because a tool is reliable does not necessarily mean that it is valid. You would not use a meat thermometer to measure a patient's temperature; nor would you use a patient satisfaction survey to measure the outcomes of diabetes teaching.

A valid tool measures what it is designed to measure.[15] For example, a thermometer measures temperature; it cannot be used to measure blood pressure.

A valid indicator identifies situations in which quality is lacking, e.g., that the number of nosocomial infections is on the rise or that the number of unsupported patient falls resulting in injury is escalating. A valid indicator would identify that practitioners are not turning high-risk patients every 2 hours or that diabetic patients remain unable to recognize the signs and symptoms of hypoglycemia and intervene appropriately even after instruction.

Indicators must be measurable. The promotion of a safe environment is not a measurable indicator, whereas the number of unsupported patient falls not involving injury is. You cannot manage what you cannot measure. Key processes must be translated into measurable, quantifiable variables.

Indicators must be specific and definite. Specificity relates to the precision with which the indicator measures the event. Indicators must apply to, characterize, or denote a particular issue or event. They are an exact written description of a specification. For example, an indicator related to chemotherapy is specific to cancer patients, whereas an indicator related to fetal monitoring characterizes care given only to obstetric patients.

Indicators must be relevant to service, practice, or governance. They should focus on the critical processes of the service, practice, or governance, not the marginal issues, and touch on every subsystem within the organization. For example, on a surgical unit, indicators should relate to preoperative preparation, the surgery itself, and postoperative recovery as well as the equipment, supplies, and interdisciplinary coordination and cooperation.

THE INDICATOR INFORMATION SET
Indicators and Report Cards

Indicators are the basic criteria of report cards. Although the role of national report cards was discussed in Chapter 2, this chapter will more fully explore the performance measures developed by the Joint Commission on Accreditation of Healthcare Organizations (JCAHO) and the National Council for Quality Assurance (NCQA).

More than 250 organizations are currently developing performance measures.[10] These organizations hope that these indicators will be used to set industry-wide standards that will serve as external benchmarks of performance.

THE JOINT COMMISSION'S DEVELOPMENT OF INDICATORS

In the fall of 1986, the Joint Commission launched a major initiative called the Agenda for Change. The project was implemented to improve the Joint Commission's ability to evaluate the clinical and organizational performance of health care organizations. Its goal was to develop an outcome-focused performance assessment that assists organizations in improving the quality of care they provide.

Developing Clinical Indicators

One of the chief aspects of this developmental program was the design and testing of clinical indicators that relate to key functions. These indicators were to be used to monitor diagnostic and treatment activities rel-

evant to the processes and outcomes. It was projected that information related to these indicators would be pooled, and the institution as well as patients and third-party payers would be able to compare the institution's results with those of comparable institutions. It would be similar to the comparisons made in other industries. For example, in the airline industry, comparisons are made of the on-time arrival record or the frequency and volume of luggage being lost.

Initially, three areas were chosen for indicator development. Task forces were assigned to study obstetrics, anesthesia, and hospital-wide care. The task force members and the Joint Commission project specialists soon found that the literature provided little assistance in defining indicators because of the virtual absence of professional consensus. Eventually, however, 48 indicators were developed in the 3 areas and pilot-tested in 17 hospitals across the country.

The purpose of the testing was to identify and assess problems in data collection and to improve the efficiency of the process for data collection. Refinement or abandonment of the initial indicators was contingent on the feedback from the pilot sites.

Initially there were 70 areas for hospital-wide indicator development. These were condensed in seven major groups: mortality; medication errors; complications and unanticipated procedures related to surgery and other procedures; readmission within 30 days of scheduled surgery; hospital-acquired pressure sores; nosocomial infections; and assessment of antibiotic therapy. Feedback from the pilot sites sent the Joint Commission Task Force "back to the drawing board," because many of these initial indicators did not apply hospital-wide but were more specialty specific. For example, proper timing of antibiotic prophylaxis for specified surgical procedures had no relevance for medical units. Likewise, development of pneumonia in patients treated in special care units by definition applied only to critical care.

Two areas were defined as "key functions" in hospital care. These were the appropriate and effective use of medications and the prevention, detection, and control of infections. These functions involve more than one department within the hospital; their results depend on the performance of clinical management and support services. The role of specific disciplines in each of these key functions is being outlined through task analysis. For example, administration, nursing, medicine, pharmacy, clerical staff, and vendors play a role in medication administration. A task analysis would reveal the relevant activities of each discipline and the relationship among them.[2]

Task forces were assembled to develop indicators on the key functions of medication use and infection control. The medication use task force held its first meeting in March 1989. Initially, a flow chart was developed to outline key tasks and the relationships among specific disciplines and departments (Figure 9-1). Indicators were then developed based on the key processes. Thirteen potential target areas for indicator development were identified. Recommended key processes for measurement included:

Correct drug selection
Dosage individualization for the patient
Drug preparation
Medication administration to the right patient
Patient education about medications

The box on p. 112 lists the medication use indicators in alpha testing.

The infection control task force met for the first time in January 1990. The focus of their work was nosocomial infections. The process of infection control did not readily lend itself to flowcharts. However, since nosocomial infection rates have been monitored since the 1970s, it was felt that this database in conjunction with extensive field experience in surveillance practices would serve as a foundation for indicator development. These indicators are expected to foster better use of current data in an effort to reduce the risks of nosocomial infections.[8] The box on p. 113 lists the infection control indicators in alpha testing.

Five major aspects of care were selected as the basis for the obstetrical indicators. These include prenatal care, maternal complications, cesarean sections, neonatal complications, and obstetrical-related mortality. The box at the top of p. 114 lists the 21 initial obstetrical indicators. Feedback from alpha testing led to revisions (see box at the bottom of p. 114).

Eight important aspects of care formed the basis for the anesthesia indicators. These include anesthesia-related mortality; neurological deficits; cardiovascular complications; pulmonary complications; technical problems including mechanical trauma; protocol changes; transfusion and renal problems; and laboratory indications of anesthesia-related difficulties. The box on p. 115 (left) lists the original 14 anesthesia indicators. The box on p. 115 (right) lists the revised indicators that resulted from alpha testing.

Both obstetric and anesthesia indicators became available for use in 1991. Their use, however, remains optional.

New sets of indicators have been developed in cardiovascular, oncology, and trauma care. Sixty indicators that include process and outcome, appropriateness, and effectiveness have been designed. Alpha testing at new pilot sites began in 1990. Beta testing began in the spring of 1991.

Cardiovascular indicators included angioplasty, coronary artery bypass graft, myocardial infarction, and congestive heart failure.

The trauma indicators encompassed prehospital care, emergency department care, operating room, and intensive care unit.

Oncology indicators focused on the three most common tumor sites in adults: breast, colorectal region, and lung. In October 1990 a core group met to define the function of home infusion therapy and to delineate the scope of care for indicator development. The development of home care indicators was the first project that was nonhospital based.[8] The flowchart in Figure 9–2 depicts home infusion therapy as a system.

By 1994 ten indicators were included in the Joint Commission's indicator measurement system, which had officially been titled *IMSystem,* or *IMS.* The IMS is an indicator-based performance monitoring system for accredited organizations. The focus was on three patient populations: patients who underwent a surgical procedure, received anesthesia, and had an inpatient stay; delivered mothers; and newborns. The box on p. 117 lists these 10 indicators.

Cardiovascular, oncology, and trauma indicators were soon added. The box on pp. 118-119 lists these indicators. These indicators included continuous variable indicators.[9]

The Board of Commissioners formally approved three infection control indicators and five medication use indicators for inclusion in the IMSystem in 1996. A complete list of the 33 indicators currently accepted by the IMSystem can be found in Appendix 9-2.

In 1995 the primary focus of the IMSystem changed dramatically. Rather than focusing on the development of indicators to be used in its accreditation process, the Joint Commission announced a redesign of its indicator selection process in hopes of rapidly creating an expanded array of good performance measures in addition to those indicators already developed and accepted by the Joint Commission. In the new process, an independent council on performance measurement will review systems developed by any of the organizations involved in indicator development. Systems that meet predetermined criteria will be included in the IMSystem.[10]

In the new process, a series of requests for indicators (RFI) will be issued to professional organizations, academic institutions, and others involved in creating health care performance measures. Specific information submitted for each indicator will include the following:

- definition (calculation of numerator and denominator)
- intent or rationale
- setting(s) of care to which it is applicable
- nature and extent of testing

Key Function: Appropriate, Safe, Effective, and Efficient Use of Medications

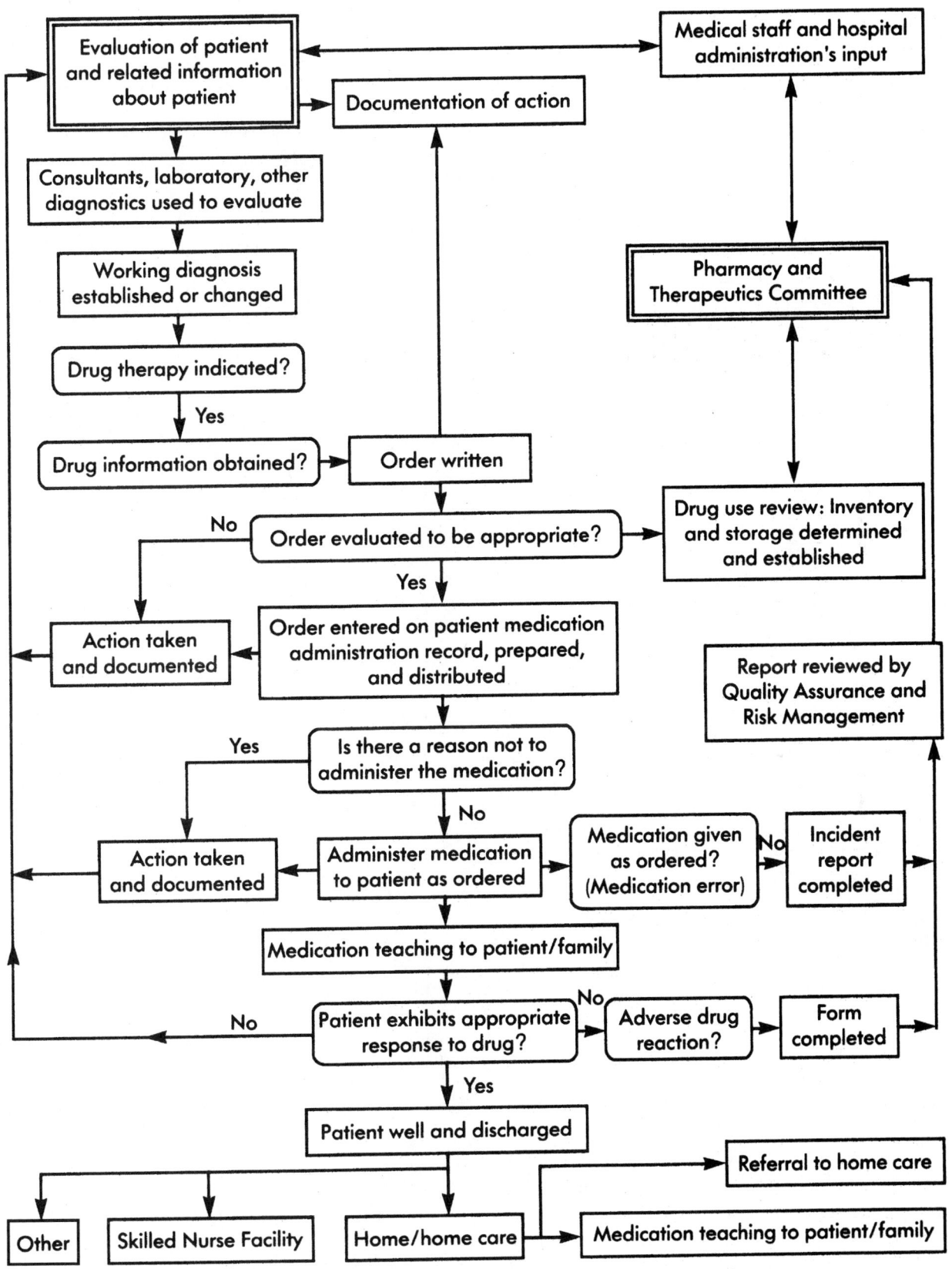

Figure 9-1 Example of medication usage flow diagram. (Copyright 1990 by the Joint Commission on Accreditation of Healthcare Organizations, Oakbrook Terrace, Ill. Reprinted from *Primer on indicator development and application,* with permission.)

MEDICATION USE INDICATORS FOR ALPHA TESTING: SUMMARY LIST

MU-1

INDICATOR FOCUS: Individualizing dosage

Indicator (Numerator): Inpatients over 65 years old in whom creatinine clearance has been estimated.

MU-2

INDICATOR FOCUS: Individualizing dosage

Indicator (Numerator): Inpatients under 1 year old receiving parenteral aminoglycosides who have a measured aminoglycoside serum level.

MU-3

INDICATOR FOCUS: Reviewing the order

Indicator (Numerator): New medication orders prompting consultation by the pharmacist with physician or nurse subcategorized by orders changed.

MU-4

INDICATOR FOCUS: Timing of medication administration

Indicator (Numerator): Inpatients receiving intravenous prophylactic antibiotics within 2 hours before the first surgical incision.

MU-5

INDICATOR FOCUS: Accuracy of medication dispensing and administration

Indicator (Numerator): Number of reported significant medication errors.

MU-6

INDICATOR FOCUS: Informing the patient about the medication

Indicator (Numerator): Inpatients with principal and/or other diagnoses of insulin-dependent diabetes mellitus who demonstrate self blood glucose monitoring and self-administration of insulin before discharge, subcategorized by referral for postdischarge evaluation.

MU-7

INDICATOR FOCUS: Monitoring patient response

Indicator (Numerator): Inpatients receiving digoxin, theophylline, phenytoin, or lithium who have no corresponding measured drug levels or whose highest measured level exceeds a specific limit.

MU-8

INDICATOR FOCUS: Monitoring patient response

Indicator (Numerator): Inpatients over 65 years old receiving tricyclic antidepressants who fall.

MU-9

INDICATOR FOCUS: Monitoring patient response

Indicator (Numerator): Inpatients receiving anticoagulant therapy who also receive vitamin K, protamine sulfate, or fresh frozen plasma, subcategorized by ADRs reported to the ADR reporting system for the patients above.

MU-10

INDICATOR FOCUS: Reporting adverse drug reactions

Indicator (Numerator): ADRs reported through the hospital's ADR reporting system subcategorized by method of reporting (concurrent or retrospective medical record abstraction) and by type of ADR (dose related or non-dose related).

MU-11

INDICATOR FOCUS: Reviewing complete therapeutic drug regimen

Indicator (Numerator): Inpatients receiving more than one type of benzodiazepine simultaneously.

MU-12

INDICATOR FOCUS: Reviewing complete therapeutic drug regimen

Indicator (Numerator): Inpatients with seven or more prescribed medications on discharge.

MU-13

INDICATOR FOCUS: System/management control

Indicator (Numerator): Inpatients who have an allergy to penicillin recorded in the medical record and who receive penicillin.

MU-14

INDICATOR FOCUS: Appropriate prescribing

Indicator (Numerator): Pediatric inpatients with febrile viral illness receiving aspirin (ASA).

MU-15

INDICATOR FOCUS: Overall performance of medication use system

Indicator (Numerator): Patients with a principal diagnosis of bronchoconstrictive pulmonary disease, who are readmitted to the hospital or visit the emergency department within 15 days of discharge due to an exacerbation of their principal diagnosis.

From Joint Commission on Accreditation of Healthcare Organizations: *Joint Commission Perspectives*, Oakbrook Terrace, Ill, March/April 1991.

INFECTION CONTROL INDICATORS FOR ALPHA TESTING: SUMMARY LIST

IC-1

INDICATOR FOCUS: Surgical wound infection
Indicator (Numerator): Selected surgical operations complicated by a wound infection.

IC-2

INDICATOR FOCUS: Postpartum endometritis
Indicator (Numerator): Patients who develop endometritis within 3 postoperative days following cesarean section.

IC-3

INDICATOR FOCUS: Primary bloodstream infection
Indicator (Numerator): Patients with a central or umbilical line who develop primary bloodstream infection.

IC-4

INDICATOR FOCUS: Ventilator pneumonia
Indicator (Numerator): Ventilated patients who develop pneumonia.

IC-5

INDICATOR FOCUS: Postoperative pneumonia
Indicator (Numerator): Selected surgical operations complicated by the onset of pneumonia during hospitalization but not beyond 10 postoperative days.

IC-6

INDICATOR FOCUS: Urinary catheter usage
Indicator (Numerator): Selected surgical operations on patients who are catheterized during the perioperative period.

IC-7

INDICATOR FOCUS: Employee health program
Indicator (Numerator): Hospital employees who have been immunized for measles (rubeola) or are known to be immune.

IC-8

INDICATOR FOCUS: Surveillance/Medical Record Review
Indicator (Numerator): Patients with a central or umbilical line and primary bloodstream infection identified through both medical record review *and* surveillance activities.

From Joint Commission on Accreditation of Healthcare Organizations: *Joint Commission Perspectives,* Oakbrook Terrace, Ill, March/April 1991.

A clinical advisory group will review each RFI according to specific evaluation criteria. These include the following:

- Relevance (applicability of the indicator to the services provided by affected health care organizations)
- Reliability (ability of the indicator to accurately identify the targeted events across multiple organizations)
- Validity (evidence that indicator data identify important events and provide a basis for performance improvement activities)
- Discriminatory capability (extent to which the indicator identifies variation across multiple health care organizations)
- Data collection effort (the relative effort required for, and associated cost of, collecting the data in relation to the importance of the measure)[10]

According to Dennis O'Leary, "If we are to have useful information, the performance data gathered from health plans must be comparable. Measures must also be noted, relevant to patient outcomes and reliable. Otherwise, we will waste a major investment in performance measurement and data collection activities."[11]

Most of the organizations currently developing indicators are quick to admit that a major obstacle to developing national databases is the lack of good data sources. "As the importance of indicator data grows, providers will face a corresponding burden to improve their ability to gather sound data during the course of care, in all practice settings and with the fewest possible intermediaries."[3]

The Health Plan Employer Data and Information Set

The Health Plan Employer Data and Information Set version 2.0 (HEDIS 2.0) was developed by the NCQA. Released in 1993, HEDIS 2.0 was a core set of 60 health plan performance measures covering quality, access, patient satisfaction, membership, utilization, and finance. A major aspect of HEDIS 2.0 was its effort to systematize the measurement process. HEDIS enables health plans to compare their results nationally.[1]

The Performance Assessment Committee (PAC) is a panel of experts from various types of managed care organizations including HMOs, IPOs, and PPOs. Their

OBSTETRICAL CARE INDICATORS (ORIGINAL)

1. The induction of labor for indications other than diabetes, premature rupture of membranes, pregnancy-induced hypertension, post-term gestation, intrauterine growth retardation, cardiac disease, isoimmunization, fetal demise, or chorioamnionitis with or without a cesarean section.
2. A primary cesarean section for failure to progress.
3. A successful or failed vaginal birth after cesarean section (VBAC).
4. The delivery of an infant by planned repeat cesarean section weighing less than 2500 grams or with hyaline membrane disease.
5. The delivery of an infant following the induction of labor weighing less than 2500 grams or with hyaline membrane disease.
6. Eclampsia.
7. The in-hospital initiation of antibiotics 24 hours or more after a term vaginal delivery.
8. Excessive maternal blood loss except with abruptio placenta or placenta previa as evidenced by either a red cell transfusion, a hematocrit less than 22 or a hemoglobin less than 7, or a decrease in hematocrit of more than 11 or of hemoglobin more than 3.5.
9. A maternal length of stay more than 5 days after a vaginal delivery or more than 7 days after a cesarean section.
10. A maternal readmission within 14 days of delivery.
11. A maternal death up to and including 42 days postpartum.
12. The in-hospital intrapartum death of a fetus weighing 500 grams or more.
13. The perinatal death of an infant weighing 500 grams or more.
14. The neonatal death of an infant with a birth weight of 750-999 grams born in a hospital with a NICU.
15. The delivery of an infant weighing less than 1800 grams in a hospital without a NICU.
16. The transfer of a neonate to a NICU at another hospital.
17. A term infant admitted to a NICU.
18. An Apgar score of 3 or less at 5 minutes.
19. The diagnosis of massive aspiration syndrome referenced as ICD9-CM code 770.1.
20. The diagnosis of birth trauma referenced as ICD-9-CM code 767.
21. A term infant having a clinically apparent seizure prior to discharge from the delivery hospital.

From Joint Commission on Accreditation of Healthcare Organizations: *Agenda for Change UPDATE* 2(1), June 1988.

OBSTETRICAL CARE INDICATORS (REVISED)

1. Patients with primary cesarean section for failure to progress.
2. Patients with attempted vaginal birth after cesarean section (VBAC), subcategorized by success or failure.
3. Patients with excessive maternal blood loss defined by either post-delivery red blood cell transfusion or a low post-delivery hematocrit or hemoglobin (Hct less than 22%, Hgb less than 7 gms) or a significant pre- to post-delivery decrease in hematocrit (decrease ≥ 11%) or hemoglobin (decrease ≥ 3.5 gms), excluding patients with abruptio placenta or placenta previa.
4. Patients with diagnosis of eclampsia.
5. The delivery of infants weighing less than 2500 grams, following either induction of labor or repeat cesarean section without medical indications.*
6. Term infants admitted to a neonatal intensive care unit (NICU) within 24 hours of delivery and with NICU stay greater than 24 hours excluding admissions for major congenital anomalies.*
7. Neonates with an Apgar score of 3 or less at 5 minutes and a birthweight greater than 1500 grams.
8. Neonates with a discharge diagnosis of significant birth trauma.*
9. Term infants with a diagnosis of hypoxic encephalopathy or clinically apparent seizure prior to discharge from the hospital of birth, excluding newborns with a diagnosis of fetal alcohol syndrome, and other drug reactions and withdrawal syndromes.
10. Deaths of infants weighing 500 grams or more subcategorized by intrahospital neonatal deaths, total stillborns and intrapartum stillborns.

Reprinted with permission of Joint Commission on Accreditation of Healthcare Organizations.

*A list of the specific diagnoses and appropriate ICD-9-CM diagnostic codes for medical indications for induction of labor and repeat cesareans, for major congenital anomalies, and for significant birth trauma will be provided with the data element specifications for the obstetrics indicators.

ANESTHESIA CARE INDICATORS (ORIGINAL)

1. Mortality within a specified time* following anesthesia care.
2. Failure to emerge from general anesthesia within a specified time.
3. Development of injury to the brain or spinal cord within a specified time following anesthesia care.
4. Development of a peripheral neurologic deficit within a specified time following anesthesia care.
5. Cardiac arrest within a specified time following anesthesia care.
6. Clinically apparent acute myocardial infarction within a specified time following anesthesia care.
7. Fulminant pulmonary edema within a specified time following anesthesia care.
8. Respiratory arrest within a specified time following anesthesia care.
9. Aspiration of gastric contents with development of typical x-ray findings of aspiration pneumonitis within a specified time following anesthesia care.
10. Development of postdural puncture headache within a specified time following anesthesia care.
11. Dental injury during anesthesia care.
12. Ocular injury during anesthesia care.
13. Unplanned hospital admission within a specified time following an outpatient procedure involving anesthesia.
14. Unplanned admission to an intensive care unit within a specified time following administration of an anesthetic.

From Joint Commission on Accreditation of Healthcare Organizations: *Agenda for Change UPDATE* 2(1), June 1988.

*All time ranges will be specified following evaluation and analysis of pilot-site empirical data.

ANESTHESIA CARE INDICATORS SUMMARY LIST

1. Patients developing a CNS complication occurring during or within 2 post-procedure days of procedures involving anesthesia administration, subcategorized by ASA-PS class, patient age, and CNS vs. non-CNS related procedures.
2. Patients developing a peripheral neurologic deficit during or within 2 post-procedure days of procedures involving anesthesia administration.
3. Patients developing an acute myocardial infarction during or within 2 post-procedure days of procedures involving anesthesia administration, subcategorized by ASA-PS class, patient age, and cardiac vs. noncardiac procedures.
4. Patients with a cardiac arrest during or within 1 postprocedure day of procedures involving anesthesia administration, excluding patients with required intraoperative cardiac arrest, subcategorized by ASA-PS class, patient age, and cardiac vs. noncardiac procedures.
5. Patients with unplanned respiratory arrest during or within 1 postprocedure day of procedures involving anesthesia administration.
6. Death of patients during or within 2 postprocedure days of procedures involving anesthesia administration, subcategorized by ASA-PS class and patient age.
7. Unplanned admission of patients to the hospital within 1 postprocedure day following outpatient procedures involving anesthesia administration.
8. Unplanned admission of patients to an intensive care unit within 1 postprocedure day of procedures involving anesthesia administration and with ICU stay greater than 1 day.

Reprinted with permission of Joint Commission on Accreditation of Healthcare Organizations.

goal was to develop an integrated performance measurement system that

- could be used by employees and others (widespread use)
- is composed of elements that both health care plans and purchasers of health care services can effectively utilize to promote better understanding of the services purchased and to improve those provided
- has all performance measures defined and collected in a manner to facilitate comparability among health plans and to define benchmarks for improvement purpose
- considers existing information in order to contain costs and avoid duplication of effort
- continues to evolve with the incorporation of new performance measures and the revision of existing measures
- respects patient confidentiality[1]

The HEDIS measures address a broad spectrum of health services including preventive services, such as childhood immunization, cholesterol screening, mammography, and cervical cancer screening; prenatal care; care for acute and chronic illnesses such as asthma and diabetes; and mental health services. The box on p. 119 lists the major categories of the HEDIS standards for accreditation.

For each quality measure, the PAC has specified two measurement strategies: chart review and administrative data.

In addition to measures of the technical quality of care, there are two other major dimensions: access to services and enrollee satisfaction. The Institute of Medicine, IOM, defines access as a term related to a broad set of concerns that centers on the degree to which individuals and groups are able to obtain needed services from the medical care system.

Satisfaction relates to the ability of the health plan to meet the expectations of its enrollees. Standardization

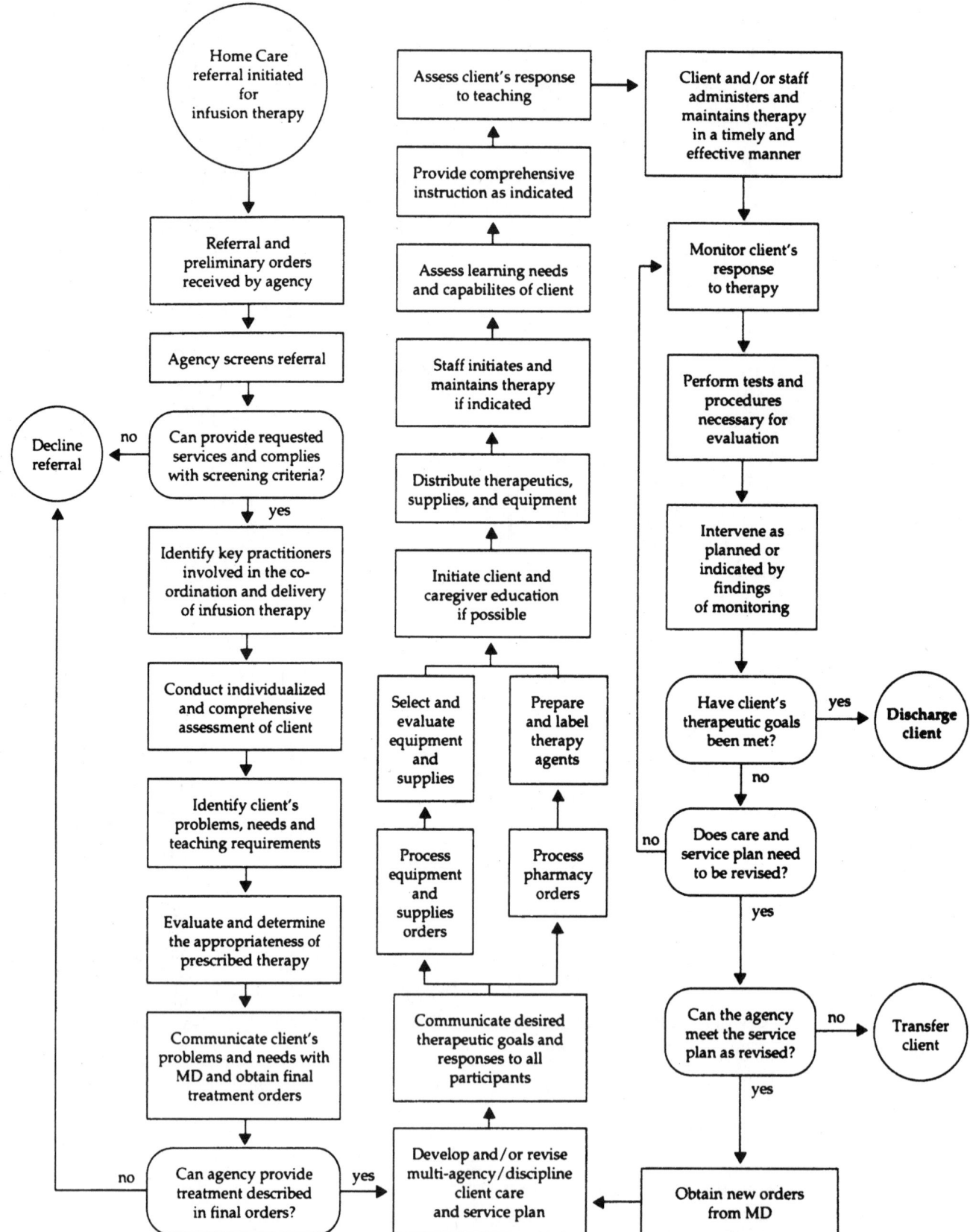

Figure 9-2   Infusion therapy in the home care setting. (Copyright 1991 by the Joint Commission of Accreditation of Healthcare Organizations, Oakbrook Terrace, Ill. Reprinted with permission from the March/April 1991 Joint Commission Perspectives.)

IMSYSTEM INDICATORS FOR 1994

1. **Numerator:** Patients developing a central nervous system (CNS) complication within two postprocedure days of procedures involving anesthesia administration procedures.
2. **Numerator:** Patients developing a peripheral neurological deficit within two postprocedure days of procedures involving anesthesia administration.
3. **Numerator:** Patients developing an acute myocardial infarction (AMI) within two postprocedure days of procedures involving anesthesia administration.
4. **Numerator:** Patients with a cardiac arrest within two postprocedure days of procedures involving anesthesia administration.
5. **Numerator:** Intrahospital mortality of patients within two postprocedure days of procedures involving anesthesia administration.
6. **Numerator:** Patients delivered by cesarean section.
7. **Numerator:** Patients with vaginal birth after cesarean section (VBAC).
8. **Numerator:** Live born infants with a birthweight of less than 2500 grams.
9. **Numerator:** Live born infants with a birthweight greater than or equal to 2500 grams who have at least one of the following: an Apgar score of less than 4 at five minutes, a requirement for admission to the NICU within one day of delivery for greater than 24 hours, a clinically apparent seizure or significant birth trauma.
10. **Numerator:** Live born infants with a birthweight greater than 1000 grams and less than 2500 grams who have an Apgar score of less than 4 at five minutes.

From Joint Commission on Accreditation of Healthcare Organizations: *Joint Commission Perspectives*, Nov/Dec 1993.

of satisfaction data would provide more meaningful comparisons to employers.

Descriptive information regarding membership and utilization is also collected. This provides employers with information on the enrolled population and resource allocation. Financial measurements provide information on premium trends and summary statistics related to revenues, reserves, short-term liquidity, capital structure, and others.

The title of the PAC has recently been changed to the Committee on Performance Measurement. This new committee is charged with updating the HEDIS performance measures. According to the NCQA, the next generation of HEDIS will include an increased number of outcome measures, will emphasize both acute and chronic care, and will address the needs of the poor and elderly enrollees.[5] "The best use of this information by health plans lies in their capitalizing on opportunities for improvement."[1] Currently about 300 HMOs and other health plans use the HEDIS performance measures. In addition, the new set will likely become a standard for the proliferation of managed care companies and a "quality check for HCFA's ambitious moves into managed care."[5]

DEVELOPING PRACTICE AND GOVERNANCE INDICATORS

Along with the clinical indicators, the Joint Commission determined that there must be mechanisms to ensure that the organization is able to facilitate the delivery of quality care. "Since management effectiveness is one of the prerequisites for improving an organization's clinical performance, the Joint Commission set out to identify those principles of organizational and management effectiveness that could be used to guide standards revision as well as indicator development."[7] These principles focus on innovative leadership, system-wide assessment based on feedback from internal and external customers or users of the institution's services, and total organizational commitment to continuous improvement in quality of care.

Organizational indicators are being developed related to the leadership functions and those that address support and operations. They demonstrate the organization's commitment to continual improvement. The box on p. 119 lists the 12 principles upon which indicators may be developed. These indicators will help an institution to analyze objectively how their organization and management affect its performance. These principles emphasize the following points:

- The organization—not its individual units—is accountable for performance.
- Commitment to continual improvement should be pervasive in day-to-day organizational function.
- Effective internal coordination and collaboration among governance, management, practitioners, and other staff members are essential to the support of quality improvement activities.
- The payoff is performance. Structural requirements should largely be an organizational prerogative and should be designed to support organizational performance objectives.
- Performance must be rigorously monitored through the application of effective measures that examine clinical care, management, and vital internal processes.[12]

With the change in emphasis of the IMSystem, it remains to be seen if other organizations will consider practice and governance indicators to be as significant

CARDIOVASCULAR, ONCOLOGY, AND TRAUMA INDICATORS

- **Focus:** Extended postoperative stay as a means of assessing multiple aspects of coronary artery bypass graft (CABG) care.
  *Indicator Statement:** Patients undergoing isolated CABG procedures: number of days from initial surgery to discharge.

- **Focus:** Diagnostic accuracy.
  *Numerator:** Patients with a principal discharge diagnosis of congestive heart failure with documented etiology.

- **Focus:** Extended post-procedure stay as a means of assessing multiple aspects of percutaneous transluminal coronary angioplasty (PTCA) care.
  Indicator Statement: Patients undergoing a PTCA: number of days from procedure to discharge.

- **Focus:** Intrahospital mortality as a means of assessing multiple aspects of CABG patient care.
  Numerator: Intrahospital mortality of patients undergoing an isolated CABG.

- **Focus:** Intrahospital mortality as a means of assessing multiple aspects of PTCA patient care.
  Numerator: Intrahospital mortality of patients undergoing a PTCA.

- **Focus:** Intrahospital mortality as a means of assessing multiple aspects of acute myocardial infarction (AMI) patient care.
  Numerator: Intrahospital mortality of patients with a principal discharge diagnosis of AMI.

- **Focus:** Availability of data for diagnosis and staging.
  Numerator: Patients undergoing resection for primary cancer of the female breast, lung or colon/rectum for whom a surgical pathology consultation report is present in the medical record.

- **Focus:** Use of staging by managing physicians.
  Numerator: Patients undergoing resection for primary cancer of the female breast, lung or colon/rectum with stage of tumor designated by a managing physician.

- **Focus:** Use of tests critical for any of the following: diagnosis, prognosis, and clinical management.
  Numerator: Female patients with Stage I or greater primary breast cancer who, after initial biopsy or resection, have estrogen receptor analysis results in the medical record.

- **Focus:** Effectiveness of preoperative diagnosis and staging.
  Numerator: Patients with non-small cell primary lung cancer undergoing thoracotomy with complete surgical resection of tumor.

- **Focus:** Comprehensiveness of diagnostic workup.
  Numerator: Patients with resection for primary cancer of the colon/rectum whose preoperative evaluation, by a managing physician, included examination of the entire colon.

- **Focus:** Ongoing monitoring of trauma patients.
  Numerator: Trauma patients with systolic blood pressure, pulse rate, and respiratory rate documented on arrival to the emergency department (ED) and at least hourly for three hours or until ED disposition, whichever is earlier.

- **Focus:** Ongoing monitoring of trauma patients.
  Numerator: Trauma patients with selected intracranial injuries with Glasgow coma scale (GCS) score documented on arrival to ED and at least hourly for three hours or until ED disposition, whichever is earlier.

- **Focus:** Airway management of comatose trauma patients.
  Numerator: Comatose trauma patients with selected intracranial injuries discharged from the ED prior to endotracheal intubation or cricothyrotomy.

- **Focus:** Timeliness of diagnostic testing.
  Indicator Statement: Trauma patients with head computerized tomography (CT) scan performed: time from ED arrival to initial CT scan.

- **Focus:** Timeliness of surgical intervention for selected head injuries.
  Indicator Statement: Trauma patients undergoing selected neurosurgical procedures: time from ED arrival to procedure.

- **Focus:** Timeliness of surgical intervention for selected orthopedic injuries.
  Indicator Statement: Trauma patients undergoing selected orthopedic procedures: time from ED arrival to procedure.

From Joint Commission on Accreditation of Healthcare Organizations: *Joint Commission Perspectives,* 14(2) March/April, 1994.

Continued.

CARDIOVASCULAR, ONCOLOGY, AND TRAUMA INDICATORS—cont'd

- **Focus:** Timeliness of surgical intervention for selected abdominal injuries.
  Indicator Statement: Trauma patients undergoing selected abdominal surgical procedures: time from ED arrival to procedure.

- **Focus:** Clinical decision making for potentially preventable deaths.
  Numerator: Intrahospital mortality of trauma patients with a diagnosis of pneumothorax or hemothorax who did not undergo a thoracostomy or thoracotomy.

- **Focus:** Clinical decision making for potentially preventable deaths.
  Numerator: Intrahospital mortality of trauma patients with a systolic blood pressure of less than 70 mmHg within two hours of emergency department arrival who did not undergo a laparotomy or thoracotomy.

*An Indicator Statement is used when the measure is a continuous variable. A Numerator is used when the measure is rate-based.

MAJOR CATEGORIES OF HEDIS STANDARDS FOR ACCREDITATION

- HEDIS standards for accreditation
- Quality management and improvement
- Utilization management
- Credentialing
- Members' rights and responsibilities
- Preventive health services
- Medical records

PRINCIPLES OF ORGANIZATIONAL AND MANAGEMENT EFFECTIVENESS

- Mission
- Culture
- Strategic, program, and research plans
- Organizational change
- Role of governing body and management and clinical leadership
- Leadership qualifications, development, and assessment
- Resources
- Clinical competence of independent practitioners
- Recruitment, development, evaluation, and retention policies and practices
- Evaluation and improvement of patient care
- Organizational integration and coordination
- Continuity and comprehensiveness of care

From Joint Commission on Accreditation of Healthcare Organizations, *Agenda for Change UPDATE* 2(1), June 1988.

as the Joint Commission. HEDIS 2.0 does focus on fiscal indicators. To date most performance measures have been clinically focused.

Service delivery staff members are committed to measuring service indicators, whereas managers are drawn to organizational indicators. One example of this is at St. Joseph Medical Center in Wichita; the departments are measuring indicators in three areas in addition to clinical or service: fiscal, human resources, and image. Fiscal indicators measure department income or expenses. These are governance indicators. Examples of fiscal indicators include lost central supply charges, length of stay, late charges, IV charges, and overtime reduction. Human resource indicators include staff competency, turnover, staff satisfaction, staff coping skills, and skills for stress management. Human resource indicators focus on personnel competency and productivity. These are practice indicators. Image indicators measure customer perceptions and include customer satisfaction and complaints.[14]

LINKING STANDARDS AND INDICATORS

We believe that the generic indicators developed nationally serve as umbrella indicators. Each disci-

pline will then be responsible for evaluating its contribution to the structure, process or outcome and designating subindicators for internal performance measurement. For example, one obstetrical indicator is primary cesarean section for failure to progress in labor. Although nursing does not make the ultimate decision regarding the necessity of the cesarean section, nursing does participate significantly in the ultimate outcome because of the nursing interventions aimed at facilitating progress in labor. Nursing may identify specific patient outcomes related to labor progress, such as:

- Three contractions within a 10-minute period. For the internally monitored patient: contractions over 55 mm of pressure and 5 to 15 mm resting tone

- For the externally monitored patient: firm contractions lasting 45 to 60 seconds
- Absence of complications/emergencies

Then practice guidelines would be developed to outline the structure and processes standards necessary to achieve those outcomes. Staff members would then select structure, process or outcome indicators from the standards written for that particular patient situation.

Externally developed performance measures is one approach to standards-based performance measurement. However, a standards-based performance measurement system can be derived from purely an internal focus or need. Although no national performance database exists for impaired mobility, it is a critical factor for a rehabilitation facility.

Physical therapy plays a significant role in this area. However, it is not sufficient merely to record the numbers of patients that develop impaired mobility. As we have seen in the past, volume indicators alone do not provide enough information to pinpoint problems or improve care. That general indicator must be translated into specific standards related to impaired mobility. These might include practice guidelines for the management of impaired mobility and procedures for range of motion exercises or mobility equipment. Appendix 9-1 is an example of a practice guideline for the management of impaired mobility.

In reality an organization's performance measurement system should be standards-based and reflect a blend of externally and internally developed performance measures. Regardless of how the indicators are generated, there are some key points to consider when developing indicators.

DEVELOPING GOOD INDICATORS

Well-developed written standards are the key to good indicators. If standards are reliable, valid, measurable, specific, and relevant, then indicators will be also. For instance, well-developed practice guidelines for the management of failure to progress in labor will define the desired outcomes and the nursing process necessary to achieve those results. Structure, outcome or process indicators can be chosen from the information provided in that standard. The stated outcomes can be translated directly into service, practice, or governance performance indicators.

For example, using the practice guideline for the management of impaired mobility, any one or all of the following clinical outcomes could be measured.

$$\frac{\text{The number of patients who perform mobility tasks requiring assistance no more than 25\% of the time}}{\text{The total number of patients with stage 1 or greater impaired mobility}}$$

$$\frac{\text{The number of patients who demonstrate the use of assistive devices according to procedure}}{\text{The total number of patients with stage 1 or greater impaired mobility}}$$

$$\frac{\text{The number of patients with stage 4 impaired mobility who maintain range of motion}}{\text{The total number of patients with stage 4 impaired mobility}}$$

Professional and administrative indicators are developed in much the same way as the clinical ones. An example of a practice outcome related to this guideline might include this equation:

$$\frac{\text{The number of staff members able to identify stage 4 impaired mobility}}{\text{The total number of staff members}}$$

An example of a governance outcome related to this guideline might include this equation:

$$\frac{\text{The number of times a physical/occupational therapy consultation occurs within 24 hours of written referral on a patient with stage 4 impaired mobility}}{\text{The total number of patients with stage 4 impaired mobility}}$$

In designing indicators for a given process of service, practice, or governance, it is important to determine the true or potential problems that impede the pursuit of improvement. These are the issues requiring the greatest attention in measurement. Focusing on these issues will ensure that the measurement activities are relevant.

Developing indicators can be an overwhelming task. Where does one start? How does one decide what is an indicator? To assist in the design of indicators and to ensure that they are linked to written standards, we designed the indicator development form (see Figure 10-5). Based on the Joint Commission prototype Clinical Indicator Development Form, this form facilitates indicator development.

Determining an indicator and setting its performance targets are parts of the same process. This chapter focuses on indicator development. Setting performance targets is the focus of Chapter 10. Since the indicator development form includes both of these processes, it is described in detail at the end of that chapter.

Indicators provide order within our lives. They keep us on track and provide clues that prod us to act both positively and negatively. Indicators in health care serve the same function. They are the "red flags" that indicate when performance falls below a predetermined acceptable level.

Good indicators are derived from well written standards. Without well written standards, it is impossible to design relevant indicators.

REFERENCES

1. Corrigan JM, Nielsen DM: Toward the development of uniform reporting standards for managed care organizations: the health plan employer data and information set (version 2.0), *Jt Comm J Qual Improv* 19(12):566-575, 1993.

2. Joint Commission on Accreditation of Healthcare Organizations: Characteristics of clinical indicators, *Qual Rev Bulletin* 15(11):330-339, 1989.

3. Lansky D: The new responsibility: measuring and reporting on quality, *Jt Comm J Qual Improv* 19(12):545-551, 1993.

4. *The measurement mandate*, Oakbrook Terrace, Ill, 1993, The Joint Commission on Accreditation of Healthcare Organizations.

5. NCQA assembles panel to refine HEDIS measures, *Modern Health Care*, p 60, Dec 18-25, 1995.

6. O'Leary D: President's column, *Joint Commission Perspectives*, pp 2-3, July/Aug 1989.

7. O'Leary D: President's column, *Joint Commission Perspectives*, 10(1):6-7, 1990.

8. O'Leary D: President's column, *Joint Commission Perspectives*, 10(6):1, 1990.

9. O'Leary D: President's column, *Joint Commission Perspectives*, 13(6):1, 1993.

10. O'Leary D: President's column, *Joint Commission Perspectives*, 15(2):1, 1995.

11. O'Leary D: President's column, *Joint Commission Perspectives*, 15(3):2, 1995.

12. O'Leary D: President's column, *Joint Commission Perspectives*, pp 2-3, Jan/Feb 1994.

13. Olivas G et al: Case management: a bottom line care delivery model, *J Nurs Admin* 19(11):16-20, 1989.

14. Swindle DN, Wetta-Hall R: Beyond clinical indicators, *Quality Connection* 3(1):6-7, 1993.

15. Treece E, Treece J: *Elements of research in nursing*, ed 3, St. Louis, 1982, Mosby.

Appendix 9-1   Practice Guideline for Management of Impaired Mobility

Severity Index

STAGE 0: At risk

1. Independence with bed mobility, all transfers, ambulation on all surfaces, and stairs
2. Activities performed with or without assistive device or modifications

STAGE 1: Minimal

1. Performance of mobility tasks requiring hands-on assistance for up to 25% of the task(s):
   - bed mobility: occasional contact assistance required to position extremities or facilitate weight shift when moving from the supine to the sitting position; intermittent contact may be required to assist an involved extremity
   - transfers: occasional assistance required for anterior weight shift and/or pelvic guidance; assistance required for sliding board placement
   - wheelchair: occasional assistance required for management of legrests; assistance required for propulsion over uneven surfaces
   - ambulation: occasional hands-on assistance required to maintain balance and stability
   - stairs: occasional assistance required for facilitation of weight shift or control of lower extremity/foot placement
2. Possible requirement of assistive device(s)

STAGE 2: Moderate

1. Performance of mobility tasks requiring hands-on assistance for 25% to 75% of the task(s):
   - bed mobility: frequent manual contact with two extremities and trunk assistance required
   - transfers: frequent manual contact required for facilitation and maintenance of anterior weight shift and pelvic guidance; lower extremity stabilization may be required
   - wheelchair: frequent assistance required for management of legrests; assistance required for maneuvering through doorways, over uneven surfaces, and for distances greater than 150 feet over level surfaces
   - ambulation: manual contact required to ensure proper sequencing for gait; proper weight shift and frequent manual facilitation required at pelvis and lower extremities
   - stairs: frequent assistance required for facilitation of weight shift and stabilization through lower extremities with assistance to advance to the next step
2. Possible requirement of assistive device(s)

STAGE 3: Maximal

1. Performance of mobility tasks requiring hands-on assistance for greater than 75% of the task(s):
   - bed mobility: patient able to initiate or partially assist with task but requires constant manual contact to maintain position and complete task
   - transfers: constant manual contact required to facilitate and maintain weight shift and control of lower extremities; constant manual contact required for completion of task; manual contact required for sliding board transfers for trunk stability and pelvic guidance as well as board placement
   - wheelchair: constant cuing/physical assistance required to propel 50 feet; total assistance required for parts management; dependent for propulsion over uneven surfaces
   - ambulation: constant physical assistance required to maintain erect trunk position; stability for ambulation up to 50 feet
   - stairs: unable to negotiate
2. Requirement of assistive device(s)
3. Inability to attain/maintain upright posture with less than 75% assistance

---

STAGE 4: Dependent

1. Performance of mobility tasks requiring total assistance:
   - bed mobility: patient unable to perform or assist with bed mobility tasks
   - transfers: total lift or Hoyer lift required to transfer patient
   - wheelchair: patient unable to propel wheelchair
   - ambulation/stairs: patient nonambulatory
2. Requirement of assistive device(s)
3. Inability to attain/maintain upright posture with less than total assistance or external support

INDICATIONS

1. Amputation
2. Burns
3. Demyelinating disease
4. Cerebrovascular accident
5. Spinal cord injury
6. Head injury
7. Cardiopulmonary complications
8. Orthopedic injury
9. Arthritis
10. Surgical intervention
11. Elderly patient
12. Prolonged bed rest
13. Sensory impairment
14. Cognitive impairment

DEFINITION OF TERMS

1. Ambulation: the ability to walk about
2. Assistive device: a tool used to facilitate safe achievement of a task (e.g., overhead trapeze, bed rails, Hoyer lift, sliding board, wheelchair, reacher, walker, cane, crutches, stair rail, orthosis, and prosthesis)
3. Bed mobility: the ability to change position in bed by rolling side to side, bridging, or moving up in bed; the ability to make the transition from the supine to the sitting position and back
4. Independent: not requiring or relying on somebody else
5. Mobility: the ability of persons to move about effectively in their surroundings (modes of mobility include bed mobility, wheelchair mobility, transfers, and ambulation)
6. Procedure: a series of steps followed in a regular order
7. Sequelae: pathological consequences of immobility
8. Transfers: the ability to move from one surface to another (e.g., sit to stand; movement in and out of bed, chair, commode, tub/shower, or car/van)
9. Wheelchair mobility: the ability to maneuver a wheelchair safely on level surfaces, through doorways, and up and down ramps

AUTHORS

Jacqueline Katz, MS, RN
Eleanor Green, BSN, RN
Anne-Marie J. Caron, PT
Nancy M. Koenig, MS, PT

References

Eisenberg MG, Grzesiak RC, editors: *Advances in clinical rehabilitation,* vol 1, New York, 1987, Springer-Verlag New York Inc.

Granger CV, Gresham GE, editors: *Functional assessment in rehabilitation medicine,* Baltimore, 1984, Williams & Wilkins.

Haley SM et al: *Pediatric evaluation of disability inventory: development, standardization & administration manual,* Boston, 1992, PEDI Research Group, New England Medical Center Hospitals.

Lewis CB: *Improving mobility in older persons: a manual for geriatric specialists,* Rockville MD, 1989, Aspen Publishers Inc.

APPROVAL BY

DATE

REVIEW DATE

REVISE DATE

DISTRIBUTION

Impaired Mobility

STAGE 0: At risk

1. Independence with bed mobility, all transfers, ambulation on all surfaces, and stairs
2. Activities performed with or without assistive device or modifications

COMPETENCIES:

In order to manage patients in this stage the individual must be able to:
1. Identify patients at risk for impaired mobility
2. Perform processes outlined in this stage
3. Identify complications associated with this stage
4. Achieve outcomes outlined in this stage
5. Identify factors that produce impaired mobility

Credentialing: None

ASSESSMENT:

1. Obtain history of mobility:
   - living environment (e.g., stairs, railings, bed and bath accessibility, and ramps)
   - assistive devices
   - activities of daily living (ADL)
2. Assess bed mobility per routine
3. Assess transfers per routine
4. Assess ambulation/wheelchair mobility on all surfaces per routine
5. Assess for potential risk factors that cause impaired mobility
6. Collect information regarding patient's/significant others' knowledge concerning impaired mobility
7. Monitor therapeutic effects of prescribed medications
8. Identify risk factors that may affect patient's mobility
9. Assess patient's compliance

DIAGNOSIS:

1. Stage patient's level of impaired mobility
2. Determine patient's ability to communicate mobility limitations
3. Determine patient's and/or significant others':
   - involvement in care
   - communication and support needs
   - knowledge base and readiness to learn
4. Determine level of compliance and desire to be physically and independently mobile

OUTCOMES IDENTIFICATION:

Patient

1. Maintains independent mobility level

Staff

1. Identifies and stages patients at risk for impaired mobility
2. Utilizes processes outlined in this stage
3. Identifies signs and symptoms of worsening condition and restages patient status
4. Maintains communication regarding the patient's clinical condition and treatment plan with all involved persons

System

1. A qualified staff member is available to care for this patient
2. An environment conducive to independent mobility is maintained

3. Equipment necessary to implement stage 0 processes is available as needed:
   - teaching materials
   - assistive devices

PLANNING:

In-House

1. Develop a daily mobility–activities plan
2. Modify the interventions outlined in this stage as indicated by patient condition or physician order
3. Modify the patient education outlined in this stage based on patient's readiness to learn
4. Modify the outcomes outlined in this stage based on assessment data

Discharge

1. Design an at-home daily mobility–activities plan
2. Develop an at-home plan for use of assistive devices

EDUCATION:

1. Reinforce care of assistive devices according to procedure
2. Provide patient with all the information necessary to make informed health care decisions
3. Teach patient importance of physical mobility
4. Discuss daily mobility–activities plan

INTERVENTIONS:

1. Encourage patient to be out of bed as much as possible if condition permits
2. Implement daily mobility–activities plan
3. Provide portable devices to allow for patient independence (e.g., IV poles, leg bags, and portable oxygen tanks)
4. Discourage use of devices/procedures that contribute to immobility:
   - wheelchairs
   - tight covers on bed
5. Initiate indicated stage of noncompliance practice guideline

Complications

1. Mobility impairment:
   - implement indicated stage of this practice guideline

EVALUATION:

1. Analyze patient's progress toward outcomes
2. Analyze patient's response to interventions, treatments, and medications
3. Evaluate effectiveness of teaching
4. Analyze patient's understanding and cooperation with the plan of care
5. Evaluate effectiveness of the daily mobility–activities plan

COMMUNICATION:

Verbal

1. Report:
   - any signs of impaired mobility

Written

1. Record initiation and specific stage of the practice guideline on the Careprint
2. Note any modifications to the stage on the Careprint and rationale for each modification as it occurs
3. Chart all baseline data, ongoing monitoring data, interventions taken, and the patient's response on the patient care flowsheet
4. Record evaluation of patient outcomes on the progress record
5. Record all patient teaching

Impaired Mobility

STAGE 1: Minimal

1. Performance of mobility tasks requiring hands-on assistance for up to 25% of the task(s):
   - bed mobility: occasional contact assistance required to position extremities or facilitate weight shift when moving from the supine to the sitting position; intermittent contact may be required to assist an involved extremity
   - transfers: occasional assistance required for anterior weight shift and/or pelvic guidance; assistance required for sliding board placement
   - wheelchair: occasional assistance required for management of legrests; assistance required for propulsion over uneven surfaces
   - ambulation: occasional hands-on assistance required to maintain balance and stability
   - stairs: occasional assistance required for facilitation of weight shift or control of lower extremity/foot placement
2. Requirement of assistive device(s)

COMPETENCIES:

In order to manage patients in this stage the individual must be able to:
1. Identify signs and symptoms of stage 1 impaired mobility
2. Perform mobility techniques according to procedure
3. Use terms the patient understands
4. Perform all procedures associated with assistive devices
5. Perform processes outlined in this stage
6. Identify complications associated with this stage
7. Achieve outcomes outlined in this stage
8. Identify factors that contribute to impaired mobility
9. Identify resources for referral

Credentialing:

Physical Assessment
Body Mechanics

ASSESSMENT:

1. Obtain history of mobility:
   - living environment (e.g., stairs, elevator, railings, bed and bath accessibility, and ramps)
   - assistive devices
   - ADL
2. Ascertain patient's knowledge of assistive device(s) used
3. Assess level/degree of mobility
4. Collect information regarding patient's/significant others' knowledge about impaired mobility and necessary assistive devices
5. Assess for signs and symptoms of potential problems caused by impaired mobility:
   - pressure sores
   - increased risk of falls
   - contractures
   - secondary cardiopulmonary complications
   - circulatory compromise
   - prolonged healing time
6. Monitor therapeutic effects of prescribed medications
7. Identify additional risk factors:
   - prolonged bed rest
   - sensory impairment
   - strength limitation
   - range-of-motion limitation
   - decreased endurance
   - pain
8. Assess level of compliance to increased mobility regimen
9. Assess for anxiety

10. Assess for pain during mobility activities
11. Assess for activity intolerance
12. Assess skin integrity
13. Assess risk for falls

DIAGNOSIS:

1. Stage patient's level of impaired mobility
2. Determine patient's ability to communicate mobility limitations
3. Determine patient's and significant others':
   - involvement in care
   - communication and support needs
   - knowledge base and readiness to learn
4. Determine falls risk
5. Determine level of activity intolerance
6. Determine level of pain (acute or chronic)
7. Determine level of altered skin integrity
8. Determine level of anxiety
9. Determine level of noncompliance

OUTCOMES IDENTIFICATION:

Patient

1. Performs mobility tasks, requiring assistance no more than 25% of the time
2. Demonstrates use of assistive devices according to procedure

Staff

1. Identifies patients with stage 1 impaired mobility
2. Utilizes processes outlined in this stage
3. Identifies signs and symptoms of worsening or improving condition and restages patient status
4. Maintains communication regarding the patient's clinical condition and treatment plan with all involved persons

System

1. A qualified staff member is available to care for this patient
2. Physical/occupational therapy consultation occurs within 24 hours of written referral
3. An environment conducive to patient's level of mobility is maintained
4. Equipment necessary to implement stage 1 processes is available as needed:
   - teaching material
   - assistive devices

PLANNING:

In-House

1. Obtain a physical/occupational therapy consultation
2. Design a daily mobility–activities plan to be performed in conjunction with the therapy staff
3. Develop a risk factor–modification plan
4. Modify the interventions outlined in this stage as indicated by patient condition or physician order
5. Modify the patient/caregiver education outlined in this stage based on patient's/caregiver's readiness to learn
6. Modify the outcomes outlined in this stage based on assessment data

Discharge

1. Develop at-home plan for use of assistive devices
2. Design at-home daily mobility–activities plan
3. Refer to community/outpatient services as indicated

EDUCATION:

1. Reinforce care of assistive devices according to procedure
2. Review modified mobility level as designated by physician
3. Provide patient with all the information necessary to make informed health care decisions
4. Teach patient the importance of physical mobility
5. Discuss daily mobility–activities plan
6. Discuss risk factor–modification plan

INTERVENTIONS:

1. Ensure patient accessibility to communicate need for assistance (e.g., call light, bell, intercom, and routine visits)
2. Encourage patient to be out of bed as much as possible if condition permits
3. Implement daily mobility–activities plan in conjunction with therapy staff
4. Provide portable devices to allow for patient mobility (e.g., IV poles, leg bags, and portable oxygen tanks)
5. Discourage use of devices/procedures that contribute to immobility:
   - wheelchairs
   - tight covers on bed
   - restrictive garments
6. Initiate indicated stage of falls prevention practice guideline
7. Initiate indicated stage of activity intolerance practice guideline
8. Initiate indicated stage of acute or chronic pain practice guideline
9. Initiate indicated stage of altered skin integrity practice guideline
10. Initiate indicated stage of anxiety practice guideline
11. Initiate indicated stage of noncompliance practice guideline
12. Implement risk factor–modification plan

Complications

1. Moderate mobility impairment:
   - implement stage 2 of this practice guideline

EVALUATION:

1. Compare patient's mobility status to baseline
2. Analyze patient's progress towards outcomes
3. Analyze patient's response to interventions, treatments, and medications
4. Evaluate effectiveness of teaching
5. Analyze patient's understanding and cooperation with the plan of care
6. Evaluate effectiveness of the daily mobility–activities plan
7. Evaluate effectiveness of the risk factor–modification plan

COMMUNICATION:

Verbal

1. Report:
   - any changes in mobility status
   - all noncompliance with treatment regimen

Written

1. Record initiation and specific stage of the practice guideline on the Careprint
2. Note an modifications to the stage on the Careprint and rationale for each modification as it occurs
3. Chart all baseline data, ongoing monitoring data, interventions taken, and patient's responses on the patient care flowsheet
4. Record evaluation of patient outcomes on the progress record
5. Record all patient/caregiver teaching

Impaired Mobility

STAGE 2: Moderate

1. Performance of mobility tasks requiring hands-on assistance for 25% to 75% of the task(s):
   - bed mobility: frequent manual contact with two extremities and trunk assistance required
   - transfers: frequent manual contact required for facilitation and maintenance of anterior weight shift and pelvic guidance; lower extremity stabilization may be required
   - wheelchair: frequent assistance required for management of legrests; assistance required for maneuvering through doorways, over uneven surfaces, and for distances greater than 150 feet over level surfaces
   - ambulation: frequent manual contact required to ensure proper sequencing for gait; proper weight shift and frequent manual facilitation required at pelvis and lower extremities
   - stairs: frequent assistance required for facilitation of weight shift and stabilization through lower extremities with assistance to advance to the next step
2. Possible requirement of assistive device(s)

COMPETENCIES:

In order to manage patients in this stage the individual must be able to:
1. Identify signs and symptoms of stage 2 impaired mobility
2. Perform mobility techniques according to procedure
3. Use terms the patient understands
4. Perform all procedures associated with assistive devices
5. Identify complications associated with this stage
6. Perform processes outlined in this stage
7. Achieve outcomes outlined in this stage
8. Identify factors that contribute to impaired mobility
9. Identify resources for referral

Credentialing:

Physical Assessment
Body Mechanics

ASSESSMENT:

1. Obtain history of mobility:
   - living environment (e.g., stairs, elevators, railings, bed and bath accessibility, and ramps)
   - assistive devices
   - ADL
2. Ascertain patient's knowledge of assistive device(s) used
3. Assess vital signs prior to assisting patient into upright position
4. Obtain baseline gross motor strength/range-of-motion
5. Assess level/degree of mobility
6. Collect information regarding caregiver's ability to assist with mobility tasks
7. Collect information regarding patient's/significant other's knowledge about impaired mobility
8. Assess for signs and symptoms of potential problems caused by impaired mobility:
   - pressure sores
   - increased risk of falls
   - increased risk of contracture
   - secondary cardiopulmonary complications
   - circulatory compromise
   - prolonged healing time
9. Monitor therapeutic effects of prescribed medications
10. Identify additional risk factors:
    - sensory impairment
    - decreased strength
    - decreased range-of-motion
    - decreased endurance

- decreased balance
- pain
- cognitive changes
11. Assess level of compliance to increased mobility regimen
12. Assess for anxiety
13. Assess for pain during mobility activities
14. Assess for activity intolerance
15. Assess skin integrity
16. Assess risk for falls

DIAGNOSIS:

1. Stage patient's level of impaired mobility
2. Determine patient's ability to communicate mobility limitations
3. Determine patient's and significant others':
   - involvement in care
   - communication and support needs
   - knowledge and readiness to learn
4. Determine falls risk
5. Determine level of activity tolerance
6. Determine level of pain (acute or chronic)
7. Determine level of altered skin integrity
8. Determine level anxiety
9. Determine level of noncompliance
10. Determine level of competence of caregivers to use assistive devices/techniques with patient

OUTCOMES IDENTIFICATION:

Patient

1. Performs mobility tasks with 25% to 75% assistance
2. Demonstrates use of assistive device(s) according to procedure

Staff

1. Identifies patients with stage 2 impaired mobility
2. Utilizes processes outlined in this stage
3. Identifies signs and symptoms of worsening or improving condition and restages patient status
4. Maintains communication regarding the patient's clinical condition and treatment plan with all involved persons

System

1. A qualified staff member is available to care for this patient
2. Physical/occupational therapy consultation occurs within 24 hours of written referral
3. An environment conducive to patient's mobility level is maintained
4. Equipment necessary to implement stage 2 processes is available as needed:
   - teaching material
   - assistive devices

PLANNING:

In-House

1. Obtain a physical/occupational therapy consultation
2. Design a daily mobility–activities plan to be performed in conjunction with therapy staff
3. Assist the patient to set realistic compliance goals
4. Develop a risk factor modification plan
5. Modify the interventions outlined in this stage as indicated by patient condition or physician order
6. Modify the patient/caregiver education outlined in this stage based on patient's/caregiver's readiness to learn
7. Modify the outcomes outlined in this stage based on assessment data

Discharge

1. Develop at-home plan for use of assistive devices
2. Design at-home daily mobility–activities plan
3. Refer to community/outpatient services as indicated

EDUCATION:

1. Reinforce care of assistive devices according to procedure
2. Review modified mobility level as designated by physician
3. Educate patient/caregiver on monitoring skin integrity, turning schedule, range-of-motion, and use of assistive devices
4. Provide patient with all the information necessary to make informed health care decisions
5. Teach patient the importance of physical mobility

INTERVENTIONS:

1. Ensure patient accessibility to communicate need for assistance (e.g., call light, bell, intercom, and routine visits)
2. Encourage patient to be out of bed as much as possible if condition permits
3. Implement a daily mobility–activities plan in conjunction with therapy staff
4. Perform range-of-motion activities throughout daily care within medical limits
5. Provide wheelchair appropriate to patient need with emphasis on therapeutic positioning
6. Provide portable devices to facilitate patient mobility (e.g., IV poles, leg bags, and portable oxygen tanks)
7. Initiate indicated stage of falls prevention practice guideline
8. Initiate indicated stage of activity intolerance practice guideline
9. Initiate indicated stage of acute or chronic pain practice guideline
10. Initiate indicated stage of altered skin integrity practice guideline
11. Initiate indicated stage of anxiety practice guideline
12. Initiate indicated stage of noncompliance practice guideline
13. Implement risk factor–modification plan

Complications

1. Maximal mobility impairment:
   - implement stage 3 of this practice guideline

EVALUATION:

1. Compare patient's mobility status to baseline
2. Analyze patient's progress toward outcomes
3. Analyze patient's response to interventions, treatments, and medications
4. Evaluate effectiveness of teaching
5. Analyze patient's understanding and cooperation with the plan of care
6. Evaluate effectiveness of daily mobility–activities plan
7. Evaluate effectiveness of risk factor–modification plan

COMMUNICATION:

Verbal

1. Report:
   - any additional changes in mobility status

Written

1. Record initiation and specific stage of practice guideline on the Careprint
2. Note any modifications to the stage on the Careprint and rationale for each modification as it occurs
3. Chart all baseline data, ongoing monitoring data, interventions taken, and patient's responses on the patient care flowsheet
4. Record evaluation of patient outcomes on the progress record
5. Record all patient/caregiver teaching

Impaired Mobility

STAGE 3: Maximal

1. Performance of mobility tasks requiring hands-on assistance for greater than 75% of the task(s):
   - bed mobility: patient able to initiate or partially assist with task but requires constant manual contact to maintain position and complete task
   - transfers: constant manual contact required to facilitate and maintain weight shift and control of lower extremities; constant manual contact required for completion of task; manual contact required for sliding board transfers for trunk stability and pelvic guidance as well as board placement
   - wheelchair: constant cuing/physical assistance required to propel 50 feet; total assistance required for parts management; dependent for propulsion over uneven surfaces
   - ambulation: constant physical assistance required to maintain erect trunk position, stability for ambulation up to 50 feet
   - stairs: unable to negotiate
2. Requirement of assistive device(s)
3. Inability to attain/maintain upright postures with less than 75% assistance

COMPETENCIES:

In order to manage patients in this stage the individual must be able to:
1. Identify signs and symptoms of stage 3 impaired mobility
2. Perform mobility techniques according to procedure
3. Use terms the patient understands
4. Perform all procedures associated with assistive devices
5. Perform processes outlined in this stage
6. Identify complications associated with this stage
7. Achieve outcomes outlined in this stage
8. Identify factors that contribute to impaired mobility
9. Perform range-of-motion activities according to procedure
10. Identify resources for referral
11. Calculate intake and output
12. Take vital signs and interpret the results

Credentialing:

Physical Assessment
Body Mechanics
Range-of-Motion
   Techniques

ASSESSMENT:

1. Obtain history of mobility:
   - living environment (e.g., stairs, elevators, railings, bed and bath accessibility, and ramps)
   - assistive devices
   - ADL
2. Ascertain patient's/caregiver's knowledge of assistive device(s) used
3. Assess vital signs prior to assisting patient into upright position
4. Obtain baseline gross motor strength/range-of-motion
5. Assess level/degree of mobility
6. Collect information regarding caregiver's ability to assist with mobility task
7. Collect information regarding patient's/significant others' knowledge about impaired mobility
8. Assess for signs and symptoms of potential problems caused by impaired mobility:
   - pressure sores
   - increased risk of falls
   - increased risk of contracture
   - secondary cardiopulmonary complications

- circulatory compromise
- prolonged healing time

9. Monitor therapeutic effects of prescribed medications
10. Identify additional risk factors:
    - sensory impairment
    - decreased strength
    - decreased range-of-motion
    - decreased endurance
    - decreased balance
    - pain
    - cognitive changes
11. Assess level of compliance to increased mobility regimen
12. Assess for anxiety
13. Assess for pain during mobility activities
14. Assess for activity intolerance
15. Assess skin integrity
16. Assess risk for falls
17. Assess lung sounds each shift for:
    - adventitious sounds (crackles, wheezes)
18. Obtain baseline weight and weigh the same time each day using the same scales and the same clothing
19. Assess nutritional status every 24 hours
20. Obtain bowel history regarding normal bowel routine
21. Assess ADL needs

DIAGNOSIS:

1. Stage patient's level of impaired mobility
2. Determine patient's ability to communicate mobility limitations
3. Determine patient's and significant other's:
    - involvement in care
    - communication and support needs
    - knowledge and readiness to learn
4. Determine falls risk
5. Determine level of activity intolerance
6. Determine level of pain (acute or chronic)
7. Determine level of altered skin integrity
8. Determine level of anxiety
9. Determine level of noncompliance
10. Determine level of constipation
11. Determine altered nutritional status: more or less than body requirements
12. Determine level of fluid volume excess or deficit
13. Determine level of impaired gas exchange
14. Determine level of competence of caregivers to use assistive devices/techniques with patient
15. Determine level of self-care deficit
16. Determine bowel and bladder routine

OUTCOMES IDENTIFICATION:

Patient

1. Performs mobility tasks with 25% to 75% hands-on assistance
2. Demonstrates use of assistive device(s) according to procedure

Staff

1. Identifies patients with stage 3 impaired mobility
2. Utilizes processes outlined in this stage
3. Identifies signs and symptoms of worsening or improving condition and restages patient status
4. Maintains communication regarding the patient's clinical condition and treatment plan with all involved persons

System

1. A qualified staff member is available to care for this patient
2. Physical/occupational therapy consultation occurs within 24 hours of written referral
3. Dietary consultation occurs within 24 hours of written referral
4. An environment conducive to patient's mobility level is maintained
5. Equipment necessary to implement stage 3 processes is available as needed:
   - teaching materials
   - assistive devices
   - bed scales
   - stethoscope

PLANNING:

In-House

1. Obtain a physical/occupational therapy consultation
2. Obtain a dietary consultation
3. Design a daily mobility–activities plan to be performed in conjunction with therapy staff
4. Assist the patient to set realistic goals
5. Develop a risk factor–modification plan
6. Modify the interventions outlined in this stage as indicated by patient condition or physician order
7. Modify the patient/caregiver education outlined in this stage based on patient's/caregiver's readiness to learn
8. Modify the outcomes outlined in this stage based on assessment data

Discharge

1. Develop at-home plan for use of assistive devices
2. Design at-home daily mobility–activities plan
3. Refer to community/outpatient services as indicated

EDUCATION:

1. Reinforce care of assistive devices according to procedure
2. Review modified mobility level as designated by physician
3. Educate patient/caregiver on monitoring skin integrity, turning schedule, range-of-motion, and use of assistive devices
4. Educate patient/caregiver regarding signs and symptoms of intolerance to mobility activities
5. Provide patient with all the information necessary to make informed health care decisions
6. Teach patient the importance of physical mobility
7. Discuss daily mobility–activities plan
8. Discuss risk factor–modification plan

INTERVENTIONS:

1. Ensure patient accessibility to communicate need for assistance (e.g., call light, bell, intercom, and routine visits)
2. Encourage patient to be out of bed as much as possible if condition permits
3. Implement a daily mobility–activities plan in conjunction with therapy staff
4. Perform range-of-motion activities throughout daily care within medical limits
5. Provide wheelchair appropriate to patient need with emphasis on therapeutic positioning
6. Provide portable devices to facilitate patient mobility (e.g., IV poles, leg bags, and portable oxygen tanks)
7. Initiate indicated stage of falls prevention practice guideline
8. Initiate indicated stage of activity intolerance practice guideline
9. Initiate indicated stage of acute or chronic pain practice guideline
10. Initiate indicated stage of altered skin integrity practice guideline
11. Initiate indicated stage of anxiety practice guideline
12. Initiate indicated stage of noncompliance practice guideline
13. Initiate indicated stage of constipation practice guideline

14. Initiate indicated stage altered nutritional status: more or less than body requirements practice guideline
15. Initiate indicated stage of fluid volume excess or deficit practice guideline
16. Initiate indicated stage of impaired gas exchange practice guideline
17. Implement risk factor–modification plan
18. Implement indicated stage of self-care deficit practice guideline

Complications:

1. Dependent mobility:
   - implement stage 4 of this practice guideline

EVALUATION:

1. Compare patient's mobility status to baseline
2. Analyze patient's progress toward outcomes
3. Analyze patient's response to interventions, treatments, and medications
4. Evaluate effectiveness of teaching
5. Analyze patient's understanding and cooperation with the plan of care
6. Evaluate effectiveness of daily mobility–activities plan
7. Evaluate effectiveness of risk factor–modification plan

COMMUNICATION:

Verbal

1. Report:
   - any additional changes in mobility status to all members of the care team

Written

1. Record initiation and specific stage of practice guideline on the Careprint
2. Note any modifications to the stage on the Careprint and rationale for each modification as it occurs
3. Chart all baseline data, ongoing monitoring data, interventions taken, and patient's response on the patient care flowsheet
4. Record evaluation of patient outcomes on the progress record
5. Record all patient/caregiver teaching

Impaired Mobility

STAGE 4: Dependent

1. Performance of mobility tasks requiring total assistance:
   - bed mobility: patient unable to perform or assist with bed mobility tasks
   - transfers: total lift or Hoyer lift required to transfer patient
   - wheelchair: patient unable to propel wheelchair
   - ambulation/stairs: patient nonambulatory
2. Requirement of assistive device(s)
3. Inability to attain/maintain upright posture with less than total assistance or external support

COMPETENCIES:

In order to manage patients in this stage the individual must be able to:
1. Identify signs and symptoms of stage 4 impaired mobility
2. Perform mobility techniques according to procedure
3. Use terms the patient understands
4. Perform all procedures associated with assistive devices
5. Perform processes outlined in this stage
6. Identify complications associated with this stage
7. Achieve outcomes outlined in this stage
8. Identify factors that contribute to impaired mobility
9. Perform range-of-motion activities according to procedure
10. Identify resources for referral
11. Calculate intake and output
12. Take vital signs and interpret the results

Credentialing:

Physical Assessment
Body Mechanics
Range-of-Motion
   Techniques

ASSESSMENT:

1. Obtain history of mobility:
   - living environment (e.g., stairs, railings, bed and bath accessibility, and ramps)
   - assistive devices
   - ADL
2. Ascertain patient's/caregiver's knowledge of assistive device(s) used
3. Assess vital signs prior to assisting patient into upright position
4. Obtain baseline gross motor strength/range-of-motion upon initial assessment
5. Assess level and degree of mobility
6. Collect information regarding caregiver's ability to assist with mobility task
7. Collect information regarding patient's/significant others' knowledge about impaired mobility
8. Assess for potential sequelae caused by impaired mobility:
   - pressure sores
   - increased risk of falls
   - increased risk of contracture
   - secondary cardiopulmonary complications
   - circulatory compromise
   - prolonged healing time
   - gastrointestinal complications
   - sensory impairment
   - decreased strength
   - decreased range-of-motion
   - decreased endurance

- decreased balance
- pain
- cognitive changes
9. Monitor therapeutic effects of prescribed medications
10. Assess level of compliance to increased mobility regimen
11. Assess level of anxiety
12. Assess for pain during mobility activities
13. Assess for activity intolerance
14. Assess skin integrity
15. Assess risk for falls
16. Assess lung sounds each shift for:
    - adventitious sounds (crackles, wheezes)
17. Obtain baseline weight and weigh the same time each day using the same scale and the same clothing
18. Assess nutritional status every 24 hours
19. Obtain bowel history regarding normal bowel routine
20. Assess ADL needs

DIAGNOSIS:

1. Stage patient's level of impaired mobility
2. Determine patient's and significant others':
   - involvement in care
   - communication and support needs
   - knowledge and readiness to learn
3. Determine falls risk
4. Determine level of activity tolerance
5. Determine level of pain (acute or chronic)
6. Determine level of altered skin integrity
7. Determine level of anxiety
8. Determine level of noncompliance
9. Determine level of constipation
10. Determine level of altered nutritional status: more or less than body requirements
11. Determine level of fluid volume excess or deficit
12. Determine level of impaired gas exchange
13. Determine communication needs
14. Determine level of competence of caregivers to use assistive devices/techniques with patient
15. Determine level of self-care deficit
16. Determine bowel and bladder routine

OUTCOMES IDENTIFICATION:

Patient

1. Performs mobility tasks with total assistance
2. Maintains range-of-motion

Staff

1. Identifies patients with stage 4 impaired mobility
2. Utilizes processes outlined in this stage
3. Identifies signs and symptoms of improving condition and restages patient status
4. Maintains communication regarding the patient's clinical condition and treatment plan with all involved persons

System

1. A qualified staff member is available to care for this patient
2. A physical/occupational therapy consultation occurs within 24 hours of written referral
3. A dietary consultation occurs within 24 hours of written referral
4. An environment conducive to patient's mobility level is maintained

5. Equipment necessary to implement stage 4 processes is available as needed:
   - teaching materials
   - assistive devices
   - bed scales
   - stethoscope

PLANNING:

In-House

1. Obtain physical/occupational therapy consultation
2. Obtain dietary consultation
3. Design daily mobility–activities plan to be performed in conjunction with therapy staff
4. Assist patient to set realistic goals
5. Develop risk factor–modification plan
6. Modify interventions outlined in this stage as indicated by patient condition or physician order
7. Modify patient/caregiver education outlined in this stage based on patient's/caregiver's readiness to learn
8. Modify outcomes outlined in this stage based on assessment data

Discharge

1. Develop at-home plan for use of assistive devices
2. Design at-home daily mobility–activities plan
3. Refer to community/outpatient services as indicated

EDUCATION:

1. Reinforce care of assistive devices according to procedure
2. Review modified mobility level as designated by physician
3. Educate patient/caregiver on monitoring skin integrity, turning schedule/pressure relief, range-of-motion, and use of assistive devices
4. Educate patient/caregiver regarding signs and symptoms of intolerance to mobility activities
5. Provide patient with all information necessary to make informed health care decisions
6. Discuss daily mobility–activities plan
7. Discuss risk factor–modification plan

INTERVENTIONS:

1. Ensure patient accessibility to communicate need for assistance (e.g., call light, bell, intercom, and routine visits)
2. Encourage patient to be out of bed as much as possible if condition permits
3. Implement daily mobility–activities plan in conjunction with therapy staff
4. Perform range-of-motion activities throughout daily care within medical limits
5. Provide wheelchair appropriate to patient need with emphasis on therapeutic positioning
6. Provide special cushions/mattresses as indicated by circulatory need and mobility level (consult physical/occupational therapy)
7. Provide portable devices to facilitate patient mobility (e.g., IV poles, leg bags, and portable oxygen tanks)
8. Initiate indicated stage of falls prevention practice guideline
9. Initiate indicated stage of activity intolerance practice guideline
10. Initiate indicated stage of acute or chronic pain practice guideline
11. Initiate indicated stage of altered skin integrity practice guideline
12. Initiate indicated stage of anxiety practice guideline
13. Initiate indicated stage of noncompliance practice guideline
14. Initiate indicated stage of constipation practice guideline
15. Initiate indicated stage of altered nutritional status: more or less than body requirements practice guideline
16. Initiate indicated stage of fluid volume excess or deficit practice guideline
17. Initiate indicated stage of impaired gas exchange practice guideline
18. Implement risk factor–modification plan
19. Initiate indicated stage of self-care deficit practice guideline

Complications

1. Contractures
2. Sequelae development

EVALUATION:

1. Compare patient's mobility status to baseline
2. Analyze patient's progress toward outcomes
3. Analyze patient's response to interventions, treatments, and medications
4. Evaluate effectiveness of teaching
5. Analyze patient's understanding and cooperation with the plan of care
6. Evaluate effectiveness of daily mobility–activities plan
7. Evaluate effectiveness of risk factor–modification plan

COMMUNICATION:

Verbal

1. Report:
   - any additional changes in mobility status to all members of the care team

Written

1. Record initiation and specific stage of practice guideline on the Careprint
2. Note any modifications to the stage on the Careprint and rationale for each modification as it occurs
3. Chart all baseline data, ongoing monitoring data, interventions taken, and patient's response on the patient care flowsheet
4. Record evaluation of patient outcomes on the progress record
5. Record all patient/caregiver teaching

Appendix 9-2

Joint Commission Indicators for the Indicator Measurement System and Hospital Use

The Joint Commission plans to incorporate outcomes and other performance measures into its accreditation process to improve evaluation of the performance of accredited health care organizations. These performance measures will supplement and guide the standards-based survey process by providing:

- A more targeted basis for your regular accreditation survey.
- A basis for measuring your organization's performance between triennial on-site surveys.
- A basis for guiding and stimulating continuous improvement in your health care organization, with the Joint Commission's ongoing support.

Once performance-measurement data are used in the accreditation process (currently anticipated to be no sooner than 1997), every accredited hospital will be required to participate in an approved performance measurement system(s).

To offer your organization a choice of performance measurement systems, the Joint Commission will be collaborating with other leading performance measurement systems. A Council on Performance Measurement, composed of nationally recognized experts, will make recommendations to the Joint Commission's Board of Commissioners about which performance measurement systems should be approved as fulfilling the requirements for accreditation. To make these recommendations, the Council will

- identify the criteria (for example, relevance, cohort size, willingness to share data) used to evaluate the applicant measurement systems.
- establish the criteria necessary for approval.
- evaluate the measurement systems against these criteria.

Therefore, while your organization will be required in the future to participate in a performance measurement system, you will be able to choose any of the approved measurement systems, of which the Joint Commission's Indicator Measurement System (IMSystem) will be one.

The IMSystem is an indicator-based, performance-measurement system. In 1996, the IMSystem includes the following indicators for acute care hospitals:

- Obstetrical care
- Perioperative care
- Oncology care
- Cardiovascular care
- Trauma care
- Medication use
- Infection control.

Expert task forces developed these indicators, and each indicator's relevancy, reliability, and validity were rigorously assessed through extensive testing activities in volunteer hospitals.

In 1994, hospitals that enrolled in the IMSystem began submitting indicator data to the IMSystem and receiving quarterly performance reports. An organization can use these data to

- assess and improve its performance.
- better understand its processes of care.
- identify problems with current processes.
- manage risk.
- meet the demands of patients, payers, and others who want to make informed health care decisions.

If you would like more information about the IMSystem, please call the Department of Indicator Measurement at 708/916-5220.

This appendix contains two sections: the indicators selected for the Joint Commission's IMSystem, and other indicators tested by the Joint Commission and recommended for hospital's internal use (but not as a part of the IMSystem).

SECTION 1: 1996 IMSYSTEM INDICATORS

The Joint Commission's Board of Commissioners approved the inclusion of the indicators in this section in the IMSystem. The decision to include indicators in the IMSystem is based on specific criteria and the health care environment. The IMSystem became operational in 1994 with perioperative and obstetrical care indicator sets. Based on field-testing results and recommendations from expert task forces, the Board of Commissioners approved the addition of trauma, oncology, and cardiovascular indicators in the IMSystem in 1995, and the medication-use and infection-control indicators in 1996.

1. **Focus:** Preoperative patient evaluation, intraoperative and postoperative monitoring, and timely clinical intervention
   Numerator: Patients developing a central nervous system (CNS) complication within 2 postprocedure days of procedures involving anesthesia* administration
2. **Focus:** Preoperative patient evaluation, appropriate surgical preparation, intraoperative and postoperative monitoring, and timely clinical intervention
   Numerator: Patients developing a peripheral neurological deficit within 2 postprocedure days of procedures involving anesthesia administration
3. **Focus:** Preoperative patient evaluation, intraoperative and postoperative monitoring, and timely clinical intervention
   Numerator: Patients developing an acute myocardial infarction within 2 postprocedure days of procedures involving anesthesia administration
4. **Focus:** Preoperative patient evaluation, intraoperative and postoperative monitoring, and timely clinical intervention
   Numerator: Patients with a cardiac arrest within 2 postprocedure days of procedures involving anesthesia administration
5. **Focus:** Preoperative patient evaluation, intraoperative and postoperative monitoring, and timely clinical intervention
   Numerator: Intrahospital mortality of patients within 2 postprocedure days of procedures involving anesthesia administration
6. **Focus:** Prenatal patient evaluation, education, and treatment selection
   Numerator: Patients delivered by cesarean section
   Denominator: All deliveries
7. **Focus:** Prenatal patient evaluation, education, and treatment selection
   Numerator: Patients with vaginal birth after cesarean section (VBAC)
   Denominator: Patients delivered with a history of previous cesarean section
8. **Focus:** Prenatal patient evaluation, intrapartum monitoring, and clinical intervention
   Numerator: Live-born infants with a birth weight less than 2,500 grams
   Denominator: All live births
9. **Focus:** Prenatal patient evaluation, intrapartum monitoring, neonatal patient evaluation, and clinical intervention
   Numerator: Live-born infants with a birth weight greater than or equal to 2,500 grams, who have at least one of the following: an Apgar score of less than four at 5 minutes, a requirement for admission to the neonatal intensive care unit within one day of delivery for greater than 24 hours, a clinically apparent seizure, or significant birth trauma
   Denominator: All live-born infants with a birth weight greater than 2,500 grams

---

*For the indicators related to perioperative care, the population of interest (denominators) includes all patients undergoing procedures involving anesthesia and an inpatient stay. **Anesthesia** is defined as the administration to any patient, in any setting, for any purpose, by any route, general, spinal, or other major regional anesthesia or sedation (with or without analgesia) for which there is a reasonable expectation that, in the manner used, the sedation or analgesia will result in the loss of protective reflexes.

10. **Focus:** Prenatal patient evaluation, intrapartum monitoring, neonatal patient evaluation, and clinical intervention
    Numerator: Live-born infants with a birth weight greater than 1,00 grams and less than 2,500 grams who have an Apgar score of less than four at 5 minutes
    Denominator: All live-born infants with a birth weight greater than 1,000 grams and less than 2,500 grams

11. **Focus:** Extended postoperative stay as a means of assessing multiple aspects of coronary artery bypass graft (CABG) care
    Indicator Statement:* Patients undergoing isolated CABG procedures: number of days from surgery to discharge

12. **Focus:** Timing of thrombolytic therapy administration
    Indicator Statement: Patients admitted through the emergency department with a principal discharge diagnosis of acute myocardial infarction (AMI) receiving thrombolytic therapy: time from emergency department arrival to administration of thrombolytic therapy

13. **Focus:** Diagnostic accuracy
    Numerator: Patients with principal discharge diagnosis of congestive heart failure (CHF) with documented etiology
    Denominator: Patients with principal discharge diagnosis of CHF

14. **Focus:** Extended postprocedure stay as a means of assessing multiple aspects of percutaneous transluminal coronary angioplasty (PTCA) care
    Indicator Statement: Patients undergoing PTCA: number of days from procedure to discharge

15a. **Focus:** Intrahospital mortality as a means of assessing multiple aspects of coronary artery bypass graft (CABG) patient care
    Numerator: Intrahospital mortality of patients undergoing an isolated CAGB
    Denominator: Patients undergoing an isolated CABG

  b. **Focus:** Intrahospital mortality as a means of assessing multiple aspects of percutaneous transluminal coronary angioplasty (PTCA) patient care
    Numerator: Intrahospital mortality of patients undergoing a PTCA
    Denominator: Patients undergoing a PTCA

  c. **Focus:** Intrahospital mortality as a means of assessing multiple aspects of acute myocardial infarction (AMI) patient care
    Numerator: Intrahospital mortality of patients with a principal discharge diagnosis of AMI
    Denominator: Patients with a principal discharge diagnosis of AMI

16. **Focus:** Availability of data for diagnosis and staging
    Numerator: Patients undergoing resection for primary cancer of the female breast, lung, or colon/rectum for whom a surgical pathology consultation report is present in the medical record
    Denominator: Patients undergoing resection for primary cancer of the female breast, lung, or colon/rectum

17. **Focus:** Use of staging by managing physicians
    Numerator: Patients undergoing resection for primary cancer of the female breast, lung, or colon/rectum with stage of tumor designated by a managing physician
    Denominator: Patients undergoing resection for primary cancer of the female breast, lung, or colon/rectum

18. **Focus:** Use of tests critical for prognosis and clinical management of female breast cancer
    Numerator: Female patients with Stage 1 or greater primary breast cancer who, after initial biopsy or resection, have estrogen receptor analysis results in the medical record
    Denominator: Female patients with Stage 1 or greater primary breast cancer undergoing initial biopsy or resection

19. **Focus:** Effectiveness of preoperative diagnosis and staging
    Numerator: Patients with nonsmall cell primary lung cancer undergoing thoracotomy with complete surgical resection of tumor
    Denominator: Patients with nonsmall cell primary lung cancer undergoing thoracotomy

20. **Focus:** Comprehensiveness of diagnostic workup
    Numerator: Patients undergoing resection for primary cancer of the colon or rectum whose preoperative evaluation by a managing physician included examination of the entire colon
    Denominator: Patients undergoing resection for primary cancer of the colon or rectum

---

*An **Indicator Statement** (as contrasted with a numerator) is used when the measure is a continuous variable.

21a. **Focus:** Ongoing monitoring of trauma patients
Numerator: Trauma patients with systolic blood pressure, pulse rate, and respiratory rate documented on arrival to the emergency department (ED) and at least hourly for 3 hours or until ED disposition, whichever is earlier
Denominator: All trauma patients

  b. **Focus:** Ongoing monitoring of trauma patients
Numerator: Trauma patients with selected intracranial injuries with Glasgow coma scale (GCS) score documented on arrival to emergency department (ED) and at least hourly for 3 hours or until ED disposition, whichever is earlier
Denominator: Trauma patients with selected intracranial injuries

22. **Focus:** Airway management of comatose trauma patients
Numerator: Comatose trauma patients with selected intracranial injuries discharged from the emergency department prior to endotracheal intubation or cricothyrotomy
Denominator: Emergency department comatose trauma patients with selected intracranial injuries

23. **Focus:** Timeliness of diagnostic testing
Indicator Statement: Trauma patients with head computerized tomography (CT) scan performed: time from emergency department arrival to initial CT scan

24a. **Focus:** Timeliness of surgical intervention for selected head injuries
Indicator Statement: Trauma patients undergoing selected neurosurgical procedures: time from emergency department arrival to procedure

  b. **Focus:** Timeliness of intervention for selected orthopedic injuries
Indicator Statement: Trauma patients undergoing selected orthopedic procedures: time from emergency department arrival to procedure

  c. **Focus:** Timeliness of surgical intervention for selected abdominal injuries
Indicator Statement: Trauma patients undergoing selected abdominal surgical procedures: time from emergency department arrival to procedure

25a. **Focus:** Clinical decision-making for potentially preventable deaths
Numerator: Intrahospital mortality of trauma patients with a diagnosis of pneumothorax or hemothorax who did not undergo a thoracostomy or thoracotomy
Denominator: Intrahospital mortality of trauma patients with a diagnosis of pneumothorax or hemothorax

  b. **Focus:** Clinical decision making for potentially preventable deaths
Numerator: Intrahospital mortality of trauma patients with a systolic blood pressure of less than 70 mm Hg within two hours of emergency department arrival who did not undergo a laparotomy or thoracotomy
Denominator: Intrahospital mortality of trauma patients with a systolic blood pressure of less than 70 mm Hg within two hours of emergency department arrival

26. **Focus:** Individualizing dosage
Numerator: Inpatients 65 years of age or older in whom creatinine clearance has been estimated
Denominator: Inpatients 65 years of age or older

27. **Focus:** Timing of medication administration
Indicator Statement: Patients with selected surgical procedures receiving intravenous prophylactic antibiotics: timing of prophylactic antibiotic administration

28. **Focus:** Informing the patient about the medication
Numerator: Inpatients with a discharge diagnosis of insulin-dependent diabetes mellitus who demonstrate self-blood-glucose monitoring and self-administration of insulin before discharge or are referred for postdischarge follow-up for diabetes management
Denominator: Inpatients with a discharge diagnosis of insulin-dependent diabetes mellitus

29a. **Focus:** Monitoring patient response
Numerator: Inpatients receiving digoxin who have no corresponding measured drug level or whose highest measured level exceeds a specific limit
Denominator: Inpatients receiving digoxin

  b. **Focus:** Monitoring patient response
Numerator: Inpatients receiving theophylline who have no corresponding measured drug level or whose highest measured level exceeds a specific limit
Denominator: Inpatients receiving theophylline

  c. **Focus:** Monitoring patient response
Numerator: Inpatients receiving phenytoin who have no corresponding measured drug level or whose highest measured level exceeds a specific limit
Denominator: Inpatients receiving phenytoin

   d. **Focus:** Monitoring patient response
      Numerator: Inpatients receiving lithium who have no corresponding measured drug level or whose highest measured level exceeds a specific limit
      Denominator: Inpatients receiving lithium
30. **Focus:** Reviewing complete drug regimen
    Indicator Statement: Inpatients: number of prescribed medications at discharge
31. **Focus:** Surgical site infection
    Numerator: Selected inpatient and outpatient surgical procedures complicated by a surgical site infection
    Denominator: Number of selected inpatient and outpatient surgical procedures
32. **Focus:** Ventilator pneumonia
    Numerator: Ventilated inpatients who develop pneumonia
    Denominator: Inpatient ventilator days
33. **Focus:** Concurrent surveillance of primary bloodstream infection
    Numerator: Inpatients with a central or umbilical line who develop primary bloodstream infection
    Denominator: Inpatient central or umbilical line days

SECTION II: ADDITIONAL INDICATORS APPROVED FOR HOSPITAL USE

The following indicators have undergone testing in the Joint Commission indicator-development and testing process, and are recommended for hospital use, if appropriate. Indicators in the IMSystem are useful for interhospital comparisons. However, testing showed that for the following indicators, there were difficulties with present technologies in collecting comparable data across many hospitals. While not included in the IMSystem, these indicators may be useful for internal hospital use. Your hospital may find these indicators valuable in trending your performance and identifying opportunities to improve your performance.

Additional Anesthesia-Related Perioperative Indicators

- Patients with a discharge diagnosis of fulminant pulmonary edema developed during procedures involving anesthesia administration or within one postprocedure day of a procedure's conclusion
- Patients diagnosed with an aspiration pneumonitis occurring during procedures involving anesthesia administration or within 2 postprocedure days of a procedure's conclusion
- Patients developing a postural headache within 4 postprocedure days following procedures involving spinal or epidural anesthesia administration
- Patients experiencing a dental injury during procedures involving anesthesia care
- Patients experiencing an ocular injury during procedures involving anesthesia care
- Unplanned admission of patients to the hospital within 2 postprocedure days following outpatient procedures involving anesthesia
- Unplanned admission of patients to an intensive care unit within two postprocedure days of procedures involving anesthesia administration and with intensive care unit stay greater than 1 day

Additional Obstetric Indicators

- Intrahospital neonatal deaths of infants with a birth weight of 750 to 999 grams born in a hospital with a Neonatal Intensive Care Unit (NICU)
- Maternal readmissions within 14 days of delivery
- Intrahospital maternal deaths occurring within 42 days postpartum
- Infants with a birth weight less than 1,800 grams delivered in a hospital without an NICU
- Neonates transferred from a non-NICU hospital to an NICU hospital
- Patients with excessive maternal blood loss

Additional Cardiovascular Indicators

- **Focus:** Specific complication of CABG as a means of assessing the management of CABG patients
  Numerator: Patients undergoing isolated CABG procedures returning to the operating room for treatment of postoperative thoracic bleeding subcategorized by presence or absence of thrombolytic therapy received within 48 hours prior to CABG

- **Focus:** Specific complication of CABG as a means of assessing multiple aspects of CABG care
  Numerator: Intraoperative or postoperative cerebrovascular accident in patients undergoing isolated CABG procedure
- **Focus:** Effectiveness of PTCA
  Numerator: Patients with repeat PTCA of the same lesion occurring within 72 hours of the most recent PTCA subcategorized by emergent and nonemergent status of original PTCA
- **Focus:** Specific complication of PTCA as a means of assessing multiple aspects of PTCA care
  Numerator: Patients with post-PTCA complications at femoral or brachial artery insertion site subcategorized by thrombolytic therapy within 48 hours prior to PTCA
- **Focus:** Management of thrombolytic therapy in patients with acute MI
  Numerator: Hemorrhagic complications in patients receiving thrombolytic therapy for acute MI, subcategorized by complications occurring to patients prior to discharge from the institution initiating therapy and post-transfer complications occurring to patients receiving therapy prior to transfer
- **Focus:** Effectiveness of PTCA
  Numerator: Patients undergoing attempted or completed PTCA during which any lesion attempted is not dilated

Additional Oncology Indicators

- **Focus:** Availability of specific data needed for diagnosis
  Numerator: Presence of a written pathology report in the medical record of the treating institution documenting the pathologic diagnosis of patients receiving initial treatment for primary lung, colorectal, or female breast cancer
- **Focus:** Symptomatic or palliative care
  Numerator: Systematic initial assessment of pain for all patients hospitalized due to metastic lung, colorectal, or female breast cancer with pain
- **Focus:** Use of clinical staging
  Numerator: Presence of documented American Joint Commission on Cancer (AJCC) clinical staging in the medical record prior to the first course of therapy for female patients with primary breast cancer
- **Focus:** Use of multimodal therapy in treatment and follow-up
  Numerator: Treatment of female patients with primary invasive AJCC clinical Stage I or II breast cancer by excision biopsy, segmental mastectomy, or quadrantectomy without radiation therapy
- **Focus:** Use of psychosocial support for patient follow-up
  Numerator: Referral to support or rehabilitation groups or provision of psychosocial support for female patients with primary breast cancer
- **Focus:** Patient education
  Numerator: Patients undergoing resection for primary colorectal cancer with enterostomy present at discharge who demonstrate understanding of enterostomy care and management instructions
- **Focus:** Use of multimodal therapy in treatment and follow-up
  Numerator: Female patients with Stage II pathologic lymph node positive primary breast cancer treated with systemic adjuvant therapy
  Denominator: Female patients with Stage II pathologic lymph node positive primary breast cancer
- **Indicator Focus:** Specific clinical events as a means of assessing multiple aspects of surgical care for lung cancers
  Numerator: Patients undergoing pulmonary resection for primary lung cancer with postoperative complications of bronchopleural fistula, reoperation for postoperative bleeding, mechanical ventilation greater than five days postoperatively, or intrahospital death
  Denominator: Patients undergoing pulmonary resection for primary lung cancer

Additional Trauma Indicators

- **Focus:** Communication between Emergency Medical Service (EMS) and Emergency Department (ED)
  Numerator: Copy of ambulance run report(s) not present with ED medical record for trauma patients transported by prehospital EMS personnel
- **Focus:** Trauma patient assessments in the emergency department
  Numerator: Trauma patients admitted through the ED with inpatient discharge diagnosis of cervical spine injury not indicated in admission diagnosis

- **Focus:** ED decision making
  Numerator: Death of trauma patients with discharge diagnosis for closed pelvic fracture who receive transfusions of greater than six units of blood
- **Focus:** Clinical decision making for surgical intervention
  Numerator: Trauma patients receiving initial abdominal, thoracic, vascular, or cranial surgery (excluding orthopedic, plastic, and hand surgery) more than 24 hours after ED arrival
- **Focus:** Use of blood products
  Numerator: Transfusion of platelets or fresh frozen plasma within 24 hours of ED arrival in adult trauma patients receiving less than eight units of packed red blood cells or whole blood
- **Focus:** Effectiveness of surgical intervention
  Numerator: Return of trauma patients to the operating room within 48 hours of completion of initial surgery
- **Focus:** Clinical decision making for femoral shaft fractures
  Numerator: Trauma patients with femoral diaphyseal fractures that are not associated with other injuries who do not receive physical therapy or rehabilitation therapy
- **Focus:** Efficiency of emergency medical services
  Numerator: Trauma patients transported by prehospital emergency medical services: scene time
- **Focus:** Systems necessary for obtaining autopsies for trauma victims
  Numerator: Trauma patients who expired within 48 hours of ED arrival for whom an autopsy was performed

Additional Medication Use Indicators

- **Focus:** Individualizing dosage
  Numerator: Inpatients receiving parenteral aminoglycosides who have a measured aminoglycoside serum level
- **Focus:** Reviewing the order
  Numerator: New medication orders prompting consultation by the pharmacist with physician or nurse subcategorized by orders changed
- **Focus:** Accuracy of medication dispensing and administration
  Numerator: Number of reported significant medication errors
- **Focus:** Monitoring patient response
  Numerator: Inpatient receiving warfarin or intravenous therapeutic heparin who also receive Vitamin K, protamine sulfate, or fresh frozen plasma
- **Focus:** Reporting adverse drug reactions (ADRs)
  Numerator: ADRs reported through the hospital's ADR-reporting system analyzed by method of reporting (spontaneous or retrospective medical record abstraction), type of ADR (dose related or nondose related), and time of occurrence (before admission or during hospitalization)
- **Focus:** Reviewing complete drug regimen
  Numerator: Inpatients receiving more than one type of oral benzodiazepine simultaneously
- **Focus:** Overall performance of medication use system
  Numerator: Patients less than 25 years old with a principal discharge diagnosis of bronchoconstrictive pulmonary disease, who are readmitted to the hospital or visit the emergency department within 15 days of discharge due to an exacerbation of their principal diagnosis

Additional Infection Control Indicator

- **Focus:** Postoperative pneumonia
  Numerator: Selected inpatient surgical procedures complicated by the onset of pneumonia during hospitalization, but not beyond 10 postoperative days

Modified from *1996 Comprehensive accreditation manual for hospitals.* Oakbrook Terrace, Ill: Joint Commission on Accreditation of Healthcare Organizations, 1995, pp. 579-587. Reprinted with permission.

Chapter 10

Setting Performance Targets

Quality is a matter of perception and, like beauty, lies in the eyes of the beholder.

Ellie Green

Torrential rain cascaded over John's shoulders from his ranger's hat. As he inched his way along the catwalk of the dam, he was grateful for the almost constant lightning that acted as backup to his flashlight.

At last he reached the gauges. Carefully he leaned over the edge of the dam to read the water level indicator. At midnight it had risen an inch above the yellow warning line, and according to policy, he had alerted the mayor to the possible need for an emergency evacuation of the town below.

At 1 AM, as the storm continued to rage, John again was peering at the gauges to see whether the water level had reached the red danger line. If so, he would initiate the evacuation plan adopted by the town council 6 months earlier. He hoped it would not be necessary. He knew how frightened his wife Mary would be if the evacuation alarm were sounded on such a stormy night.

In this story, John's targets were clearly established: when the water level reached the yellow line, the mayor was notified of the problem. If the rain had continued, causing the water level to rise to the red line, the town would be evacuated.

The target clearly delineated the acceptable level of safety or tolerance; exceeding that level would be

John's signal to initiate immediate action. The yellow line served as a caution point. The red line served as the danger point—the point at which immediate action would be taken.

In other words, John relied upon preestablished targets—the yellow and red lines—to provide the data necessary for the decision-making process.

DEFINITION OF TARGETS

There are many targets in health care organizations. These targets are so common they often go unnoticed. For example, the blood pH target parameters are 7.35 to 7.45. If a patient's pH deviates from this acceptable range, then a physician is notified at once. Insulin has a target relating to its shelf-life, which specifies the amount of time the solution is viable. In the coronary care department, targets for patients' heart rate and rhythm alarms are routinely set. In labor and delivery patients, fetal heart monitor alarm ranges are also set. Such targets are used daily by staff members in all health care organizations in making decisions about patient care. Similarly, there are practice and governance targets related to such areas as documentation and budgeting.

Obviously, the concept of targets is neither new nor mysterious, but rather part of the daily work experience of all employees.

CHARACTERISTICS OF TARGETS

A target is the border between performance and nonperformance with written process standards. Performance is a positive factor. It signifies adherence or conformance to written standards. When staff members are performing, they deliver customer service in accordance with the structure, process, and outcome standards preestablished by the organization. Performance is composed of those controllable factors that affect quality outcomes. These might include the patient's understanding of the treatment plan, the staff's competence, or the availability of system resources. When all customer, staff, and governance system variables are controlled that can be, performance is optimal. When customer, staff, and governance variables are not fully controlled—i.e., they are not up to standard—performance decreases and quality suffers.

Nonperformance is the result of the lack of adherence or conformance to written standards. Nonperformance is a negative factor. When staff does not deliver services according to the structure process, and outcome standards set by the organization, nonperformance exists. A portion of nonperformance is caused by customer, staff, and governance variables that are less than optimal. When these variables are not fully controlled, nonperformance increases. A portion of nonperformance is also the result of chance or individual differences. This is the portion of nonperformance that is not controllable under any circumstances. For example, the patient's anatomy, the staff's critical thinking abilities, or the physical plant may be uncontrollable variables. The portion of nonperformance allowable in aggregate data is the portion that is not controllable.

As stated, the point that separates performance from nonperformance is the target. Let us look at a clinical example.

The written standard states that patients' call bells will be answered within 3 minutes. In the specific department, it is determined that this standard can be adhered to 95% of the time. In other words, 95 out of 100 call bells with be answered within 3 minutes of being rung by a patient. This is a rate-based indicator and the performance target is 95%. The target measures performance, or how often something was done or achieved. Thus, if the rate of answering call bells within 3 minutes drops below 95%, further investigation of the variation would be required.

The same situation can be looked at from the opposite perspective, i.e., how many times call bells will not be answered within 3 minutes. This perspective focuses on nonperformance or how often something is not done or achieved. In this example, we would expect that no more than 5 out of 100 call bells would not be answered. The nonperformance is 5%. Should the number of call bells not answered exceed 5%, further investigation of the variation would be indicated.

Performance and nonperformance are two sides of the same coin, and the target is the dividing line. One hundred percent minus the percentage of nonperformance equals the percentage of performance. Alternatively, one hundred percent minus the percentage of performance equals the percentage of nonperformance.

If adherence to standards is being measured, targets will be written that are high, i.e., closer to 100%. If, however, negative occurrences (nonperformance) are being monitored, targets will be written that are low, i.e., closer to 0%.

Targets are also dynamic. They change with continual improvement. Like performance, targets should improve over time. However, there comes a point in continual improvement when all the variables have been controlled that can be controlled. There may always be some variables that cannot be controlled. When service is at its optimum level of performance, the emphasis is then placed on maintaining that level of performance while streamlining the process.

Targets also must be realistic. That is, they need to be feasible given the range of customer, staff, or system capabilities. Setting unachievable targets can quickly undermine performance improvement efforts. When establishing targets, keep in mind the uncontrollable factors that affect achievement. Many staff members have difficulty accepting a target lower than 100% or greater than 0%. Except for sentinel events, such extremes may be noble but are not realistic for most indicators.

To set absolute targets for every indicator being measured is to program the system for failure. Staff members become frustrated with the amount of review required, since an inquiry is needed for all deviations from 100% or 0%. The system becomes administratively unmanageable because of the additional paperwork required; performance measurement becomes a tedious exercise rather than the vital tool it was intended to be.

Lastly, targets are objective. They are the unbiased signs that mark the need for further investigation of a critical process. They are the benchmark against which current and future performance is and will be evaluated.

SETTING TARGETS

There are two types of occurrences for which targets are set: sentinel events and rate-based indicators. Sentinel events are negative, unpredictable occurrences. At best there is a conscientious attempt by management and all employees to make the system error-proof. This is accomplished through many mechanisms, such as employee orientation and education, developing and adhering to standards, and preceptor programs. There is no tolerance for sentinel events; the target for compliance is 0%. Because the target is 0%, each sentinel event must be evaluated immediately upon occurrence. Examples of sentinel events include administration of incompatible blood, sponges left in the abdomen postoperatively, amputating the wrong body part, and a hazardous waste spill.

Targets for rate-based indicators, on the other hand, are not so easily measured. Rate-based indicators will never be 100% because too many variables exist in an organization's delivery of service as well as in staff member practices and governance processes.

Targets may not be set arbitrarily by a gut feeling, hunch, or guess. For example, a manager may not mandate a 98% target for pre-discharge diabetic education and expect all practitioners to "hit the bull's-eye." Before a target can be set, data must be collected over a period of time to find the mean of the process as it is being carried out by workers. Only then may upper and lower control limits be set based on standard deviation. The target, then, is a range within which the manager desires staff member performance.

In the case of the pre-discharge diabetic education for a particular patient population, the indicator formed as the basis for measurement might read like this:

$$\frac{\text{The number of patients who failed to}}{\text{receive pre-discharge diabetic education}}$$

The number of patients with an order for pre-discharge diabetic education

Once the data has been collected, the mean of the process established, and the statistically derived control limits set, the manager may then track and trend staff member performance in identified critical process.

ESTABLISHING A DESIRED TARGET

Various organizations are in the process of developing national databases upon which to base the selection of targets. Health care organizations may benchmark their performance targets. These national databases will serve as precursors to the development of internal databases through which trends in performance can be noted and individual organizations can compare their performance with that of others.

Targets should never be set arbitrarily or they will have no basis in reality. Those who set targets arbitrarily frequently set a target that is unrealistic.

Making the transition to a statistically based measurement program requires that targets be set that are statistically sound. In this method, a baseline is defined as a starting point for the process of performance improvement. A retrospective analysis of a representative sample of the indicator population from the previous year is conducted to provide a baseline for the next year's target. A large representative sample increases the statistical significance of the baseline.

For example, the indicator to be evaluated might be the effectiveness of diabetic patient teaching. It may be determined that the desired outcome of insulin administration instruction is the patient's ability to administer insulin safely and correctly at home within the first 48 hours after discharge. Thus, patients with a primary diagnosis of diabetes mellitus who returned to the emergency department (ED) within 48 hours of discharge with a diagnosis of insulin shock or ketoacidosis would indicate the inability of these patients to carry out the procedure correctly. These patients become the indicator population.

An analysis of the previous year's ED admissions indicates admissions for 130 such patients. A random sample of 50 of these patients' charts is examined. Review of the charts demonstrates that in 10% of the cases, the patients either did not receive instruction in insulin administration or were unable to successfully prepare and administer the injection. Thus 10% becomes the baseline mean for measuring nonperformance. The mean performance target is 90%.

This sort of retrospective analysis should be done before the start of any measurement and should also be included as part of the annual summary report on each indicator so that the following year's target can be set using the previous year's data.

This method quickly provides a historical overview of performance and a baseline for the following year's target. The authors recognize that for high-volume indicators, the sample numbers required to obtain statistical significance may appear prohibitive when resources such as time and staff are constrained. However, the move to a statistically based performance measurement program cannot occur without the commitment of the resources necessary to provide accurate baseline data upon which to measure current practice and plan for future improvement.

TARGET PARAMETERS VERSUS ABSOLUTE TARGETS

There is variability in everything. For example, the likelihood that an expert marksman will hit the bull's-eye each time is determined by the individual's proficiency. However, the likelihood that the exact same hole in the bull's-eye will be hit each time is more uncertain. There is normal variance in performance.

Suppose we have set a performance target of 97%. Theoretically, this means that if we do not achieve that precise target each time we measure, additional analysis is necessary. The likelihood of hitting the 97% mark precisely in each of the four studies is low, just as the likelihood that the marksman will hit the same bullet hole each time is low. We aim to hit the bull's-eye, not necessarily the same bullet hole. As long as the bull's-eye is hit each time, the marksman is a winner. The bull's-eye is an area, not a pinpoint. It would be much more difficult for a marksman, no matter how skilled, to repetitively hit a bull's-eye the size of the bullet.

We want to provide staff with a targeted *area* of success to aim for, not a pinpoint target. Setting target parameters provides the limits within which it can safely be said that quality exists. It is similar to stating that a normal patient blood pressure reading is 120/80. Although 120/80 is recognized as the norm, some variation is expected. Even if an initial reading is 120/80, at a later time it may be 115/85. The medical profession, based on years of data analysis, has established parameters for blood pressure that are reasonable and safe. A blood pressure reading between 100/60 and 140/90 is generally considered acceptable, but beyond that range the physician may decide to take action.

Why? Because historically, data has proven that positive patient outcomes are associated with blood pressures within the acceptable range, whereas negative outcomes are reported when the blood pressure falls outside those parameters. In other words, there are acceptable target parameters for blood pressure readings.

Traditionally, targets have been set as absolutes. This practice places an undue burden on practitioners to "hit the mark" every time. Furthermore, it promotes unproductive and undesirable reactions: any time staff members fail to "hit the mark," they feel that they are not fully competent. Staff members can become discouraged with the process, which may hinder the entire measurement program. In their frustration over lack of achievement, their morale may suffer. Staff members do not want to participate in activities that constantly make them feel inadequate. They may become reluctant to participate in future measurement activities or recalcitrant with regard to performance improvement efforts. Worse yet, they may choose to hide (or not report) measurement results that are less than perfect. Therefore, it is far better to set statistically derived target parameters than absolute targets. Target parameters define the upper and lower limits of acceptance for the results of a study.

Thresholds for evaluation may be statistically determined control limits, specification limits, trends, or patterns. They are mechanisms used to determine when processes or outcomes of care must be further evaluated. Thresholds help determine when unexpected or possibly undesirable occurrences must be evaluated (e.g. in PM terms, "the process is out of control"). However, evaluation may (and in PM often does) occur even when thresholds are not crossed. In such circumstances, the evaluation process uses the indicator data to better understand current performance and its causes in order to develop strategies for future improvement.[2]

Statistically correct parameters are really upper and lower control limits of 1 to 3 standard deviations set above and below a desired mean. Calculating statistically accurate parameters requires a retrospective analysis of the data to determine the mean and the calculation of its standard deviation. This will provide the most accurate calculation of the target parameters and allow much more reliable prediction of the results of future studies. We again acknowledge that this type of analysis may require the commitment of resources that may not be available at the department level; however, it must be available at the organizational level. Many individual organizations look to national organizations and the development of national databases as an alternative to this analysis; however, these alternatives will not provide the same individualized data as an internal baseline.

Figure 10-1 shows a nine-step procedure for manually calculating a standard deviation and target parameters. In the example shown in Figure 10-1, the interval limits or target parameters with mean of 10 for a hypothetical data set and an upper and lower control limit of 8.1 to 11.9. Figure 10-2 is a schematic diagram of these parameters. Automated calculation of standard deviation coupled with automated data collection can streamline the process of setting statistically meaningful target parameters.

Using a statistical approach to setting target parameters aids in predicting with some degree of accuracy and confidence the probability that future results will fall within the boundaries of those parameters. That confidence interval has led some to refer to these parameters as upper and lower control limits or confidence limits. The basic statistical principles behind the development and use of control limits were developed in the early 1920s by Walter A. Shewhart. His work served as the foundation of statistical process control.[9]

Control limits are calculated by running a process untouched, taking samples, and calculating the mean and standard deviation of the sample. The normal variation that is seen in a process will form a distribution that looks like a bell-shaped curve (Figure 10-3). This is a unimodel symmetrical curve. Almost 100% (exactly 99.73%) of the data points will fall within three standard deviations (SDs) of the mean. Only 0.27% of the data will fall beyond three standard deviations.[3]

By turning the bell curve on its side (Figure 10-4), the ±3 standard deviations become the upper and lower control limits. Shewhart reckoned that 99.73% of variation from the mean in any process would fall

COL 1	COL 2	COL 3	COL 4
MONTHS	TOTAL MEDICATION ERRORS x_i	DEVIATIONS $x_i - \bar{x}$	SQUARE OF DEVIATIONS $(x_i - \bar{x})^2$
JAN	10	0	0
FEB	12	2	4
MAR	11	1	1
APR	8	−2	4
MAY	11	1	1
JUN	9	−1	1
JUL	7	−3	9
AUG	10	0	0
SEP	12	2	4
OCT	10	0	0
NOV	13	3	9
DEC	7	−3	9
	TOTAL: **120**		TOTAL: **42**

- $\bar{x} = \dfrac{\Sigma x_i}{N} = \dfrac{120}{12} = 10$

- $\sigma = \sqrt{\dfrac{\Sigma(x_i - \bar{x})^2}{N}} = \sqrt{\dfrac{42}{12}} = \sqrt{3.5} = \pm 1.9$

- Target parameters
  Upper limit: $\bar{x} + \sigma = 10 + 1.9 = 11.9$
  Lower limit: $\bar{x} - \sigma = 10 - 1.9 = 8.1$

(x_i = individual score; $\bar{x}$ = mean (or average) of scores; N = number of scores; σ = standard deviation)

1. Enter the number of medication errors reported each month in column 2.
2. Total the entries in column 2 to determine the annual total of the medication errors reported.
3. Divide the total calculated in step 2 by the number of months for which medication error data is available.
   Note: This quotient is $\bar{x}$, the mean, or average number of reported medication errors per month.
4. Subtract the calculated average ($\bar{x}$) from each reported number of monthly medication errors, and enter the deviations ($x_i - \bar{x}$) in column 3.
   Note: Values may be positive, negative, or zero.
5. Multiply each calculated deviation by itself, and enter the resultant products in column 4.
   Note: All values will be positive, or zero.
6. Add the products in column 4. To determine the sum of squared deviations [$\Sigma(x_i - \bar{x})^2$].
7. Divide the sum calculated in step 6 by the number of months for which medication error data are available.
8. Calculate the square root of the quotient determined in step 7.
   Note: This calculation yields σ, the standard deviation of the data entered in column 2.
9. Calculate:
   - the upper limit of the target parameters, $\bar{x} + \sigma$, by adding the calculated standard deviation (σ, see step 8) to the calculated average ($\bar{x}$, step 3), and
   - the lower limit of the target parameters, $\bar{x} - \sigma$, by subtracting the calculated standard deviation (σ, see step 8) from the calculated average ($\bar{x}$, step 3).

Figure 10-1   Nine-step procedure for calculating a standard deviation and confidence interval.

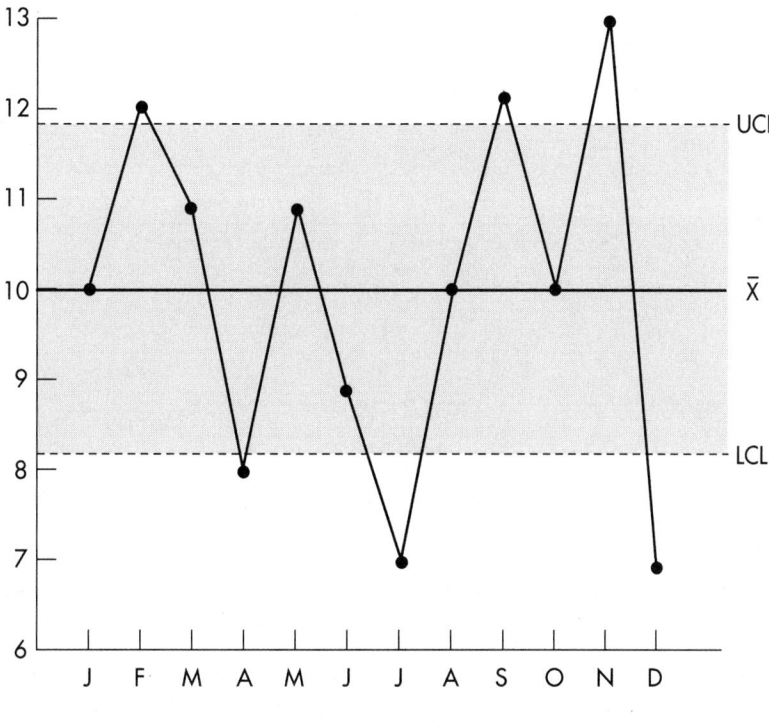

$\bar{X}$ = Mean
UCL = Upper control limit
LCL = Lower control limit

Figure 10-2   Schematic chart of upper and lower control limits.

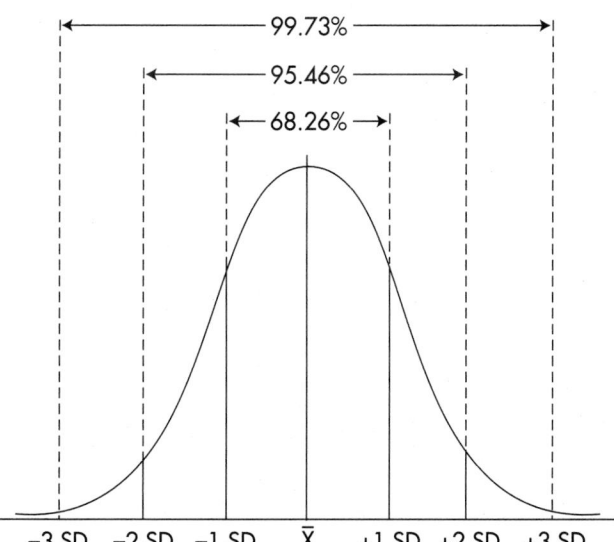

Figure 10-3   The normal distribution on the bell curve.

between these limits. Points that fall within the control limits are acceptable and are the result of normal or common process variation. These variances do not need to be evaluated further.

"The band between the control limits defines the random variation in the process. Points outside the limits indicate one or more assignable cases of variation. A process with only random causes present is said to be in 'statistical control.' Its output is considered to be as uniform as economically feasible."[5]

Any points that fall outside the upper or lower control limits are due to special causes and should be investigated to determine and correct the cause. Additional information about variation will be discussed in Chapter 12.

Manufacturing has typically used three SDs as control limits. By using less than this one runs the risk that a data point gets special investigation when in fact it is actually a normal process variation. Shewhart suggests using limits that minimize unnecessary investigation of process variation.

If data stay within the range of acceptability, the process is considered "in control." "In control" means that a process is consistent; however, it is important to remember that does not necessarily mean the product or service will meet customer needs. A process may be "in control" but not capable of meeting specifications. The goal is to get and keep key processes "in control" while constantly improving their performance. As greater consistency in the process is achieved, limits should be condensed (set closer to the mean) to further reduce process variation and to streamline operations.[8]

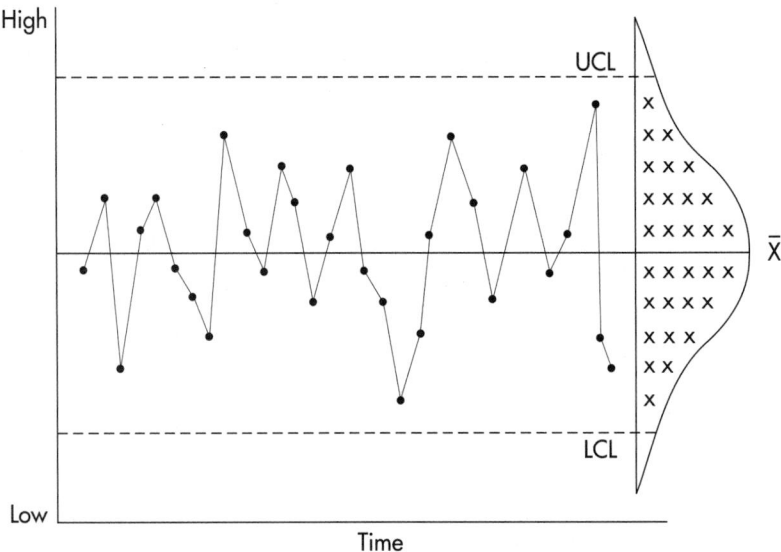

Figure 10-4   The relationship between a normal distribution and a control chart. (From Carey RG, Lloyd RC: *Measuring quality improvement in healthcare*, New York, 1995, Quality Resources.)

"The variation of any particular quality characteristic can be quantified by sampling the output of the process and estimating the parameters of its statistical distribution. Changes in the distribution can be revealed by plotting these parameters versus time."[5] This is done on a control chart, which is discussed in detail in Chapter 12. Target parameters serve as the basis for the development of a control chart.

A less desirable and less accurate way to set target parameters is to review the sample data from the baseline and determine a range that is equidistant from the target. For example, if the baseline is 80%, plus or minus 2% may be regarded as an acceptable range. If the results of a study fall within that range, they are judged to be successful and performance is maintained for that indicator. Consensus-based target parameters should allow for variation in performance that is caused by chance but should not be so wide as to be nondiscriminating. That is, they should allow for chance occurrences but should not allow for variation based on controllable service, practice, or governance variables. This method is not precise and should be used only during an initial measurement cycle (1 year). The data provided during this measurement cycle will afford the necessary information for performing the statistical analysis described earlier. We recommend that as a part of the annual summary report on each indicator, a formal statistical analysis of standard deviation be done so that the next year's target and target parameters can be set with confidence.

THE INDICATOR INFORMATION SET

The Joint Commission recommends completing the following information before using an indicator: defi-nition of terms, indicator type, rationale for use of the indicator, description of the indicator population, indi-cator data collection logic, and delineation of underlying factors that may explain variations in indicator data. This information is termed an indicator information set.[7]

Defining the terms used in the indicator ensures that everyone using the indicator is measuring the same data. Uniform operational definitions ensure uniform understanding.

Identification of indicator type means differentiating between a rate-based event versus a sentinel event or a process versus an outcome, whereas the rationale defines how or why the indicator will be beneficial. "By stating the rationale for an indicator, those considering the indicator gain a deeper understanding of its potential value and can better judge its merits."[7]

Description of the indicator population includes those customer groups or critical processes for which the indicator is relevant. For example, an indicator may be developed to measure patients who sustain a fall and have a serious injury within 2 hours of sedative administration. The indicator population may be composed of those patients receiving sedatives. Subcategories add specificity to the indicator population and permit stratification of data. For example, the subcategories of patients over the age of 75 years or ambulatory surgical patients provide homogeneous populations for stratification. Because different circumstances are at play for these populations, it is important to pinpoint specific populations so that the appropriate improvement strategies can be designed.

Indicator data logic refers to the development of data elements. Data elements are used to define the indicator event. "Terms used in the indicator are

1. Key Process of Service, Practice, Governance: _____

Developed by: _____ Date: _____

Team Leader: _____

Indicator Populations	Definitions of Terms and Tools:
1.	
2.	
3.	

Service Variables
1. _____
2. _____
3. _____

Practice Variables
1. _____
2. _____
3. _____

Governance Variables
1. _____
2. _____
3. _____

Figure 10-5 Indicator development form. (Copyright 1995 Jackie Katz and Ellie Green. Reprinted with permission.)

Continued.

155

translated into specific data elements, and corresponding data sources are identified by which data elements may be retrieved."[7] Data elements associated with the falls indicator might include the time elapsed between the administration of the sedative and the fall, and the type of sedative administered. It is from the data sources that specific information about the data elements is obtained. For example, review of the patient's progress record and the medication administration record would reveal the interval between the sedative administration and the fall. The type of sedative administered would be obtained from the physician's order sheet or the medication administration record.

Delineation of potential underlying factors refers to the identification of specific service, practice, or governance variables related to the indicator, which have a direct impact on the quality of patient outcomes for that critical process. Service variables include severity of illness, comorbid conditions, and any other nondisease factors that may affect the frequency of the event occurrence. Nondisease factors may include patient demographics. Patient variables may be beyond the control of the staff or system. Practice variables are those conditions related to the practitioner's performance that may potentially affect the quality of patient outcomes vis à vis a critical process. These factors usually relate to the practitioner's competence or productivity. Governance variables are those factors within the system that directly affect the quality of service provided and thus the outcomes for a particular process. The factors can include staffing, budgeting, or equipment availability. Unlike service variables, both practice and governance variables can be controlled.

THE INDICATOR DEVELOPMENT TOOL

In Chapter 9 we discussed the process of developing indicators. In this chapter we have considered setting targets and target parameters. Since these processes are interdependent, we designed an indicator development form that encompasses both processes. The tool is based on the Joint Commission's suggested indicator development form format. The form, depicted in Figure 10-5, integrates written standards as a basis for indicator development, the process of developing indicators, and target development.

Indicator	Target Parameters	Related Standards	Data Sources
A. Numerator: _____ Denominator:		1. 2. 3.	1. 2. 3.
B. Numerator: _____ Denominator:		1. 2. 3.	1. 2. 3.
C. Numerator: _____ Denominator:		1. 2. 3.	1. 2. 3.

Figure 10-5, cont'd.

1. Key Process of (Service) Practice, Governance: Developed by: *Pain Management Task Force*   Date: *12-17-9--*

Team Leader: *Jane Smith*

Pain Management

Indicator Populations	Definitions of Terms and Tools:
1. *Ca, breast* (*Drgs: 274,275*)	1. *McGill Pain Scale² (See attached)*
	2. *Acute Pain: intense and of short duration*
	(< 6 mos.)
2. *Ca, lung* (*Drg: 282*)	3. *Chronic pain: longer duration (> 6 mos.), continuous or*
	intermittent, can be intense
3. *Ca, colon* (*Drgs: 172,173*)	4. *PCAU: Patient Controlled Analgesia Unit*
	5. *Terminal: Predicted life expectancy < 3 months*

Service Variables
1. *Ability or will to participate in pain control i.e. the use of PCAU*
2. *Pain tolerance (affected by age, sex, duration of pain, severity of illness)*
3. *Fear and Anxiety level*

Practice Variables
1. *Personal frame of reference related to pain*
2. *Knowledge of pain theory and management*
3.

Governance Variables
1. *# of credentialed (pain) nurses/shift*
2. *# of PCAUs available*
3.

Figure 10-6   Completed indicator development form. (Copyright 1995 Jackie Katz and Ellie Green. Reprinted with permission.)

Continued.

The following are directions for completing the form.

Step 1: Key Processes of Service, Practice, or Governance. After choosing a key process of service, practice, or governance from the priority list, circle the appropriate word and write the topic in the blank provided. List the task force who developed the indicator, its team leader, and the date.

Step 2: Indicator Populations. List no more than three populations for whom this process is critical. Target populations for measurement will be chosen from this list.

Step 3: Definition of Terms and Tools. List any terms or tools associated with the key process. Define any terms that may have multiple interpretations, including acronyms and abbreviations or terms that have a specific meaning particular to a department or division. Attach a copy of any tools related to the key process (e.g., the Norton scale for pressure ulcer staging) or a classification tool for severity of medication errors. Uniform definitions ensure uniform understanding and greater accuracy and reliability in data collection.

Step 4: Service Variables (related to the key process being studied). Identify up to three variables related to the service that may have a direct impact on performance levels within the key process under investigation. These can be controllable or uncontrollable factors and might include age, sex, comorbidity, educational level, and so on.

Step 5: Practice Variables (related to key process being studied). Identify up to three variables related to the staff that may have a direct impact on the performance levels within the key process under investigation. These can be controllable or uncontrollable factors and might include years of experience, credentials, academic preparation, and so on.

Step 6: Governance Variables (related to key process being studied). Identify up to three variables related to the system that may have a direct impact on the performance levels within the key process under investigation. These can be controllable or uncontrollable factors and might include staffing, work shift differences, budget constraints, equipment availability, and so on.

Step 7: Indicators. Three boxes labeled *A, B,* and *C* provide space for the development of indicators related to the key process of service, practice, or governance identified in step 1. Use the information in steps 2 through 6 to assist in the development of specific

Indicator	Target Parameters	Related Standards	Data Sources
A. Numerator: # of Terminal Ca Patients using PCAU who express level 0-1 on McGill Pain Scale **Denominator:** Total # of Terminal Ca Patients	85-95%	1. Practice Guideline for Management of Acute Pain 2. PCAU Procedure 3.	1. Patient's progress record 2. Observation 3. Patient interview Patient's progress record
B. Numerator: # of oncology RNs certified in pain control management **Denominator:** Total # of oncology RNs	90-100%	1. Core Curriculum for Pain Management 2. 3.	1. Exam scores 2. 3.
C. Numerator: # of PCAUs in use on Terminal Ca Patients **Denominator:** Total # of Terminal Ca Patients able to participate in PCAU	90-100%	1. Goal related to resource availability 2. 3.	1. Observation 2. Unit inventory 3. Census

Figure 10-6,   cont'd.

indicators. Enter one indicator per box. Remember to write each indicator as a ratio.

Step 8: Target Parameters. Enter the target parameters that have been set for each indicator.

Step 9: Standards Identification. List the structure, process, or outcome standards that are related to the indicator to be studied as identified in step 1.

Step 10: Data Sources. List the sources for retrieval of information for each indicator. Sources can be documentation, observation, interview, and the like.

Figure 10-6 shows a completed form, using the example of pain management.

Developing process or outcome indicators for key processes of service, practice, or governance focuses the measurement activities on the three domains that control performance. Using this method to develop indicators and target parameters may be a dramatic departure from the traditional approach. This method, however, fosters a standards-based approach to the development of performance indicators and a statistical approach to setting the target parameters. The data yielded by these processes will ultimately more accurately and reliably represent the level of performance within the organization.

Once the indicator development form has been completed, the process of planning for data collection can begin.

REFERENCES

1. *Agenda for Change kit,* Chicago, 1990, Joint Commission on Accreditation of Healthcare Organizations.
2. Brassard M: *The memory jogger +,* Meuthen, Mass, 1989, GOAL/QPC.
3. Carey R, Lloyd R: *Measuring quality improvement in healthcare,* New York, 1995, Quality Resources.
4. Hospitals use M & E to improve quality, *Joint Commission Perspectives,* 11(2): 1, 1991.
5. Juran JM: *Juran's quality control handbook,* ed 4, New York, 1988, McGraw-Hill.
6. Long B, Phipps W, Cassmeyer V: *Medical-surgical nursing: a nursing process approach,* ed 3: St. Louis, 1993, Mosby.
7. *Primer on Indicator Development and Application,* Chicago, 1991, Joint Commission on Accreditation of Healthcare Organizations.
8. Schroeder P: *Improving quality and performance: tools and techniques.* In Schroeder P, editor: *Improving quality performance,* St. Louis, 1994, Mosby.
9. Shewhart WA: *Economic control of quality of manufactured product,* New York, 1931, D. Van Nostrand.

Chapter 11

Collecting and Organizing Multidisciplinary Data

In God we trust. All others must use data.

W. Edwards Deming

Well here I am, flat on my back literally and in other ways, right ankle resting on three pillows. Gravity is vital to treatment...

Dr. Sch... ordered from the drug store (in the hospital) a paste for the itch that had set in Minneapolis. The drug store was out of one of the ingredients: must order it from the wholesaler, and can not make it up till Monday. I need it tonight. On prodding from Dr. Sch... the drug store sent someone out to another drug store to fetch the missing ingredient. The paste came up that evening.

Unbelievable: the same scenario took place some days later.

I wonder why is a registered nurse making beds? It seems to me that making beds is not good use of her time. Her education and skills could be put to better use of her time. Her education and skills could be put to better use, so it seems to me.

The chair in this room is huge, would seat two people, takes up an exorbitant amount of space, heavy to move.... The coat hangers here are that maddening kind, found in most hotels....

My nurse of the moment put on a hot towel this afternoon. "I'll be back in twenty minutes, and if I don't come, please ring." Sixty-five minutes later I pressed the button. A helper came in; explained to me that this was not her kind of job, so she canceled the light for the nurse, and went off. Thirty minutes later I rang again for the nurse. The same helper came and observed again that the job was not her line of duty, so again she canceled the light and went off. The solution was simple, for me, merely discard the towel and

insulate myself with the rules or against the rules. The same event recurred another day.

What is the moral of all this? What have we learned? One answer: the superintendent of the hospital needs to learn something about supervision. Only he can make the changes in procedure and responsibility that are required.

Talks between physicians and nurses, even with the head nurse, accomplish nothing. The same problems that I have noted will continue. A physician cannot change the system. A head nurse cannot change the system. Meanwhile, who would know? To work harder will not solve the problem. The nurses couldn't work any harder.—W. Edwards Deming[3]

Dr. Deming describes his hospitalization in graphic detail. It is a scenario that is familiar to most busy health care professionals. Deming's description of his hospital care is the sort of ordinary event that never becomes part of a performance improvement study. Why? Because most of the data collected in a health care organization is directed toward process, not performance improvement. Process includes all the tasks that health care workers perform in carrying out their jobs. Process data collection begins with, "Did the employee...?" The most frequently collected data in instances like the Deming scenario likely would answer the question, "Was the treatment given?" And the answer would be yes, the treatment was given. But to the customer, Deming, the treatment was very unsatisfactory, even though it may have been medically beneficial. Therefore, the data does not reflect customer satisfaction.

So, how does a health care organization measure the many issues that irritate customers and frustrate employees and management? How is data collection transferred from the superficial, retrospective, search-for-problems style of check sheet to a meaningful gathering of information about service, practice, and governance outcomes?

There are three places in a health care organization that should use the traditional quality control style checksheets: on setup of equipment, the equipment itself, and some processes within the health care organization.

Quality control on setup of equipment. Before beginning the administration of general anesthesia, putting a patient on the heart-lung bypass machine, using the crash cart, intubating a patient, or performing diagnostic radiology, and so on, the practitioner must go through a checklist or flow chart, making sure all equipment, such as dials, gauges, hoses, lights, and drawers, is functioning properly before proceeding with the procedure. If something is not functioning properly, a correction is made *before* the procedure is performed or the equipment used.

Quality control on the equipment itself. The equipment itself must be closely controlled if performance improvement is to be maintained. This type of quality control is preventive in nature and is quite different in concept from repair of equipment breakdowns. This preventive form of equipment maintenance includes a carefully drawn set of criteria, which define the essential performance characteristics of the equipment. Then, on a schedule strictly adhered to, the equipment is checked against those criteria. For example, calibration of some machinery is essential for accurate outcomes. There is a piece of equipment in almost every department of the health care organization that falls into this category—from the glucose monitoring equipment to the radiation machinery. This control of equipment also includes mechanisms for random and regular checks of equipment that affects service, practice, and/or governance outcomes, such as refrigeration, sterilization, lab equipment, gauges, dials on the wall that deliver oxygen, and the computerized blood gas machines, the elevators, backup emergency generators, and dishwashing equipment. This is the technology measurement that is a part of THE BLUEPRINT. (See Chapter 3.)

Some processes within the health care organization. These processes include quality control on autopsies, medication administration (especially narcotic counts at the end of every shift), admissions, discharges, risk management processes such as transporting patients,

and utilization management activities such as utilization of beds. There are other processes, such as documentation, that call for quality control. For all of these processes a checksheet may be utilized, because the desired outcome is the degree of worker compliance to the policies, procedures, and practice guidelines of the organization.

These types of quality control checks that focus on what the employee does traditionally have composed the majority of the data collected in health care organizations. Today, the performance improvement initiative taking place in the health care industry is quite different from quality control. The performance improvement emphasis has been designed to support the *patient-centered,* performance-focused, functional orientation of health care organizations. Rather than evaluating specific departments and services, asking, "Did the employee . . . ," surveyors are assessing, across organizations, the performance of important patient-focused and organizational *functions.* This type of accreditation process attempts to answer these questions: (a) Were the correct processes performed? (b) Were they performed according to established standards? (c) Does the organization have an organization-wide, interdisciplinary, interactive, performance-oriented, consistent, team-based, well-planned, and open program for improving its performance?

This new approach means that health care organizations will identify processes that are troublesome, form a team to track performance of the processes over a period of time to discern trends and patterns of process "breakdowns," and then systematically "fix" each troublesome component of the process until it is working smoothly. This is the nuts and bolts of performance improvement. In the tracking phase of performance improvement there may be some checksheet "quality control style" data collection. However, these checksheets will be for a specific purpose so that they will fit into the overall picture of the process to be improved and not just exist for the sake of having an indicator or two to satisfy surveyors.

To accomplish this, health care organizations will adopt a new approach to data collection. There will be a rethinking of the traditional approach, which focused on staff members' completion of tasks. The new, more realistic, customer-focused approach utilizes meaningful data about functional outcomes and reactions to the service, practice, and governance that customers experienced while dealing with the health care organization.

For the purpose of this chapter, *data* is defined as documented observations and customer feedback, both verbal and written, over a designated period of time. This definition is useful because the methods and tools presented in this chapter are customer-focused, emphasizing methods to obtain feedback, including opinions about the health care organization's services received, staff practices witnessed, and overall satisfaction level with the management of customers' entire health care experience.

Data collection is the backbone of a performance measurement program. According to Walter Shewhart, "Knowledge begins with data and ends in other data."[3] Shewhart emphasized the importance of data to build knowledge. He especially focused on collecting and displaying data over a period of time.[6] Without accurate data, there cannot be accurate analysis or solutions.

If health care professionals desire satisfaction with their service, practice, and governance, there must be tools in place to collect not only *objective* data on checksheets but also *subjective* data. Subjective data includes feelings and perceptions about the services received. "For performance improvement, it is important not only to be concerned with ... process but also to learn about people's feelings and experiences. Customer satisfaction depends in part on how the customer feels when he or she uses the product or service."[6]

THE DEMING CREDO

In health care, both objective and subjective data are necessary. Both process and outcome must drive all data collection. It is a double-faceted approach as depicted in Figure 11-1. "Data—especially data related to customers' perceptions of quality—are useful in answering, 'What are we trying to accomplish?' Data also provide some of the background necessary to answer "How will we know that a change is an improvement?"[6]

"In God we trust. All others must use data." Mary Walton explains this Deming credo for improvement in *The Deming Management Method.* She states, "Critical to the Deming method is the need to base decisions as much as possible on accurate and timely data, not on wishes, hunches or 'experience'."[8] The bumper sticker that says, "Accountants Do It With Data," although amusing, is not far off the mark. It also endorses Deming's credo. It might be well for all health care professionals to follow the Deming credo. We should make sure that we do all of our analyses and use data to draw all our conclusions.

A training manual for Komatsu Ltd., a Japanese competitor of Caterpillar Tractor Company, states: "The first step in quality control is to judge and act on the basis of facts. Views not backed by data are more likely to include personal opinions, exaggeration and mistaken impressions."[8] If accurate data is of paramount importance in manufacturing tractors, how much more so it is in guiding health care professionals in decision-making processes about patient care, professional practice, and governance!

Unfortunately, much confusion surrounds data collection in today's health care organizations. The art of

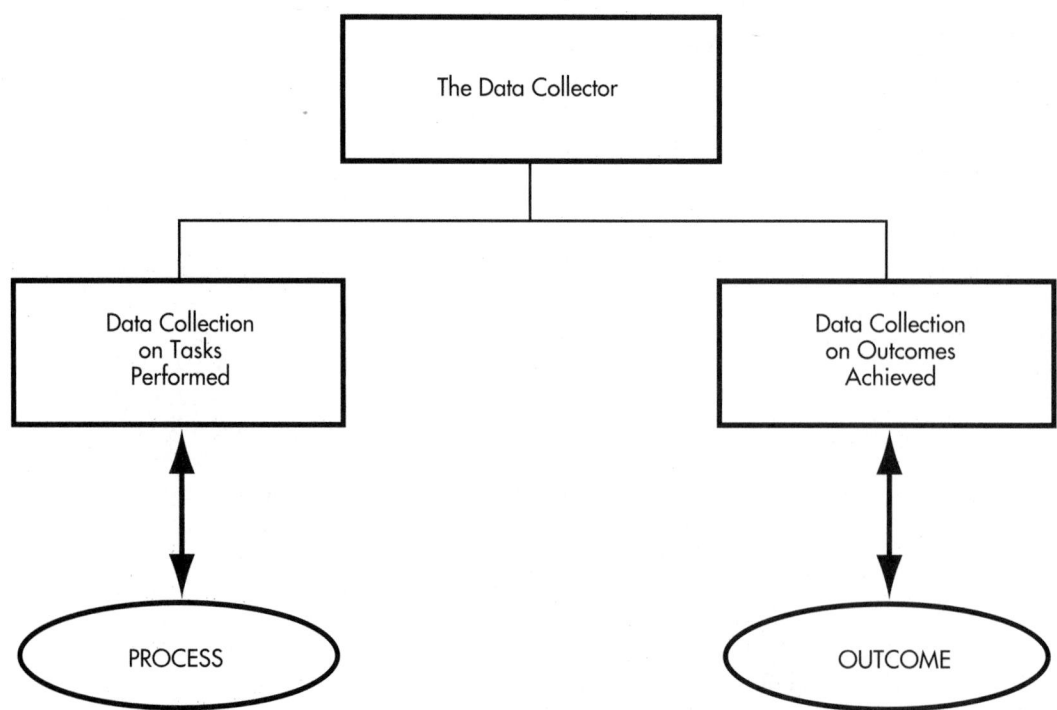

Figure 11-1   The double-faceted approach to data collection.

accurate data collection using simple statistics is new to many health care professionals. When sound decisions are made, plans are carried out correctly the first time.

PLANNING FOR DATA COLLECTION

Because it is easy for a health care organization to become swamped in useless data collection, it is necessary to establish a clear purpose for this crucial step in the performance measurement program. What is the purpose of data collection and how is it used to improve performance? Data collection is used to:

- reveal performance improvement opportunities.
- confirm the extent of variations in process performance.
- track and trend process performance.
- predict future process performance.
- confirm the success of changes.

The data collection team should pose these questions and establish answers in writing before *any* data collection is begun:

- What are the goals for collecting this data?
- Who should collect the data?
- In which domain should the data be collected?
- For what purpose should the data be collected?
- What are the data sources?
- How much data should be collected?
- What tools will be used?
- What bias exists?

All of these questions need to be answered before data collection begins. Once these questions are addressed, data collection becomes a meaningful tool in the organization's decision-making process. When sound decisions are made, plans are carried out correctly the first time. Performance management professionals can make accurate decisions about conserving or expending resources when those decisions are rooted in accurate data.

THE GOALS OF DATA COLLECTION

Because accurate data collection is the cornerstone of performance improvement, data collection plays a vital role in the performance management system. There are six key goals of data collection.

Goal one. The first goal of data collection is to set up a system to ensure accuracy of information on which to base future decisions. A poor decision made as the result of inaccurate data can result in harm to a patient, misspent funds, wasted time, improper utilization of personnel, inadequate or surplus purchases of equipment, the creation of inappropriate standards, and so on. Resources are precious in today's health care environment, and a poor decision based on inaccurate data can be extremely costly to an organization.

Goal two. The second goal of data collection is to avoid all punitive measures associated with the results of collected data. When workers feel that their jobs are threatened by the results of the data that they have collected, they may simply hide the data. This does not mean that they are bad employees. It simply means that if they feel that their job security is jeopardized by accurately reporting data, they may pursue a safe course and maintain the status quo. Dr. Deming says, "In the perception of most employees preserving the status quo is the only safe course."[7] Creating an environment of nonpunitive, safe data collection eliminates fear of repercussions and fosters accuracy and truth in reporting data results. Employees will cooperate with collecting and organizing data when they feel secure and unafraid of retaliation and negative consequences.

Goal three. The third goal of data collection is to pinpoint the exact areas of the organization that contain the performance opportunity. Once an important opportunity to improve is selected, measurement focuses on every area of the organization that "touches" this process. When this approach is used, a global picture of the improvement opportunity emerges.

Goal four. The fourth goal of data collection is to establish the degree to which improvement has occurred after the implementation of an improvement action plan. Data collection is a futile exercise unless the information is used to create improvement in service, practice, and governance of the organization. Data must be collected following the initiation of every improvement action plan to either confirm or deny expected results.

Goal five. The fifth goal is to collect data at regular intervals on all critical processes to demonstrate sustained improvement. This requires that data be used to track and discern trends or special cause variation in results.

Goal six. The sixth goal of data collection is to collect both subjective and objective data. Objective data usually fall into the category of quality control previously discussed. This means that the data collection process consists of checklists that provide yes or no answers. Quality control is a necessary part of all performance measurement programs, but it provides a very straightforward approach that does not include variables. For example, the crash cart checksheet, initialed at the beginning of every shift, shows simply that the machinery was in working order at that time. If there is a blank space indicating that the crash cart was *not* checked, there is no indication of *why* it was not checked. In other words, quality control checksheets fail to capture explanations of variables. On the other hand, subjective data provide reasons for variables. Collecting subjective data requires more time, planning, testing, and analyzing, because it deals with the customer's perceptions, thoughts, feelings, and satisfaction with service, practice, and governance of the health care organization. To meet accreditation requirements health care organizations will want a blend of both types of data collection.

SELECTING WHO COLLECTS DATA

Data collection must be planned, organized, ongoing, and systematic. Achieving this requires organization as well as delegation of accountability and responsibility. The job is too big for one person to assume. The responsibility for organization-wide data collection is enormous. Therefore, four councils, under the direction of the quality management board (QMB), serve as the performance management resource center. Teams are then appointed by the councils to assess and improve assigned processes; this includes performing the data collection for the performance improvement process that is under study. (Refer to Chapter 5 to learn how to structure an organization for performance improvement.)

This orchestration of efforts prevents duplication and waste of resources and provides structure for improvement. In order for improvement to occur, there must be a regular flow of consistent data from all departments of the organization as well as from other health care alliances and supportive services. These data are then used to track and discern trends in results over a period of time. Improvement may then be made with solid, provable data instead of hunches, guesses, or opinions.

DATA COLLECTED IN EACH DOMAIN

It is important that each process under review have a trifocus. Performance management efforts should be directed to all three domains, because the domains are interactive and each affects the whole. Collecting data from the perspective of each domain helps to present a complete picture of the situation and processes that need improving. This ensures that improvement task forces will undertake to correct or develop pertinent processes in the correct domain.

THE PURPOSE OF DATA COLLECTION

There are four important reasons to collect data:

The first reason is to validate that things are happening the way the organization plans for them to happen. Once an organization creates a standards-based system, it may then measure the standards to ensure that the standards are being adhered to by the staff members. This assessment will produce data that will confirm or deny the efficacy of the standards. Data that show positive outcomes and a high level of customer satisfaction demonstrate that the organization-wide performance management system is functioning well.

The second reason for data collection is to provide a basis for change or improvement in the service, practice, or governance of the organization. Positive change or improvement is neither happenstance nor instantaneous. The Ford Motor Company did not go from producing the Model T to manufacturing the Taurus instantly or by chance. Without continuous research—data collection and development—and without acting on the data, the automobile industry might still be using a crank to start its engines. Health care also must continue to change, develop, and improve. Accurate data will lay the foundation for necessary change and continual improvement.

The third reason to collect data is to provide a rationale for increasing or decreasing resources or maintaining the same level of resources within the organization. Health care organizations lack resources to hire, fire, purchase, plan, or govern based on a "hunch." Sound data collection can prevent the carrying out of inappropriate, costly "hunches." Accurate data ensure that the organization makes decisions based on factual information grounded in the realities of current health care practices.

The fourth reason to collect data is to provide a basis for the development of reliable performance targets for evaluation to be used in tracking and discerning trends or special cause variation of service, practice, and governance of the organization. Without a historic database gathered over a period of months to years, target parameters are, at best, guesses. Performance targets will never be reliable until sound scientific and statistical methods are employed in their development. Accurate data are needed for targets to evolve into meaningful statistics that are beneficial to organizations.

SOURCES OF DATA

Data come from three types of sources, which reflect the three domains of health care: the consumer of the service, the deliverer of the service, and the management of the service. Some examples of consumer sources include the patient who receives the service, the family and significant others, third-party payers, and the community. Some examples of practice sources, or deliverers of service, include health care workers, physicians, and allied personnel beyond the walls of the organization, such as vendors and contractors who must interact in the organization's continuum of care. Management sources include department managers, supervisors, the top management team, and the board of directors.

All three domains contain important data sources and each domain should be considered when designing the performance management system. Limiting data collection to one source will narrow the scope of the collection process and restrict its usefulness. Similarly, utilizing only one type of collection tool will limit the scope and narrow the focus of the collection process. Many different tools should be used.

AMOUNT OF DATA TO BE COLLECTED

The volume of data to be collected will vary, depending on the type of study being undertaken. As part of THE BLUEPRINT, we established the guidelines that appear in the box below to assist in determining appropriate sample sizes. Using these guidelines or developing similar guidelines of its own will help an organization establish some fundamental operating rules for measurement. As would be expected, a query review requires a larger sample than a routine review, and a sentinel event necessitates investigation of every incident.

We recommend a sample size of 5% or 30, whichever is the larger for a routine review. The study may involve 30 charts, patients, nurses, doctors, and so on, depending on its focus.

A query review occurs when data demonstrate a variance outside the established target parameters that cannot readily be explained or justified. For a query review, we recommend a sample size of 10% or 60, whichever is greater. The study may involve 60 charts, patients, nurses, doctors, procedures, and so on, depending on its focus.

An intensive review is conducted when unusual occurrences or trends within the organization demonstrate a negative impact on patient outcomes. We recommend that intensive reviews use a sample size of 15% or 90, whichever is greater. The study may involve 90 charts, patients, nurses, doctors, procedures, and so on, depending on its focus.

The sentinel event review is conducted when adverse happenings extend a patient's length of stay in the facility, compromise a patient's quality of life, or cause death. Examples include exsanguination, airway obstruction, electrical hazards, medication errors resulting in death, administering the wrong blood type to a patient, and the like. Sentinel events require 100% target and investigation of every event.

TOOLS USED IN DATA COLLECTION

Seven different types of tools are typically used to collect data. They are:

- Data collection tools
- Tools for management rounds
- End-of-shift reports
- Suggestion boxes
- Satisfaction surveys
- Hot lines
- Focus groups

Data Collection Tools

Essential to any good performance management system is a data collection tool that is simple to understand, contains necessary data when completed, and is flexible enough to be used throughout the organization. THE BLUEPRINT contains a data collection tool that has been widely tested in health care facilities and has met the criteria of understandability, pertinence, and flexibility (Figure 11-2). It has been designed to be used in conjunction with the indicator development tool (see Figure 10-5). The indicator development tool is always completed first, then the data collection tool is filled in. Together, these tools provide a comprehensive yet easy-to-use data collection format for the improvement team. An explanation of how the data collection tool is used follows. The numbers in the explanation correspond to the sections identified by number in Figure 11-2.

1. Fill in the date when data collection begins.
2. Fill in the date when the study ends.
3. Enter a study number. Assigning study numbers permits easy comparison of data on graphic displays.
4. Enter the name of the department in which the study is being conducted.
5. Identify the name of the person(s) collecting the data.
6. Enter the key process about which data are to be collected. Note that this will also have been designated on the indicator development tool.

KATZ-GREEN GUIDELINES FOR DATA COLLECTION

Type of Study	Sample Size
Routine review	5% or 30 (whichever is greater)
Query review	10% or 60 (whichever is greater)
Intensive review	15% or 90 (whichever is greater)
Sentinel event	100% (every event)

DATA COLLECTION TOOL

KEY:
+ MET
− NOT MET
E EXCEPTION

1. STUDY START DATE: *Jan. 15, 1995*
2. STUDY STOP DATE: *Jan. 30, 1995*
3. STUDY NUMBER: *# 157-A*

4. DEPARTMENT NAME: *Oncology*
5. DATA COLLECTORS: 1. *Sheri Forquer, RN* 2. *Karen McClure, RN*
   3. *Angie Dennison, RN* 4. *Heidi Bowen, RN*
   5. *Laura Folkenberg, RN* 6. *Melissa Hormon, RN*

6. PROCESS: *Pain mgt. of terminal oncology patients*
7. HIGH RISK [X] HIGH VOLUME [X] PROBLEM PRONE [X] HIGH COST [X]

8. SAMPLE SIZE: *30* OUT OF *30 **

9. EXCEPTIONS: 1. *RNs employed < 3 months*
   2.
   3.

10. INFORMATION/REMARKS: *Indicator B (Staff Process)*
    * Exceptions will be eliminated and sample size lowered.

11. IDENTIFICATION #	1. 742	2. 387	3. 698	4. 259	5. 916	6. 857	7. 519	8. 174	9. 257	10. 425	11. 155	12. 928	13. 273	14. 891	15. 359	16. 792	17. 483	18. 654	19. 527	20. 941	21. 188	22. 859	23. 269	24. 839	25. 337	26. 712	27. 647	28. 499	29. 558	30. 139
13. INDICATOR: # of oncology RNs certified in pain control mgt. / Total # of oncology RNs	+	−	+	e	+	+	+	e	+	+	+	+	+	e	+	+	−	+	+	+	+	+	+	+	+	+	e	−	+	+

14. Totals: E = 4 + = 26 − = 3
15. Results: % = 88%
16. Within Limits: YES ☐ NO ✓

17. DEMOGRAPHIC DATA: RNs who did not pass c̄ 90% score on written test
18. DEMOGRAPHIC DATA: RNs who took certification test twice
19. DEMOGRAPHIC DATA: RNs who took certification test more than twice
DEMOGRAPHIC DATA:
DEMOGRAPHIC DATA:

20. 11.5% failed to pass certification on first try
21. 26.9% had to take the test twice to achieve 90% passing score
22. 7.7% had to repeat the test more than twice to achieve a passing score

Figure 11-2 Completed data collection tool. (Copyright 1995 Jackie Katz and Ellie Green. Reprinted with permission.)

7. Check the appropriate box or boxes that describe whether the process of service, practice, or governance is high volume, high risk, problem prone, or high cost.

8. Indicate the sample size. Entering the sample size helps provide a complete picture of the study. For example: 30 of 250 patient charts; 30 of 42 ventilator patients; 30 of 57 staff members.

9. List any exceptions. Exceptions are those factors that would prevent the data elements from being evaluated. For example, if patients' verbal responses to pain management were the focus of a study and the sample size included every patient, then the comatose patient would be an exception.

10. The "Remarks" section is provided for the evaluator to record any pertinent information about the study that has no designated place on the tool.

11. Identification numbers for up to 30 items in a sample are listed across the top of the tool. To maintain confidentiality of the samples, whether a customer, staff member, or system function, codes known only to the performance improvement team and the QMB may be used. For many studies, however, in which confidentiality is not an issue, patients' identification numbers or staff members' employment numbers may be used.

12. Enter the indicator from the indicator development tool. Since indicators take the form of a fraction or ratio, as a convenience to the data collector, the spaces in which to enter the numerator and denominator are clearly marked.

13. Enter a + if the response is positive to the indicator, enter a – if the response is negative to the indicator, and enter an *e* for an exception. There is a space for each response per sample. The key is located in the upper right hand corner of the form.

14. These spaces are used to total the number of positive and negative responses to the indicator and the number of exceptions. Add and enter the number of positive responses. Add and enter the number of negative responses. Add and enter the number of exceptions. Subtract the number of exceptions from the total sample size. In the example shown there were four exceptions from a sample size of 30. Subtracting the four exceptions from the sample size of 30 leaves 26 in the sample.

15. This column is used to enter the percent of compliance. To calculate compliance divide the total number of positive responses by the adjusted (i.e., excluding exceptions) sample size of 26. In the example there were 23 positive responses; 23 divided by 26 equals 0.88 or 88%.

16. This column is used in conjunction with the target parameters determined on the indicator development form. If the data fall within the established target parameters, then the box marked "yes" is checked. If the data fall outside the established parameters, then the box marked "no" is checked.

17-19. Boxes 17 to 19 with their accompanying spaces permit data collectors to record relevant demographic data. Factors that may assist in the identification of patterns or trends when data analysis occurs are considered demographic data. In the example, data were collected about the number of oncology RNs certified in pain control management on the oncology unit. Demographic data include RNs who failed to achieve the 90% mandatory passing score on the first try.

20-22. These boxes are used for a brief analysis of the demographic data. In the example, 11.5% of the RNs failed to pass the certification exam on the first try. This additional information provides an extra dimension of thoroughness to the analysis. Demographic data may include the department, the shift on which an incident occurred, or the nurse or physician involved. This portion may include information about the patient being studied, such as height, weight, sex, and room number. It may include any of the service, practice, or governance variables listed on the indicator development form.

QMB Tracking Tool

In THE BLUEPRINT, a QMB tracking tool is reproduced on the reverse side of the data collection tool. Once the data collection has been completed by the team, the data collection tool is returned to the QMB, and their review and tracking are entered on the QMB tracking tool. This form is shown in Figure 11-3. Directions for use are as follows:

1. Copy the indicator from the data collection tool to avoid the necessity of flipping back and forth each time new information is entered.

2. Enter the date.

(1) Indicator: (2) Date:

(3) I. Analysis of Initial Data (attach control chart)

(4) *Recommendations:*

      ☐ Justification of Variance required
      Route to:
         ☐ Quality Management Board (QMB)
         ☐ Service Improvement Council (SIC)
         ☐ Practice Improvement Council (PIC)
         ☐ Governance Improvement Council (GIC)
         ☐ Performance Measurement Council
    ☐ Continue Performance Measurement Plan

(5) II. Justification

(6) *Recommendations:*

      ☐ No further action needed, continue Performance Improvement Plan
      ☐ Additional assessment
         ☐ second reviewer
         ☐ query review
         ☐ intensive review

Figure 11-3   QMB tracking tool. (Copyright 1995 Jackie Katz and Ellie Green. Reprinted with permission.)

3. Enter the analysis of the initial monitoring in brief sentences.
4. If a justification of variance is required, check with the council, which must make the justification and then route the tool to it. Either the Performance Measurement Council, the Service Improvement Council, the Practice Improvement Council, or the Governance Improvement Council will receive the tool and investigate the variance. If no justification is required, check the box marked "continue performance measurement plan."
5. This space is for the council to whom the tool was routed in step 4, to write a justification of the identified variance. This justification is returned to the QMB.
6. Recommendations are then made by the QMB based on its analysis of step 5. The QMB may decide that no further action is necessary, in which case assessment will continue as planned.

If the QMB decides that an additional review is necessary, it must check the type of review that is required—either a second reviewer opinion, a query review by a department or person, or an intensive review by an appropriate council.

Tools for Management Rounds

Figure 11-4 presents a simple tool that may be used to collect data on administrative rounds. It consolidates information from a trifocus of service, practice, and governance. Once completed, it may be kept in a looseleaf binder for easy reference. When an issue or concern repeatedly surfaces, this tool helps to justify appropriate actions or expenditure of resources to solve the problem. No management round should exceed 1/2 hour of the manager's time. For this reason the tool is designed with space for interviewing a maximum of three staff members and three customers as well as space to make no more than three observations on any given round. The tool is self-explanatory. It is especially useful for novice managers.

End-of-Shift Report

Figure 11-5 is an example of an end-of-shift report. This form is one of the most popular interdisciplinary data collection tools of THE BLUEPRINT. Used successfully by many hospitals, it provides concurrent, continuous, planned, organized data collection from all three sources—consumer, deliverer, and manager—in other words, the three domains. This end-of-shift report replaces the former "generic screen" monitors. This tool is most useful in patient care services as it is designed. A similar form could be designed for non-patient care areas with specific information pertinent to individual departments.

The end-of-shift report provides a method for continuous data collection about the happenings in each department with relatively little effort. Blank copies (at least 21; one for each shift for 1 week) are hung on a clipboard in a work area visible to all personnel. Nurses, physicians, supervisors, risk managers, infection control nurses, and all other personnel are encouraged not only to use the information on the report but also to add pertinent information.

It is the duty of the supervisor or manager of the shift to oversee the completion of the report at the end of his or her shift and replace it on the clipboard. The reports accumulate for the week. At the end of the week, the data are compiled by the department manager. The information is tabulated and sent to QMB for organizational tracking.

One of the outstanding features of this end-of-shift report is the built-in tracking of "clinical outliers."

We coined the term *clinical outlier* to designate a patient care situation that extends beyond a time frame established by an interdisciplinary task force. Examples of clinical outliers include invasive devices such as IVs, arterial lines, Swan-Ganz catheters, staples, sutures, urinary catheters, and endotracheal tubes, which are not removed within the organization's designated time frames. Once the interdisciplinary task force completes its list of clinical outlier time frames, the list is posted in every nurses' station beside the end-of-shift report. When an invasive device remains in a patient beyond the time frame established by the task force, the patient is listed on the end-of-shift report as a clinical outlier. It is the duty of the charge nurse to list each outlier and the duty of the attending physician or RN to justify or explain the reason for the extended use of the device on the clinical outlier justification tool on the reverse side of the end-of-shift report. Figure 11-6 shows the justification tool that is printed on the reverse side of the end-of-shift report. Because there are no national guidelines to direct the interdisciplinary task force in creating clinical outliers, each organization's task force must establish guidelines for its own use. Some specialty organizations and some manufacturers may have suggested guidelines that might prove helpful to the task force.

The end-of-shift report obviates the need for occurrence or generic screening, because nothing "slips through the cracks" when this method is used. In fact, it not only becomes one of the organization's most valuable data collection tools but also can save the organization hundreds of dollars each year in setting up and carrying out measurement studies. Numerous small studies are unnecessary when the data are being collected already on every shift in every department in the organization.

The QMB may use the data from each department's end-of-shift report to create a division-wide picture of performance. Using this ongoing data collection method ensures that the QMB will have concurrent information that will alert it to any adverse trends and allow it to take immediate remedial action.

Here are the directions for using the end-of-shift report. The numbers on the form correspond to the following numbered explanations.

1. Enter the date, shift, and department.
2. In the spaces in this column, list the room number and acuity classification for the surgeries that occur during the shift, the patients who are admitted during the shift for a short stay, and those admitted for observation.
3. Enter the routine admissions to the department by room number and acuity classification.

DATE _____ TIME _____ DEPT. _____

EMPLOYEES INTERVIEWED	CONCERNS/ ACCOLADES	ACTIONS TO BE TAKEN	DATE OF ACTION
1.			
2.			
3.			

CUSTOMERS INTERVIEWED	CONCERNS/ ACCOLADES	ACTIONS TO BE TAKEN	DATE OF ACTION
1.			
2.			
3.			

MANAGER OBSERVATION	CONCERNS/ ACCOLADES	ACTIONS TO BE TAKEN	DATE OF ACTION
1.			
2.			
3.			

Figure 11-4   Management rounds performance data collection tool.

1. Date: Shift: Department:

Rm #/Classification	3. Admissions	4. Discharges	5. Problems related to:
Surgeries (Reg):	Rm #/Class.	Rm #/Class.	1) Bed utilization:
			2) Physicians:
Short Stays:			3) Equipment/Supplies:
			4) Assignments/Staff Members:
Observations:			
			5) Patient/Family:

(left margin bracket labeled 2.)

6.	Transferred to another facility:	
7.	Emergency Procedures/Codes/Deaths	8. Outstanding Employee:
		Why?
		9. Outstanding Physician:
		Why?

10.	Pace/Workload: Quiet Steady Busy Very Busy Short-staffed by acuity Specify:

11.	Report patients who: Name/Rm#
	1. Develop a decubitus not present on admission
	2. Have a decubitus present on admission
	3. Develop Pulmonary Edema not present on admission
	4. Develop CHF not present on admission
	5. Aspirate within the hospital
	6. Develop post-op respiratory problems
	7. Develop IV complications
	8. Fall/Injuries
	9. Temps > 100° F
	10. Develop post-op wound infection
	11. Hemorrhage

12.	Also report department clinical outliers
	1.
	2.
	3.
	4.
13.	Comments:
	14. Signature(s):

Figure 11-5   The end-of-shift report. (Copyright 1991 Roane General Hospital. Reprinted with permission.)

JUSTIFICATION
OF CLINICAL OUTLIERS

DEPT _____

SHIFT _____

DATE _____

Key

1 - acceptable performance
no recommendations
2 - acceptable nonperformance
with recommendations
3 - unacceptable nonperformance

PATIENT	CLINICAL OUTLIERS	JUSTIFICATION BY MD/RN	RATING		
			1	2	3

Figure 11-6 Justification tool. (Copyright 1995 Jackie Katz and Ellie Green. Reprinted with permission.)

4. Enter the room number and acuity classification of the patients discharged from the department during this shift.

5. Enter a brief description of each problem related to:

   a. Bed utilization—problems such as boarding patients in the emergency department because beds are filled to capacity and difficulty transferring patients to another area are examples of bed utilization problems that should be noted.

   b. Physicians—when physicians have problems locating supplies, make requests for special instruments or equipment, or have a dissatisfaction with anyone or anything within the department, it should be noted in this space.

   c. Equipment and supplies—all broken equipment or missing supplies from the department should be noted.

   d. Assignments and staff members—reasons for refusing an assignment should be noted. Any staff member problem such as an injury or leaving the department owing to sudden illness or emergency should be recorded in this space.

   e. Patient or family—any problems relating directly to the patient or the family should be noted in this space. Examples include a family that is abusive to patient or staff, and a patient who habitually screams, attempts to get out of bed, or is combative.

6. Enter the name of any patient who is transferred to another facility during this shift.

7. List any emergency procedures, codes, or deaths that occur on this shift. Also, enter the patient's name and room number.

8. Enter the name of any staff member who exhibited outstanding behavior during this shift. Explain why this behavior was so appreciated by the other staff members.

9. Enter the name of any physician who extended himself or herself on behalf of the staff members during this shift. Explain why the physician's behavior was appreciated.

10. This space is used to track the pace of the department. Any shift that is not staffed correctly by acuity should be noted on the end-of-shift report. This information can be used to justify the need for increased staffing.

11. Enter the names and room numbers of all patients who exhibit any of the indicators listed. QMB uses such continuously collected data to create an overall analysis of the services within the organization.

12. List in this section department outliers as they occur on each shift. Use the list created by the multidisciplinary task force that is posted in the department.

13. Add comments that help explain any of the collected data in this space. Important comments from families or patients may also be noted in this space.

14. The person in charge of the department on this shift is responsible for the report and should sign his or her name in this space.

This end-of-shift report has proven valuable to many organizations in collecting concurrent data. It may, of course, be adapted to suit any department or situation. It provides a tool for ongoing, continuous, organized, planned, systematic data collection in health care organizations.

Suggestion Boxes

Every health care organization should establish some means of open communication with visitors, staff members, physicians, and vendors; in short, anyone from within or outside the organization who has a problem, suggestion, or desire to communicate information with the organization's administration. To foster communication, suggestion boxes can be prominently displayed in highly visible areas and suggestions can be solicited from all three sources of data: the customer, the staff, and management.

Shady Grove Adventist Hospital in Rockville, Maryland, established a very successful suggestion system called "The Sounding Board." The "Sounding Board" form shown in Figure 11-7 is visible in a plastic container near every elevator in the building. A sign encourages all who pass by to share constructive suggestions and comments with the administration of the hospital. Commitments are made to maintain confidentiality and to channel the question to the person in the organization who can best answer it. A personal interview may also be scheduled upon request. The organization reports that many staff members and visitors take advantage of this forum for communicating with the administration.

Satisfaction Surveys

It is critical that health care organizations establish adequate measures of patient satisfaction with their care and services. There must be an effective means for quickly identifying complaints and problems. The satisfaction of all three of the domains is vital to a well-rounded performance management system.

Figure 11-8 is an example of a patient satisfaction survey from Ballard Community Hospital in Seattle, Washington. Once the questionnaire is developed and distributed to patients, it must be treated as a serious method of data collection. The data must be compiled

SOUNDING BOARD

Sounding Board provides opportunity for you, as an employee of Shady Grove Adventist Hospital, to have a voice—to "sound-off" about any subject related to your work specifically, or the hospital program in general.

We encourage constructive suggestions and comments, and will attempt to answer in complete confidence *bonafide* complaints or criticism regarding policies or problems. No one knows your name except the Sounding Board manager, who will channel your question to the one who can best answer it. All replies will be returned directly to you.

If you request a personal interview, Sounding Board will arrange the appointment in strict confidence.

Please use a separate
form for each subject.   Date _____

Comments: _____

_____

_____

_____

_____

☐ Check here if you want to discuss your comments or questions
     with a qualified person.

Name _____

Home address _____

Job title _____

Department _____

Sounding Board needs this information only to forward your reply. If you do not include your name and address, we will not know where to send the answer to your question.

COMPLETED FORM MAY BE SENT BY HOSPITAL INTERMAIL OR POSTAL SERVICE.

Figure 11-7   "Sounding board" form. (Used with permission of Shady Grove Adventist Hospital, Rockville, MD.)

Dear Former Patient

Recently, we were privileged to serve you as a patient at Ballard Community Hospital. We would appreciate your assistance in evaluating our services by taking a few minutes to express your thoughts regarding your stay in the hospital on this short questionnaire.

Thank you for helping us to continue to improve and thereby serve you and others more effectively.

Sincerely,

Administrator

(Please circle ONE number for each item)

ADMITTING/REGISTRATION

	Needs Improvement			Excellent		Does Not Apply
1. Waiting time before admission processing	1	2	3	4	5	____
2. Thoroughness in answering questions, explaining forms and procedures	1	2	3	4	5	____
3. Courtesy and efficiency of admitting process	1	2	3	4	5	____

Comments _____

ROOM ACCOMMODATIONS

	Needs Improvement			Excellent		Does Not Apply
4. Decor of your room	1	2	3	4	5	____
5. Cleanliness of your room	1	2	3	4	5	____
6. Temperature of your room	1	2	3	4	5	____
7. Quietness of your room	1	2	3	4	5	____
8. Telephone service	1	2	3	4	5	____

Comments _____

NURSING SERVICE

	Needs Improvement			Excellent		Does Not Apply
9. Was your admission to your room handled in a courteous, efficient manner?	1	2	3	4	5	____
10. Were you made comfortable within your first few hours here?	1	2	3	4	5	____
11. Did the nursing staff give prompt attention to your needs and requests?	1	2	3	4	5	____
12. Did the nursing staff explain your hospital routine adequately?	1	2	3	4	5	____
13. Were you taught how to care for yourself after leaving the hospital?	1	2	3	4	5	____

Comments _____

SPECIAL TESTS AND PROCEDURES

	Needs Improvement			Excellent		Does Not Apply
14. Were tests explained to you so that you were prepared for what was going to happen?	1	2	3	4	5	____
15. Was enough time allowed for you to ask questions?	1	2	3	4	5	____

Comments _____

NUTRITION/FOOD SERVICE

	Needs Improvement			Excellent		Does Not Apply
16. Were you put on a special diet? If so, what type?	1 - Yes			2 - No		
17. Attractiveness and taste of food	1	2	3	4	5	____
Hot food served hot	1	2	3	4	5	____
Cold food served cold	1	2	3	4	5	____
18. Variety and selection of food items	1	2	3	4	5	____
19. Receiving the food items ordered	1	2	3	4	5	____
20. If you received nutritional information from a dietitian, was it useful and meaningful?	1	2	3	4	5	____

Comments _____

VISITORS

	Needs Improvement			Excellent		Does Not Apply
21. Helpfulness of the hospital staff and volunteers to your visitors	1	2	3	4	5	____
22. Convenience of the visiting hours for family and friends	1	2	3	4	5	____

Comments _____

SIGNS AND DIRECTIONS

	Needs Improvement			Excellent		Does Not Apply
23. Signs and directions outside the hospital	1	2	3	4	5	____
24. Signs and directions inside the hospital	1	2	3	4	5	____

Comments _____

Figure 11-8   Patient satisfaction survey example. (Copyright 1991 Ballard Community Hospital, Seattle, WA. Reprinted with permission.)

Continued.

PARKING

	Needs Improvement			Excellent		Does Not Apply
25. Convenience of parking	1	2	3	4	5	_____
26. Directions to parking	1	2	3	4	5	_____

Comments _____

_____

_____

PATIENT BILLING/CREDIT DEPARTMENT

	Needs Improvement			Excellent		Does Not Apply
27. If you talked with the billing/credit dept., were you given a satisfactory explanation of charges and insurance coverage?	1	2	3	4	5	_____
28. Cooperation of the hospital in arranging your payment	1	2	3	4	5	_____

Comments _____

_____

_____

STAFF

	Needs Improvement			Excellent		Does Not Apply
29. How were you treated by the other staff members you came in contact with?						
A. Physicians	1	2	3	4	5	_____
B. Admissions	1	2	3	4	5	_____
C. Emergency Department	1	2	3	4	5	_____
D. Physical Therapy	1	2	3	4	5	_____
E. Laboratory	1	2	3	4	5	_____
F. Respiratory Care Dept.	1	2	3	4	5	_____
G. Housekeeping	1	2	3	4	5	_____
H. X-Ray	1	2	3	4	5	_____
I. Transportation	1	2	3	4	5	_____
J. Volunteers	1	2	3	4	5	_____
K. Business Office	1	2	3	4	5	_____
L. EKG/EEG	1	2	3	4	5	_____
M. Hospital Telephone Operator	1	2	3	4	5	_____
N. Others _____	1	2	3	4	5	_____
Specify						

GOING HOME

	Needs Improvement			Excellent		Does Not Apply
30. Please rate Ballard Community Hospital on an OVERALL basis for the service and care we gave. Please circle only one number	1	2	3	4	5	_____
31. Would you choose Ballard Community Hospital again?	1 - Yes			2 - No		_____

32. Please list the things you liked during your stay at Ballard Community Hospital.

_____

_____

_____

33. Please list the things you liked least during your stay at Ballard Community Hospital.

_____

_____

_____

34. Who completed the questionnaire:

1 - Patient   2 - Family Member   3 - Friend

35. Additional comments or suggestions:

_____

_____

_____

PATIENT PROFILE

36. Please complete the general information below:

Date of Discharge _____

Month   Day   Year

Room # _____

Length of Stay: _____
    A. 1 day
    B. 2 - 3 days
    C. 4 - 6 days
    D. 1 - 2 weeks
    E. Over 2 weeks (14 days or more)

Your age category: _____
    A. 18 - 24
    B. 25 - 34
    C. 35 - 44
    D. 45 - 54
    E. 55 - 64
    F. 65 - 74
    G. 75 and over

37. Do you want to be contacted by a hospital representative to further discuss your hospitalization .... 1 - Yes   2 - No

If yes, please note telephone number and best time(s) to call:

(   ) _____

Area Code   Telephone Number   Time(s) to call

_____

Name

Your sex is _____ A. Female   B. Male

Thank you for your cooperation in completing this questionnaire. Should you desire to remain anonymous, please remove address label and do not sign your name.

No postage required.

THANK YOU.

Figure 11-8, cont'd.

and used to create change and improvement within the organization.

Staff and administrative satisfaction surveys are useful mechanisms for evaluating the professional and management morale, a major factor in retention. These surveys may be formal or informal. They can be conducted by outside consultants or developed internally. Information can be gathered from questionnaires, in individual counseling sessions, or in group discussions.

Hot Lines

Many health care organizations have found that establishing a "hot line" works well to keep them informed of problems or complaints. Some organizations offer inpatients a phone number to call to discuss any problem, question, or gripe. Such hot lines are usually staffed by patient representatives. They serve the important function of defusing a patient's acute dissatisfaction while still in the hospital.

Administration, from the first line manager to the chief executive officer, may also have a hot line or open phone policy, whereby any staff member may call to discuss a problem or issue. These hot lines can eliminate paperwork and save the time and frustration involved in reaching the right person fast.

Focus Groups

Focus groups also can serve as an excellent mechanism for collecting information. Focus groups are an assembly of a representative sample of patient, staff, or administrators brought together to discuss a particular performance improvement opportunity.

Customer focus groups, in particular, are an essential data gathering device. In these groups, recent former patients exchange opinions and comments on their hospital experience. Such focus groups provide narrative compliments and complaints to expand upon information gathered through questionnaires. This feedback helps staff members identify and solve specific problems. Former patients are usually delighted and flattered when asked to participate in such sessions.

Staff and management groups may also be assembled for fact finding. In addition, a portion of staff and management meetings may be used for the purpose of collecting data regarding specific, important processes of professional or administrative service.

BIAS

The best of intentions are no guarantee against data collection running awry. It is up to the team conducting the performance improvement study to create data collection tools, appoint specific data collectors, and analyze data in such a way that the four types of bias are, in so far as possible, eliminated to avoid skewing the results. If the results of data collection are skewed, the performance improvement team may, without realizing it, recommend an action plan that is inappropriate.

The four common causes of bias that may negatively affect the reliability and validity of a study include the following:

Exclusion bias. If results are intended to represent an entire population or process, omitting some part may bias results. Collect data from a representative sample to ensure accuracy. (See Katz-Green Guidelines for Data Collection on p. 165.)

Perception bias. If data collectors have certain attitudes and beliefs about what the data will reveal, this may affect what they see and how they record it.

Operational bias. An improperly trained data collector or a data collection tool that has not been tested may lead to incomplete or incorrect recording of data. Transferring and processing collected data also gives rise to errors.

Nonresponse bias. Missing data can bias results. If no one responds to a question on a survey, you cannot draw conclusions about what the missing data would have been.[1]

Now the team members must ask how they can reduce the impact of factors contributing to data inconsistency or biases. They must devise a plan to ensure that measurements are consistent over time and periodically measure an identical item and determine whether any variability can be reduced.

Once data has been collected, transforming it into information to be used for performance improvement is an organizational challenge. Data alone do not provide adequate information for decision making. Data are facts that need to be summarized and displayed in a meaningful way to make them interpretable.

However, before an organization appoints a team and unleashes its energy and creativity to seek performance improvement opportunities, an overall plan or framework should be created to direct organization-wide performance improvement efforts.

One excellent example of an overall plan of performance improvement that provides direction is the one shown in Figure 11-9, created by the Living Centers of America (LCA) corporation in Houston, Texas. This is a large, national organization of more than 300 extended and subacute care facilities in the United States. At LCA all facilities follow the improvement process steps as outlined in this example.

Furthermore, employees at each facility are provided with computer equipment and training about how to gather data for their unique *Quality Information System* (QIS). Using the framework in Figure 11-9, the

The LCA Performance Improvement Process

	Step	Purpose	Procedures	Tools	Outcomes
PLAN	1 Identify your product or service	Identify a product or service for quality improvement analysis.	◆ Identify team ◆ Select a product or service for analysis	Brainstorming Multivoting Statistical tools*	◆ Name of product or service ◆ Team established ◆ Start storyboard
	2 Identify your customers, customer requirements	Understand customer requirements and what is needed to meet or exceed them.	◆ Identify customers and their requirements ◆ Collect data on how well needs are being met (baseline)	Flowchart Checksheet	◆ List of customers ◆ List of customer requirements ◆ Add to storyboard
	3 Identify your current work process	Understand what is currently done to produce the product or service.	◆ Flowchart the current work process	Flowchart	◆ Flowchart of current process ◆ Add to storyboard
	4 Identify improvement opportunities	Select an opportunity to pursue.	◆ Identify existing process complexity ◆ Use existing data to understand magnitude of complexity ◆ Prioritize improvement opportunities ◆ Select opportunity of highest common concern	Flowchart Multivoting Checksheet Stratification Statistical Tools*	◆ Prioritized list of opportunities ◆ Agreement on which opportunity to pursue ◆ Add to storyboard
	5 Establish and verify cause and effect	Ensure identification of "root cause" before process is changed.	◆ Analyze "root cause" of selected opportunity ◆ Gather data to ensure appropriate opportunity has been identified	Brainstorming Fishbone Diagram Stratification Scatter Diagram	◆ The "cause(s)" to be tackled first ◆ Add to storyboard
	6 Revise the work process	Develop plan to improve and monitor process.	◆ Develop plan to streamline, shorten, simplify or otherwise improve current process	Brainstorming Multivoting Flowchart	◆ Flowchart of revised process ◆ Add to storyboard
DO	7 Conduct a small scale test of the revised process	Test process change on a small scale before implementing throughout the system.	◆ Design a small scale test ◆ Run revised process according to test plan ◆ Collect data on new process	Flowchart Checksheet Scatter Diagram Run Chart	◆ Data on impact of process revision ◆ Add to storyboard
CHECK	8 Evaluate test results	Determine whether revised process delivers product/service to customer requirements.	◆ Confirm effects of process change, checking if root causes have been reduced ◆ Compare the problem before and after using the same indicators ◆ Go to "PLAN" if results are not satisfactory	Stratification Statistical Tools*	◆ Analysis of data ◆ Recommendation on how to proceed ◆ Add to storyboard
ACT	9 Standardize and implement the improved process	Implement the improved process throughout the system.	◆ Conduct training on new process ◆ Communicate improvement procedure and results ◆ Gather data and continuously monitor process to maintain improvement	Flowchart Checksheet Stratification Statistical Tools*	◆ Documentation of procedure and results ◆ Add to storyboard
	10 Measure and analyze customer satisfaction based on feedback	Establish ongoing feedback mechanism with customers.	◆ Develop mechanism to seek information on customer recommendations	Brainstorming Flowchart Pareto Chart Fishbone Diagram	◆ Process for collecting customer data ◆ Add to storyboard
	11 Celebrate the quality story	Free people to improve the way they do their jobs.	◆ Record team information ◆ Communicate quality story at all levels ◆ Recognize contributions ◆ Plan future improvements	Flowchart Statistical Tools*	◆ Celebration ◆ Plan for continuous improvement ◆ Share completed storyboard

*Statistical tools include Pareto Charts, Scatter Diagrams, Run and Control Charts, and Histograms.

Figure 11-9 The LCA performance improvement process. (Modified from The Pacific Bell Quality Improvement Process Handbook. In *The Portrait of Continuous Quality Improvement*, Houston, Tex, 1994, Living Centers of America.)

employees of each LCA facility are taught how to collect, enter, retrieve, analyze, and apply QIS data. Additionally they are taught how to plan and conduct ongoing self-assessment, based on the 28 core indicators collected each month.

Without a planned, organized, corporate-wide framework such as the baseline performance improvement plan, along with a corporate commitment of resources, organization-wide performance improvement would be a far-off dream. Instead it is an integral part of the daily work experience of this corporation.

The importance of accurate, meaningful data collection cannot be overstated. It is only through gathering and analyzing facts that meaningful change and improvement can occur in health care organizations. Errors and sentinel events will always occur. Although important, they can be, nevertheless, the cause of "knee jerk" reactions that waste resources and solve few problems. Health care organizations can avoid knee-jerk reactions to problems and subsequent wasted resources though the creation and management of sound systems that collect, organize, and react to data in a planned, organized, systematic way.

Tools to evaluate variations in data are the building blocks of an organization's performance measurement program. These tools are called statistical process control tools and are discussed in the next chapter.

REFERENCES

1. Bacchioni T: *Pacific Bell quality improvement process handbook*, ed 3, Washington DC, 1992, Pacific Bell Graphics.
2. Green E, Katz JM: *Clinical practice guidelines for the adult patient*, St. Louis, 1995, Mosby.
3. Juran JM: *Juran's quality control handbook*, ed 4, New York, 1988, McGraw-Hill.
4. *The Law, Medicine, and Health Care* 12(2):53-62, 1984.
5. Moen RD, Nolan TW: Process improvement, *Quality Progress*, pp 62-68, Sept. 1987.
6. Neuhauser D, McEachern JE, Headrick L: *Clinical CQI: a book of readings*, Chicago, 1995, Joint Commission.
7. Walton M: *The Deming management at work*, New York, 1990, G.P. Putnam's Sons.
8. Walton M: *The Deming management method*, New York, 1986, G.P. Putnam's Sons.

Chapter 12

Evaluating Organizational Variations

Ignorance of variation lies at the root
of many problems in health care.
Rafael Aguayo

Kay Waldo, RN, nurse manager of a 45-bed medical unit was puzzled. Another patient had developed a pressure ulcer. What was the cause of the increasing occurrence of pressure ulcers in her unit? Silently she stood, looking at the sleeping 84-year-old patient, who was her department's latest victim of "alterations in skin integrity" and wondered how he had developed the ulceration on his buttocks so quickly.

"This is the ninth case this month," she mused. "That will 'blow' our department's statistical control this quarter for skin integrity, and I'll be outside of my target parameters." She walked slowly back to her office, thinking, "This is certainly a special cause variation and it will have to be justified. If I try to 'fix' it, will I be tampering? I want to make sure that the incidence of hospital-acquired pressure sores in this department is rare, even if it is a rate-based indicator! I will submit this data about pressure ulcers in my department to QMB and request that they compare it to the data from other departments. If the organization-wide data indicate an increase in hospital acquired pressure sores, QMB will initiate a performance improvement team to study the process of pressure sore care and treatment. I wonder which statistical process control tools they will use. Our organization cannot tolerate a variance like this."

Nurse Waldo was using a thought process and language that is increasingly common among health care professionals. Words like statistical control, variance, special cause variation, target parameter, and tampering describe a scientific approach to performance management that is revolutionizing health care services. Although these words may be new to many health care professionals, they are not difficult to understand. Although many statistical concepts are quite sophisticated, the implications of the few covered in this chapter are simple.

Because the new accreditation processes of most agencies are requiring the use of statistics in data collecting and reporting, it behooves all health care professionals to seek an understanding of the requirements. The use of statistics by health care organizations comes as no surprise, given the fact that controlling process variations significantly reduces costs. This was clearly proven by Deming and Shewhart in their work with the Japanese in the early 1950s.[2] Both Deming and Shewhart designed the tools of statistical process control that are described in this chapter. Each tool is designed to either analyze or display variance data.

No longer are department managers praised for writing lengthy, narrative quarterly reports of their data with suggested corrective actions based on hunches, experience, and opinions. Rather, they are expected to use a scientific approach to performance improvement based on collected data. Why the necessity for a scientific approach?

"It's simple," says Barbara Sines, RN, MSN, an administrative assistant at Washington Adventist Hospital in Takoma Park, Maryland. "We can no longer afford 'experimental' health care. We must place our services, practices, and governance practices on a scientific basis to prevent wasted resources. Furthermore, we need to educate our staff so that they can develop performance improvement strategies that are rooted in the scientific process. When we do, staff members will find solutions that work the first time. Costs will drop and organization-wide performance will improve."[9] In other words, Nurse Sines is opposed to the traditional trial and error management style that wastes resources. She recognizes that performance improvement mechanisms that work the first time reduce costs by conserving resources and effectively managing service, practice, and governance.

THE SCIENTIFIC APPROACH

"The core of performance improvement methods is summed up in two words: scientific approach."[6] A scientific approach is simply a systematic, planned, organized method for problem solving that is understood and followed by all employees. Decisions to act are based on data rather than experience, hunches, or gut feelings. The scientific approach ensures that an organization will search for the root cause of a problem, find it, and fix it, rather than implement a quick, short-term, knee-jerk fix. Just as a band-aid may temporarily hide a malignant mole, so a "band-aid fix" may hide a problem within a health care organization for a time. Sooner or later, however, the band-aid will be insufficient to hide the greater problem. It is more cost effective and increases the chances for more positive organization-wide outcomes to address the real source of variations in processes.

Fixing the source may sometimes be difficult. It may require rethinking the health care organization's current approach to managing performance. It may also necessitate committing sufficient resources to restructure the entire organization into a shared leadership paradigm, such as the one described in Chapter 5.

However, a willingness to restructure the present organization and commit resources does not by itself ensure performance excellence. In addition, a scientific approach must be instituted and understood if performance improvement is to become the way of doing business in health care organizations.

Implementing this approach may require changing some of our traditional quality concepts, because performance management cannot occur in the traditional environment. Performance improvement involves adopting a trifocus approach to performance measurement. In other words, when a performance improvement opportunity occurs, the organization will look at every related process in each domain to identify ways to improve.

What goes on in the health care industry—even the organization-wide outcomes—is not merely the result of employees' actions. All of the processes within a health care organization affect outcomes. To affect the probability of good outcomes, health care organizations need to create an organization-wide system that fosters continuous, focused data collection to study the processes necessary to performance improvement.[3]

PROCESS VARIATIONS

There are two kinds of variations. The first is called common cause variance.[2] This involves the minor variations that occur within a health care organization, regardless of how excellent the system is. Often common cause variations can be changed only by management. Common cause variations may include minor variations in staff members' abilities, an unclear procedure, and limitations of equipment. Because resources are unavailable to detect the cause of every minor variation, they are tolerated. In addition, many variations are caused by chance. When chance is the cause of a variation, it would be futile to investigate the cause and try to fix it. Therefore, variations caused by chance are tolerated.

Organizations that do not recognize the chance phenomenon spend much time, effort, and money investigating variations in their system that could not be altered even if the reasons for them were found. Unfortunately, employees are often blamed. Management thinks that if employees would only try harder, be more efficient, work together, and be more loyal, every variance would vanish. Organizations implement elaborate mechanisms designed to educate, test, and exhort employees only to find that no improvement occurs. Employees may already be working as hard as they can, and minor variations caused by chance cannot be "fixed."

The phenomenon of chance within an organization and the futility of blaming employees for variations in process has been demonstrated by Dr. Deming in his famous red bead experiment.[10] In this exercise, Dr. Deming demonstrates the need to use acceptable parameters instead of absolute targets as a benchmark for the evaluation of processes.

Here is the exercise: Dr. Deming chooses six members of the audience. He tells them he is recruiting them to be trained to work in his factory. He appoints two of them inspectors and one chief inspector.

Deming serves as the foreman. The remaining three serve as the "workers."

This factory, Dr. Deming explains, makes white beads. Occasionally, however, it turns out red beads. The red beads are defective. The company gets paid only for white beads.

Dr. Deming instructs the workers to scoop up the white beads from one of two pans containing a mixture of white and red beads in a ratio of 4 white to 1 red. A rectangular paddle with 50 holes is used to scoop the beads and workers are expected to achieve no more than 2 red beads per scoop. The threshold for noncompliance is 4%.

Each paddleful must be reviewed by an inspector, who counts the number of red beads. This is verified by the chief inspector, who announces the count and dismisses the worker.

After the first try, a performance review is conducted. Each worker then makes three more scooping attempts. Again, after each scoop, a performance review is conducted. The results vary; a different worker achieves the best and worst results with each try. The performance of each worker varies from scoop to scoop purely by chance! There is a variation among the workers, ranging from a low of 4 red beads to a high of 18—all by chance.

Most of us assume chance plays a minor role in variations in the performance of individual workers. However, here is a case where chance is responsible for 100% of it. Suppose that management eliminates the workers with the poorest performance and keeps the top three workers. The workers with low error rates must complete two more attempts each. Once again chance comes into play and the results reflect it. In this case, the three best workers produce the worst overall performance in the company's history! "When all the variation in performance is due to chance, past performance is neither a guarantee nor an indication of future performance."[1]

In the bead factory example, individuals were held accountable for variations in their performance that were, in fact, caused by the system. The individuals had no control over their level of performance.

The second kind of variation is called special cause variance.[2] Special cause variations occur when systems and processes break down. There are several possible reasons for process breakdowns, such as employee error, lack of knowledge of the process, and breakdown of equipment. Special causes are usually easier to correct than common causes. Setting target parameters using standard deviation makes it possible to identify special cause variations while tolerating common cause fluctuations.

An organization must have a scientific method for distinguishing between common cause and special cause variation. That scientific method is statistical control and is always displayed on a control chart.

STATISTICAL CONTROL OF PROCESSES

To function effectively and efficiently, health care organizations must maintain statistical control of their processes. An organization that it is in statistical control has more certain outcomes and can begin to work toward process improvement.

Statistical control means that things are happening the way they were planned to happen—that is, the results fall within the target parameters of one, two, or three standard deviations from the mean. When a process within the organization is in statistical control, it is referred to as a stable system.[2]

In his research, Dr. Deming has demonstrated that when a variation is caused by chance, almost all of the data will fall within three standard deviations from the mean or mathematical average.[11] Within a stable system, variations occur within predetermined parameters. The parameters, or upper and lower limits of the range, are the control limits. These control limits are derived by calculating standard deviation. When all the collected data fall within the control limits, the system is considered stable, i.e., in statistical control. Variations that fall at random within the control limits are assumed to be caused by chance.

Figure 12-1 is an example of a control chart that tracks the incidence of urinary tract infections within 72 hours following insertion of a urinary catheter in a 640-bed medical center. Based on historical data, the mean is calculated at 40 with one standard deviation being ±10. Control limits are then set with the lower control limit at 30 and the upper control limit at 50.

When a result falls above or below the control limits, it is out of control. Figure 12-2 shows a control chart that demonstrates a variation out of control. When this happens, an immediate analysis of the variation is warranted. Variations outside of the control limits are called special cause variations and should be investigated.

Chance cannot be eliminated from the system. Special circumstances, however, can be corrected. For example, some patients enter hospitals with urinary tract infections (UTIs) unbeknownst to the patient, the physician, or nurse. Therefore, it is unrealistic to blame staff members for all urinary tract infections occurring in catheterized patients. However, a sudden rise in the incidence of UTIs is a special cause variance, and it must be investigated. Likewise, results that are better than expected should also be investigated to confirm reliability in the data collection process.

A system that is in statistical control is not necessarily ideal or defect-free. Rather, the system is stable and

CONTROL CHART 1

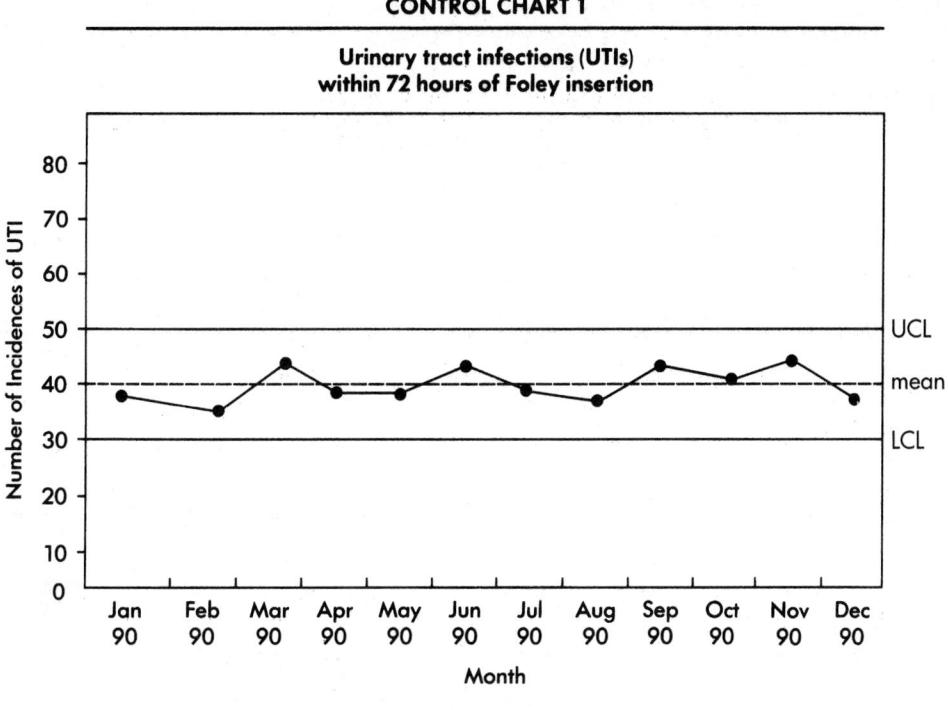

Figure 12-1   Control chart 1—urinary tract infections.

CONTROL CHART 2

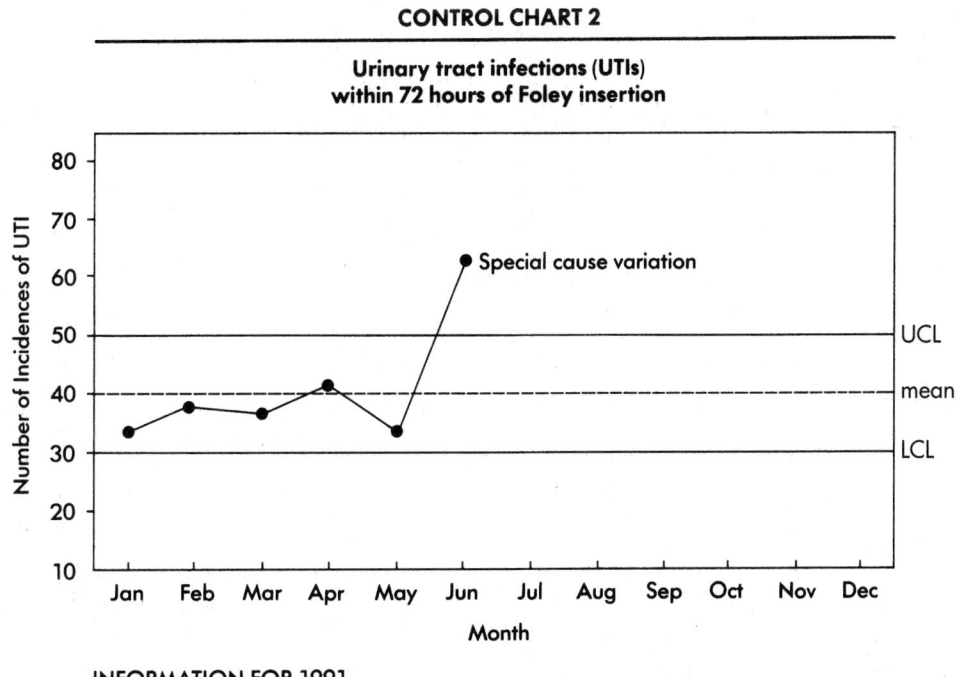

Figure 12-2   Control chart 2—urinary tract infections.

any problem may be attacked at its "root." Until statistical control is achieved, no real work can begin to find solutions to special cause variations in processes.

Furthermore, once statistical control is achieved for a process, improvement in that process can only be achieved through a change in the system—not a change in individual workers. Statistical control helps people stop needless searching for special causes when there is only a minor variation in results. It also eliminates unnecessary action to attempt to improve minor variations. Thus it controls the costs associated with improvement efforts by eliminating the possibility of tampering. Initiating corrective action aimed at improving staff performance will not result in any appreciable change in the variance and may distort the results of the next study. Also, these attempts to improve staff performance may waste scarce resources that are needed to improve the true cause of the variation.

TAMPERING WITH STABLE PROCESSES

Typically, when variations arise in the results of a study, there is an attempt to resolve the cause of the variation by changing or correcting the process. However, attempts to correct minor shifts within the target parameters may, in fact, produce worse results. Attempting to fix one part of a process distorts the other parts. As the problems resulting from the distortion start to surface, more and more steps are added to compensate.[8] This is called tampering. Tampering is a knee-jerk correction in response to a variation in data, whether the results are due to common or special causes. Tampering creates wildly fluctuating variations in processes that, in turn, yield meaningless data as a benchmark against which to measure progress.

Often when a process varies, health care professionals' attempts to fix it causes another fluctuation in data. More tampering is then necessary to correct what appears to be a greater problem. Tampering with a stable system is not productive, because it typically results in overcorrecting or undercorrecting the problem. Each correction may cost the organization thousands of dollars with no improvement noted in the processes, creating a lot of frustration in employees. The constant upheaval within the organization results in a great deal of motion but little direction. No sound improvements can occur from unstable, unexplainable, fluctuating data. Sound improvements can occur only in a stable system. As quality expert Rafael Aguayo says, "Ignorance of variation lies at the root of many problems in health care."[1]

One way for an organization to determine if tampering exists within its system is to look at the data being gathered. If it presents a roller coaster pattern, tampering is probably occurring.

When faced with negative data about outcomes of service, practice, or governance within an organization, it is easy to assume that each negative bit of information is due to one specific cause, such as the lack of effort of the staff member or poor clinical skills of the practitioner. The way to correct the situation, many people reason, is to initiate new competency checks; test staff members; implement new programs; and exhort, bribe, or, perhaps, threaten staff members with the possibility of disciplinary action. Having chosen one or more of these methods to enforce compliance, the assessment of staff members becomes intense. It is reasoned that the data will show that improvements have resulted from these efforts.

Even some of our nation's most prestigious regulatory organizations have mandated efforts to "tighten up the ship." For example, several years ago the Health Care Financing Administration (HCFA) proposed a regulation requiring organizations to certify that their professional staff was competent to perform a guaiac test on patient's stool and to perform a finger stick for machine analysis of blood glucose levels. Yet, these tests could be purchased over the counter in any drug store and performed at home. Dennis O'Leary, MD, president of the Joint Commission, commented on HCFA's proposal this way, "To characterize HCFA's proposed regulations as onerous is an understatement. HCFA had an opportunity to introduce a modicum of sanity into the statutory requirements, but such rationality was apparently not within the agency's bag of surprises this time."[7]

Inherent in HCFA's proposal was the assumption that "correcting" the employee would correct the problem. Correcting only the employee, however, instead of the system may lead to tampering and unbalance a system that is already in statistical control.

Tampering can destabilize the system and create new problems that absorb the organization's resources. It accomplishes little and is difficult to stop. An organization can improve and avoid tampering by first creating a stable system and then by eliminating special cause variations.

CREATING A STABLE SYSTEM

Creating a stable system requires tracking performance measurement results of an organization's processes over time. The control chart form shown in Figure 12-3 may be used to provide a visual display tracking of processes. Kay Waldo used the form to track the incidence of pressure ulcers in her department. Historical data showed a mean of 5%. Standard deviation was calculated at ±5; therefore, upper and lower control limits were established at 0-10%. Upper and lower limits were marked on the graph. At the completion of each monthly study, data were entered

STUDY NUMBER _____*79-4007*_____ INDICATOR NUMBER ___*#3*___

PRIMARY DATA COLLECTOR _____*Sheri Forquer and Angie Dennison*_____

TARGET PARAMETERS ___*0-10%*___

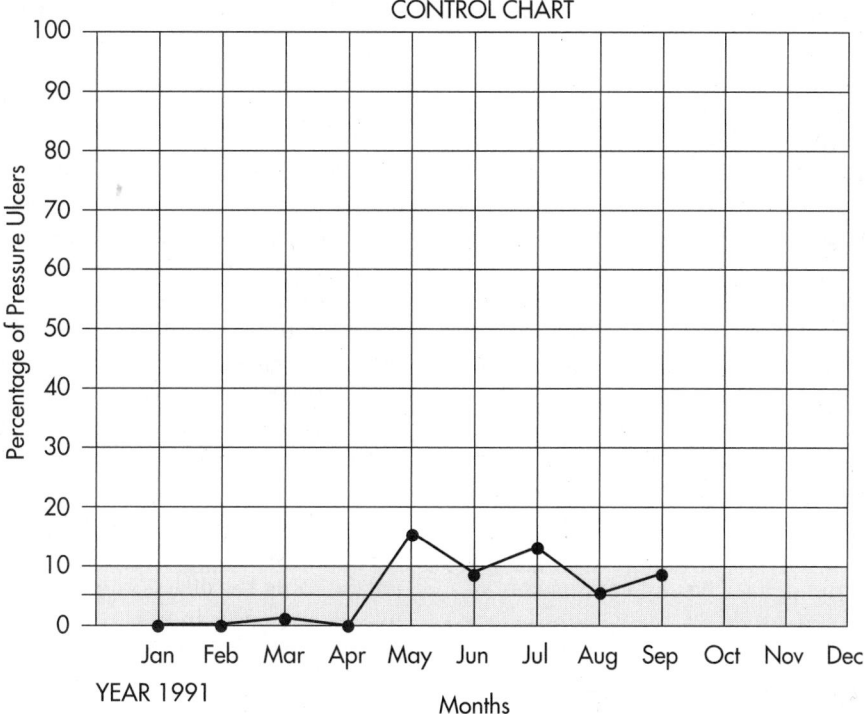

CONTROL CHART

REMARKS:

1. *No ulcers in this department this month (Jan.)*

2. *No ulcers in this department this month (Feb.)*

3. *One ulcer in this department which is on buttocks of 93-year-old incontinent pt. from extended care facility*

4. *No ulcers in this department this month*

5. *There are 12 pressure ulcers in this department this month. Investigation is underway.*

6. *There are 8 pressure ulcers in this department this month. A task force has been appointed to gather data on pt. severity of illness and co-morbidity*

7. *There are 11 pressure ulcers this month in this department. The task force has designed a pressure ulcer tracking tool.*

8. *We have reached the historical mean of 5 pressure ulcers in this unit this month.*

9. *There are 8 pressure ulcers this month. Severity of illness index indicates 7 of the patients are indigent and malnourished. 5 are on tube feedings and are cancer pts.*

10.

11.

12.

Figure 12-3   Control chart for pressure ulcers. (Copyright 1995 Jackie Katz and Ellie Green. Reprinted with permission.)

on the graph to see if the data fell within the parameters. As long as the data fell within the target parameters of 0 to 10%, statistical control was maintained. When the data fell outside of the parameters, as it did in May, this was a signal for an immediate review.

When tracking data, realize that just being within the established parameters is not always sufficient to maintain quality. If data meet the criteria discussed earlier, i.e., beyond control limits, seven consecutive points on the same side of the center line, six consecutive points increasing or decreasing little or much variation from center line, the system is also considered out of control. Whenever the system is out of control, there is cause for immediate investigation. Ishikawa's *Guide to Quality Control* specifically states that a run chart is in statistical control when "1) All the points are within the control limits, and 2) The point grouping does not assume a particular form."[5] In other words, statistical control is achieved when the data fall within the preestablished parameters in a random pattern around the mean.

Figure 12-4 shows a control chart for a system that may be out of control, even though the data remain within the established parameters. This study concerns the number of physicians' orders transcribed incorrectly. A ± standard deviation of 10, with a mean of 20% has been established. (Note that in this case the mean performance is 80%.) One glance at the graph shows that the system may be out of control, even though the data fall within the target parameters. It is also possible that the data will form an oscillating pattern and will come back down, or it may indicate the beginning of a long trend, which may continue in an "out of control" pattern. In either event, an analysis must be done to determine the cause.

Every process has variations, but the more finely tuned the process, the less deviation there is from the average.

This is the reason for standardization of structure, outcome, process, and evaluation standards within THE BLUEPRINT. Good standards eliminate much of the variance inherent in any health care organization. Once "roller coaster" variations are eliminated and a stable system is achieved, the organization can direct its resources toward improving organizational performance.

ELIMINATING SPECIAL CAUSE VARIATIONS

A system can be improved only when special causes have been eliminated after the system has been brought into statistical control. Special cause variations can often be eliminated by workers just by virtue of creating awareness of the problem. For example, compliance to handwashing routine may improve dramatically when staff members are aware that handwashing practices are being assessed. Action planning is the key to eliminating special cause variations and is described in Chapter 13.

STATISTICAL PROCESS CONTROL

Analysis of variations is accomplished through the use of specific tools designed to identify variation and to pinpoint causative factors. These tools are called statistical process control (SPC) tools. These tools are merely organized methods for describing problems and planning solutions. They help an individual or group to focus attention on a critical process of the organization that is causing difficulty, mentally "take it apart," look at it from every aspect, suggest methods to eliminate the difficulty, test the suggested methods, and then implement a permanent solution.

"Understanding quality leadership is not just rethinking where you are going," suggests Peter R. Scholtes, "it's looking at how you will get there. Paying attention to method as well as results is one of the distinguishing features of this new way [scientific approach] of doing business.[8] In other words, a scientific approach is necessary to move from the traditional methods of quality to the new approaches of performance management. If there is to be an organization-wide commitment to performance excellence, then there must be a global focus within the organization, with every process of service, practice, and governance coming under scrutiny.

Moving *from* QA *into* performance management cannot be accomplished without a knowledge of scientific tools for decision making. A movement to the use of SPC tools in a health care organization entails a new way of looking at old situations. It requires an organization to look at every process affecting service, practice, and governance to see how those processes are carried out and how they can be improved. Finding opportunities to improve service does not mean simply focusing on practitioners. In the past, QA activities often have attempted to determine: Did the health care worker do the right thing? Did nurse B do the right thing? There was little need for a scientific approach when the focus of traditional QA activities was so narrow and focused on nurses. Today the performance focuses on the entire organization.

Although many SPC tools have been developed, some key tools that may be used by health care workers in the decision-making process are the fishbone diagram, flowchart, histogram, Pareto chart, run chart, and control chart.

The Cause and Effect Diagram

A cause and effect diagram is a picture of the relationship between causes and an effect or problem. It is sometimes called the fishbone diagram because when completed, it resembles a fish skeleton. Sometimes it is called an Ishikawa diagram after its originator, Kaoru Ishikawa.[2]

Although it might appear that only one cause produces a particular effect, in fact usually many causes work together to produce a result. We need to understand these seemingly casual relationships between cause and effect.

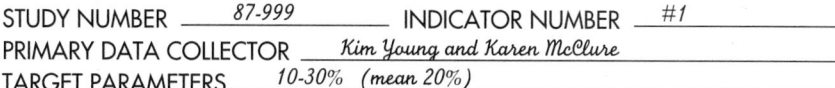

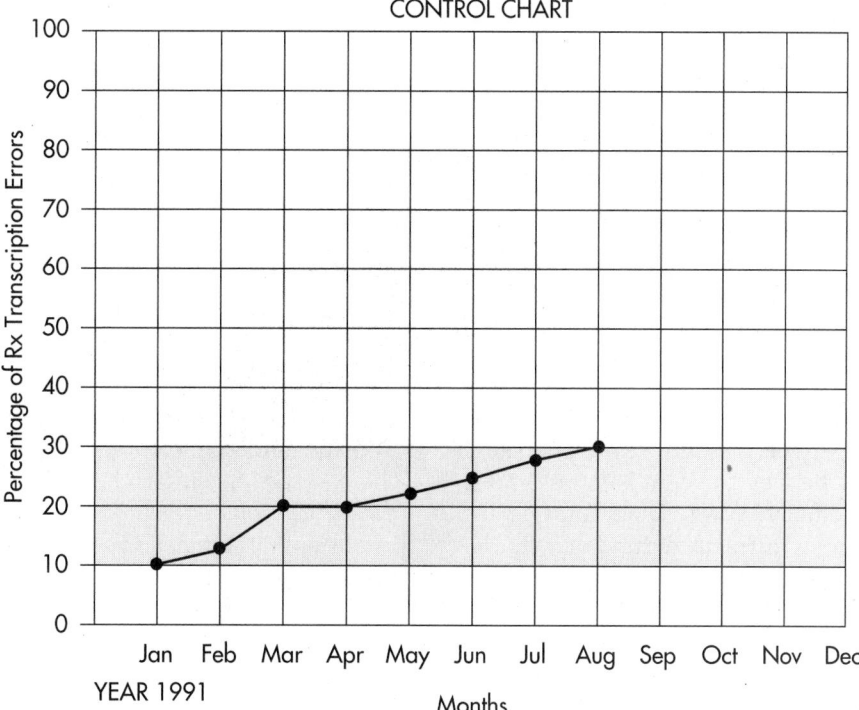

STUDY NUMBER ___87-999___ INDICATOR NUMBER ___#1___
PRIMARY DATA COLLECTOR ___Kim Young and Karen McClure___
TARGET PARAMETERS ___10-30% (mean 20%)___

CONTROL CHART

Percentage of Rx Transcription Errors

YEAR 1991

Months

REMARKS:

1. Ten charts had Rx errors in transcription-(see "folder" for breakdown)

2. Problem continues-discussed with charge nurses.

3. Problem unabated. Spoke with Nurse Manager

4. Problem stabilized

5. Problem worsened-called meeting with charge nurses and nurse managers

6. Problem worsened-Discussed at QMC.

7. Discussed problem with Director of Nurses and Nurse Manager.

8. Problem cannot be tolerated. Will call general meeting and discuss system of noting orders.

9.

10.

11.

12.

Figure 12-4   Control chart for Rx transcription errors. (Copyright 1995 Jackie Katz and Ellie Green. Reprinted with permission.)

The cause and effect diagram is used whenever a health care organization wishes to systematically analyze the cause and effect relationships between processes or identify the root causes of process complexity. It is used during team brainstorming sessions to examine every factor that may influence a given situation.

The basic construction of a cause and effect diagram includes a box in which the effect is written; a long horizontal line, or backbone, coming from the box; a series of diagonal lines representing the major categories of causes of the effect and the major categories branching out from each of the diagonal lines. The causes may be organized by standard categories such as materials, methods, equipment, and people, or by other categories suited to the types of causes generated, or by major segments of a process.

Figure 12-5 is an example of a cause and effect diagram that might be used in a problem-solving discussion focused on medication delivery. The process of administration of medication from physician's order to delivery to a patient involves many people and departments. When a team uses a cause and effect diagram, they are searching for root causes of problems. They organize the causes on each bone, drawing branch bones to show relationship among the causes. The team continues to develop causes by asking "why?" until a useful level of detail is reached.

The Flowchart

The flowchart is an extremely useful way of analyzing what is happening. One way to begin is to determine the way a process actually works. Diagramming the process can immediately turn up redundancy, inefficiency, and misunderstanding. A flowchart is a picture showing the sequence of action and decision steps that make a process work. It is used when describing the current work process or when information is needed to study, analyze, and look for ways to improve a process. It may also be used to describe improved work processes and when documenting and communicating the degree of performance improvement.

Elements of a flowchart are the ovals, used to show the first and last steps, or the beginning and ending boundaries of a process; rectangles to show action steps; and diamonds to show decision steps. Phrase each decision as a yes or no question and place in the diamonds. Show connections with a number in a small circle when a flowchart must be displayed in more than one column or on more than one page.

Figure 12-6 is a flowchart of the process of same-day surgery. Is the patient flow as desired or could it be improved? The flowchart can be used as the basis for decision making and increased precision in the flow of patients through the same-day surgery process.

The Pareto Chart

A Pareto chart is a special type of bar graph used to prioritize problems and/or data. Constructing a Pareto chart based on either checksheets or other forms of data collection helps direct attention and effort to truly important problems. The chart is arranged with the highest bar on the left and the others in decreasing order to the right. You will generally gain more by working on the tallest bar than tackling the smaller bars. Pareto charts are especially valuable as "before and after" snapshots to show what progress has been made.

The Pareto is used to identify a product or service for performance improvement, identify performance

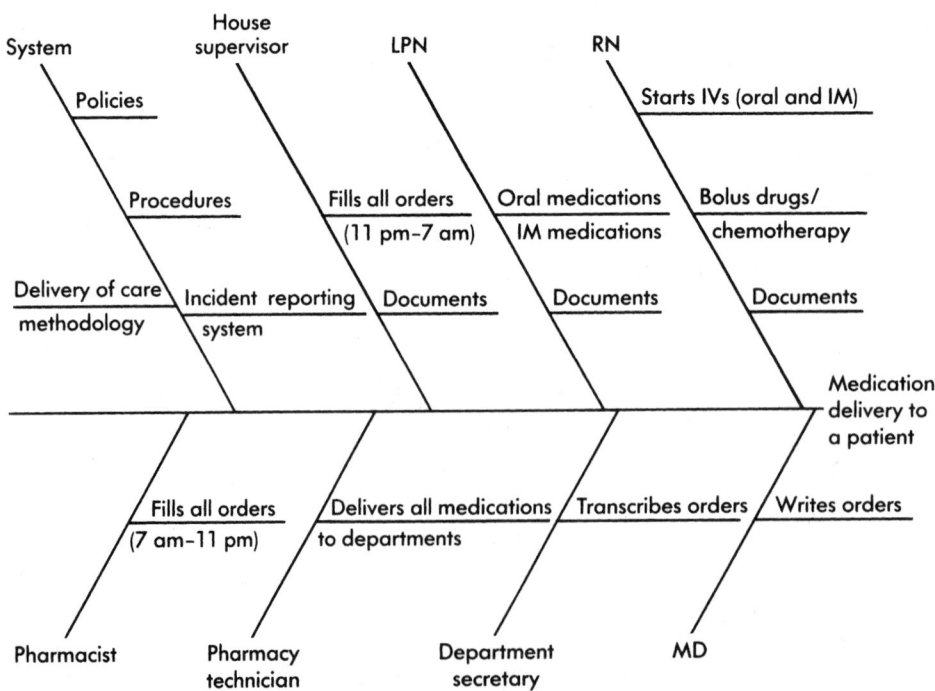

Figure 12-5   Cause-effect (fishbone) diagram of medications administration to a patient.

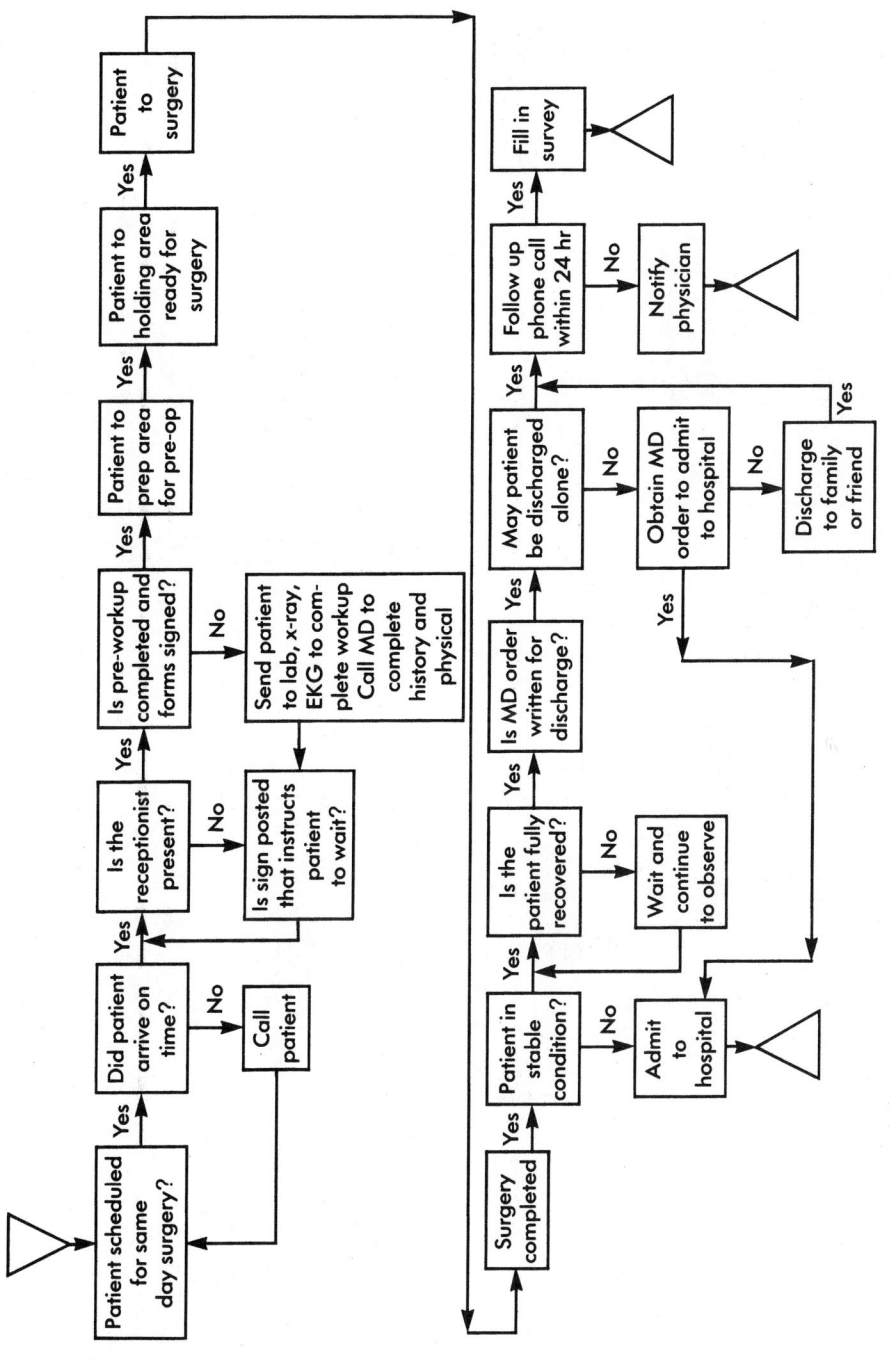

Figure 12-6 Flowchart of process of same-day surgery.

189

improvement opportunities, analyze different groups of data, prioritize solutions, and evaluate test results of changes to be made to a process.

Prepare the framework for the Pareto chart by listing the categories of errors, performance improvement opportunities, cases, employees, or whatever you are going to measure. Figure 12-7 shows categories of admissions to the emergency department. Draw a rectangle or column with a height representing the frequency or cost in that category. Figure 12-7 clearly illustrates that the top three admissions to the emergency department consisted of chest pain, chronic obstructive pulmonary disease, and asthma. Because the Pareto chart makes it clear which of the problems or categories are the "vital few," it is one of the most effective tools for both finding problems and estimating the magnitude of performance improvement possible.

THE RUN AND CONTROL CHARTS

A **run chart** is one of the simplest of the SPC tools. A run chart is used to document frequency over a period of time to illustrate trends. The example in Figure 12-8 tracks data from the number of emergency department admissions for the month of August 1995. It is evident that admissions peak on the weekends. This chart would support increased staffing during the most busy hours in the emergency department.

Possibly the most popular SPC tool is the control chart, which Dr. Deming often talks about as necessary to analyze processes. The purpose of the control chart, he emphasizes, is "to stop people from chasing down causes."[8] Properly understood and used, a control chart is a continuing guide to constant improvement. In addition, control charts are easy to use.

A control chart is simply a run chart with statistically determined upper and lower limits drawn on

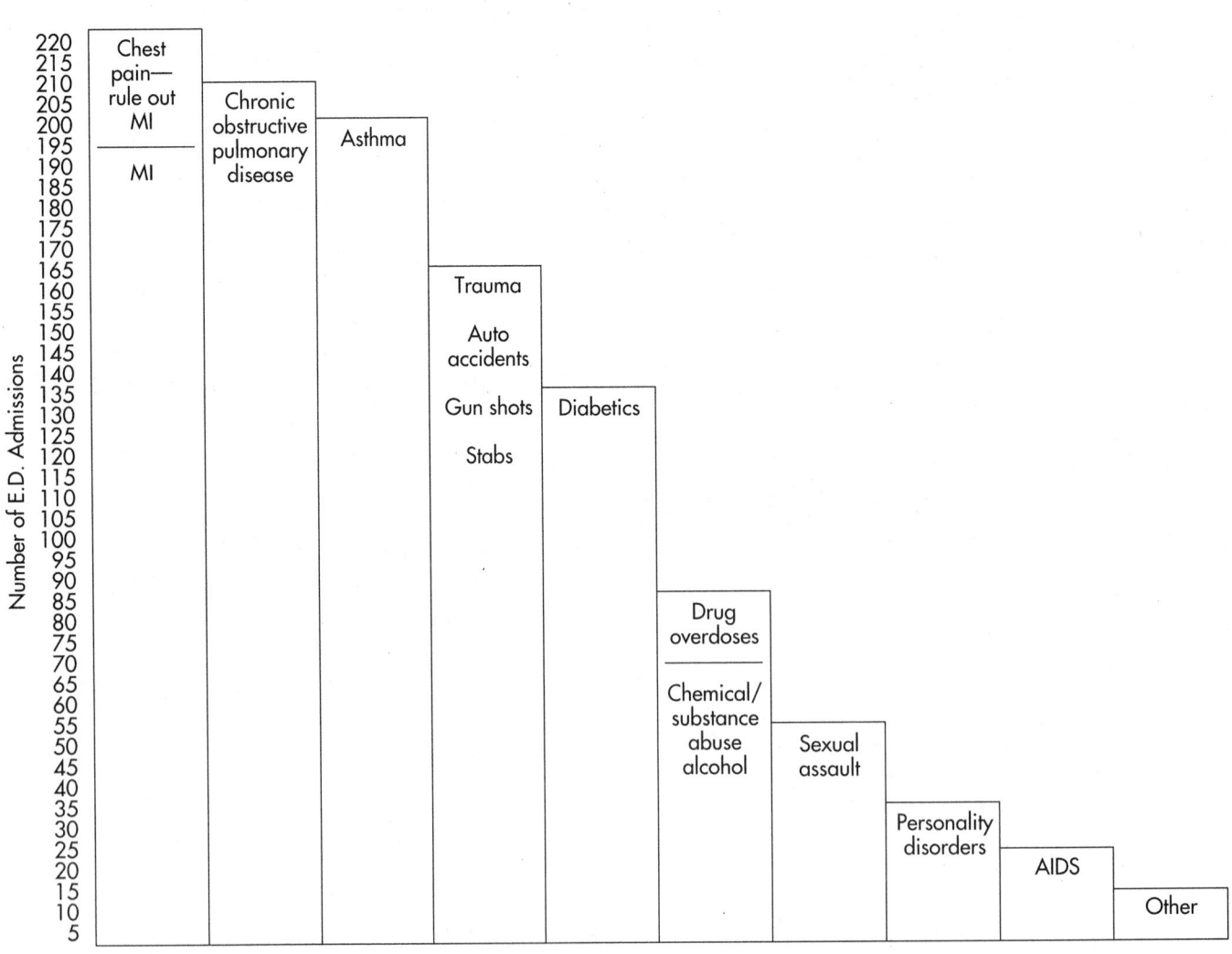

Figure 12-7   Pareto chart of emergency department admissions.

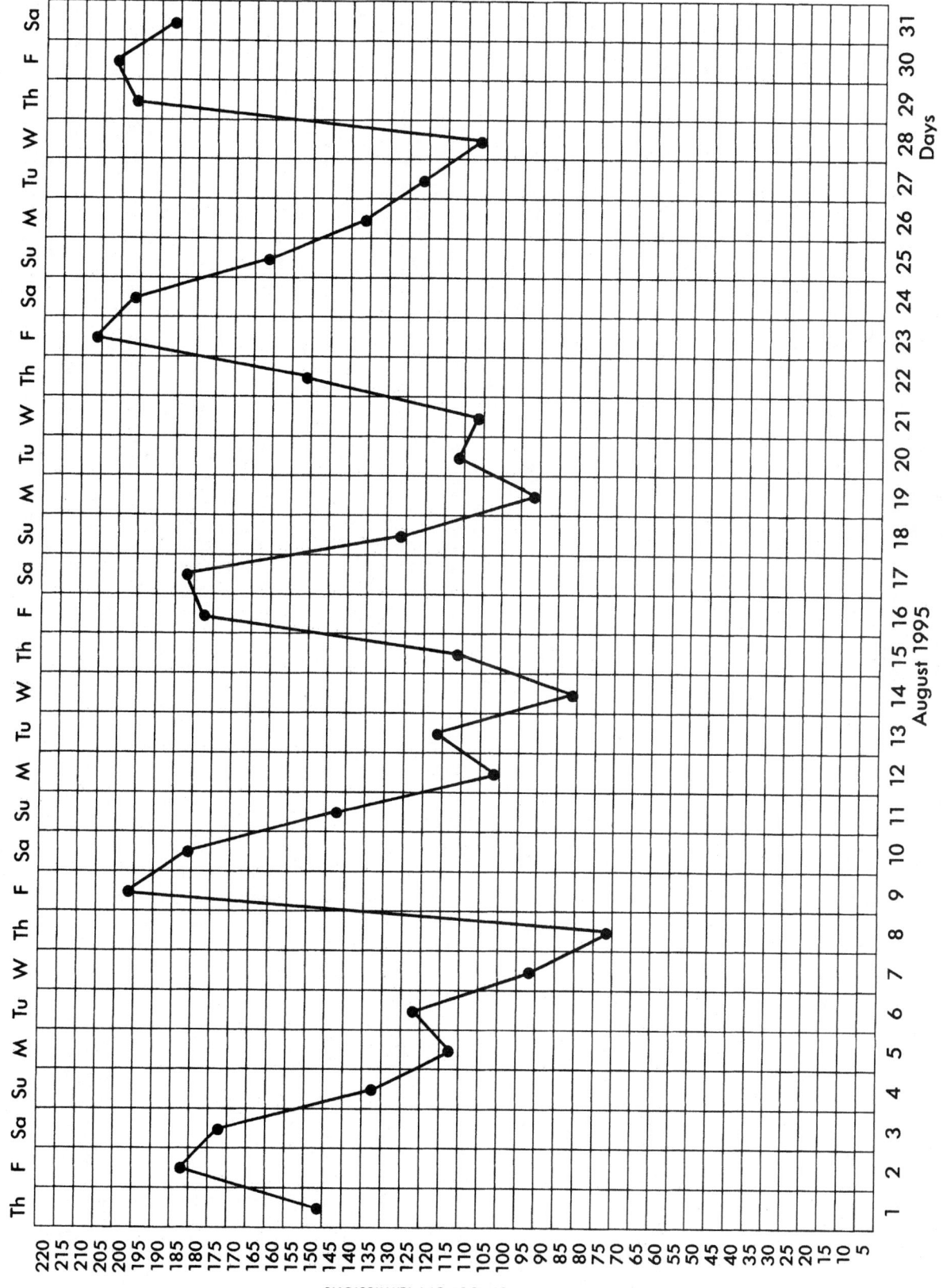

Figure 12-8 Run chart of emergency department admissions per 24 hours.

191

either side of the process average. The upper and lower control limits are determined by allowing a process to run as usual, without tampering and then analyzing the results. Every process has some variation. The more finely tuned the process, the less deviation there is from the average. Figure 12-1 is an example of a simple control chart. The target parameter forms shown in Figures 12-3 and 12-4 incorporate control charts.

Most health care organizations create control charts by computing 1 standard deviation from the mean, because they are usually working with processes that require careful monitoring and do not want a wide deviation from the standard.[4] Figure 12-9 lists the steps for developing a control chart.

There are two types of data gathered for a control chart:

Count data are qualitative data that consist of counts of observations. Examples of *count data* include the following:

- The number of admission assessment sheets completed
- The number of missed physician signatures
- The percentage of meetings starting late
- The number of pharmacy errors

Measurement data are quantitative data that yield a measurement or number for each observation (i.e., "how much" of something is present). Examples of measurement data are the following:

- Heights
- Weights
- Times
- Temperatures
- Physical dimensions

EVALUATING THE VARIATIONS

Once a variation requiring investigation is identified, it should be evaluated by those directly involved in the process to be examined. The traditional approach in health care has been to have the work of clinical staff evaluated by a "quality coordinator." This "quality coordinator" functioned like a police officer.

Eskildson and Yates state that "This policing environment encourages data-collection delays and roadblocks, game playing, and conflict between . . . departments . . ."[3] Fast feedback is essential to effective performance improvement; the lack of teamwork and the separation of "duties" has tended to erect barriers to speedy data collection and analysis. These barriers delay identification of the causes of the problem. Fast feedback requires that those who collect the data also do the analysis.

Separation of these tasks not only impedes performance management, it undermines teamwork, delays feedback and progress, increases costs of data gathering, and communicates a less than total organizational commitment to performance excellence.[3]

THE BLUEPRINT council structure (see Chapter 5) recommends a Quality Management Board chaired by the CEO, with membership drawn from every department within the organization. This board is the governing, *authoritative* body for performance management within the organization. It coordinates improvement teams and serves as the central clearinghouse for all performance management activities within the organization.

Those providing the service are involved in its measurement and improvement. The analysis of variations found during the measurement process is performed by the person(s) or team collecting the data. This analysis is then submitted to the Quality Management Board.

HOW TO ANALYZE THE VARIATIONS

Once the data have been collected and organized, the variance decision-making tree presented in Figure 12-10 can be used to analyze the variation. To begin the study analysis, staff should ask, "Do the study results fall outside the established target parameters?" If the answer is "no" and if no pattern or trend is apparent, then no corrective action is necessary and the measurement schedule should be continued. However, if the answer to the question is "yes," the specific domain(s) involved in causing the variation must be identified. If service variables are the cause of the variation, a customer action plan is necessary. This may be in the form of a practice guideline, pathway, or patient teaching plan. If service variables are not the cause, practice or governance variables are looked to as a source of the variation. (Service, practice, and governance variables were defined in Chapter 6 and are listed on the indicator development tool described in Chapter 10.) Next the determination is made concerning whether practice variables were responsible for the variance. If so, the development and implementation of an employee development plan and/or staff development plan are indicated. If practice variables are not the cause of the variance, governance or service variables are looked to as causative factors. Finally it is questioned whether governance variables are responsible for the variation in measurement results. If they are, an administrative action plan is needed to correct the variance and bring the system into control. If they are not, service and practice variables are looked to as causative factors.

In some cases, two or all three of the domains may contribute to the variance, and multiple plans may be necessary to correct the deviation. It may also be necessary to review the indicator development tool and

- *Steps in developing a control chart*:
  1. Select a series of data points measuring the process over time. It is necessary to collect data at least 15-20 times before beginning the control chart. *Fewer than 15-20 data points on a control chart provides insufficient information on which to base decisions for change.*
  2. Compute control limits using standard deviation. *An inexpensive scientific calculator may be used to compute standard deviation. Follow the directions that come with each calculator.*
  3. Construct the control chart:

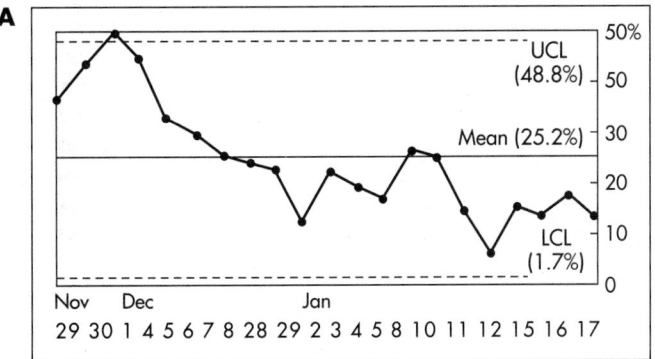

- **How do we determine "in" and "out of" statistical control? Out of statistical control occurs when:** *Points lie outside or beyond the control limit lines.*

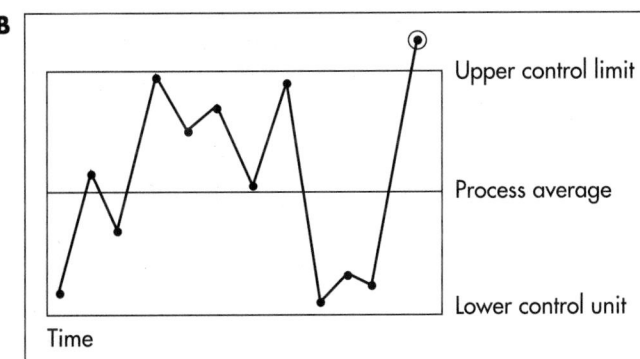

There are seven consecutive points on the same side of the centerline.

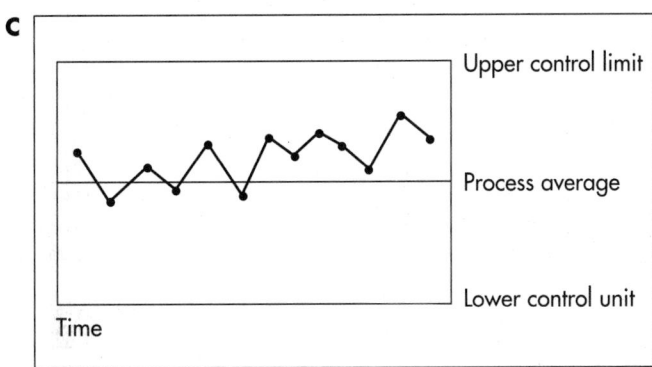

Figure 12-9   Steps in developing a control chart. (Modified from *Variation: The foundation for run charts and control charts* (Executive Learning, Inc). In *The Portrait of Continuous Quality Improvement* Houston, Tex, Living Centers of America, October 1994. Used by permission.)

Continued.

Six consecutive points increase or decrease.

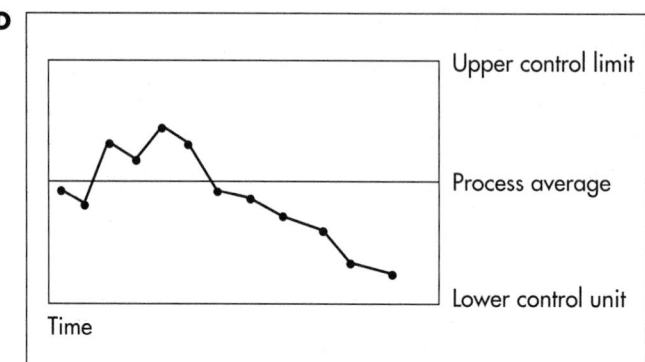

There is little variation from the center line; called stratification and indicates that the sampling process was not random.

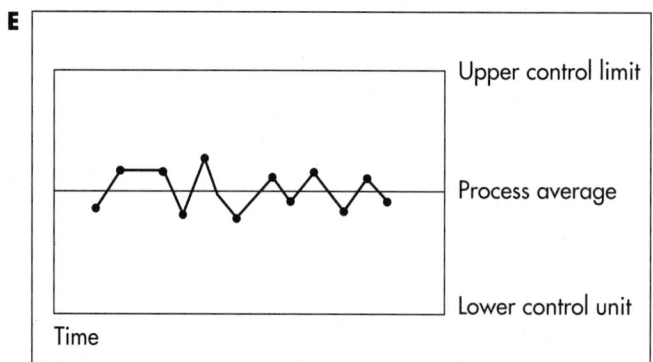

There is a lot of variation from the center line. This is called mixture and may indicate process instability or inconsistency.

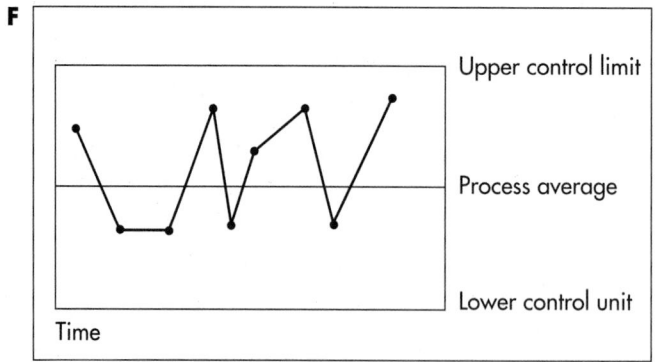

Using control charts helps us to make solid decisions based on data. It prevents us from "shooting from the hip" or from using "gut feelings" or "hunches" to manage our departments.

Figure 12-9,   cont'd.

reexamine the service, practice, and governance variables, adding additional sources of variance if the initial ones are not sufficient to fully explain the variation in results. A fishbone diagram may help in this process. In Chapter 13 the types of action planning

required in each domain to correct the problem variables are described in detail.

If the answer to the question, "Do the study results fall outside of the established target parameters?" is no, the next question becomes, "Is a trend or pattern

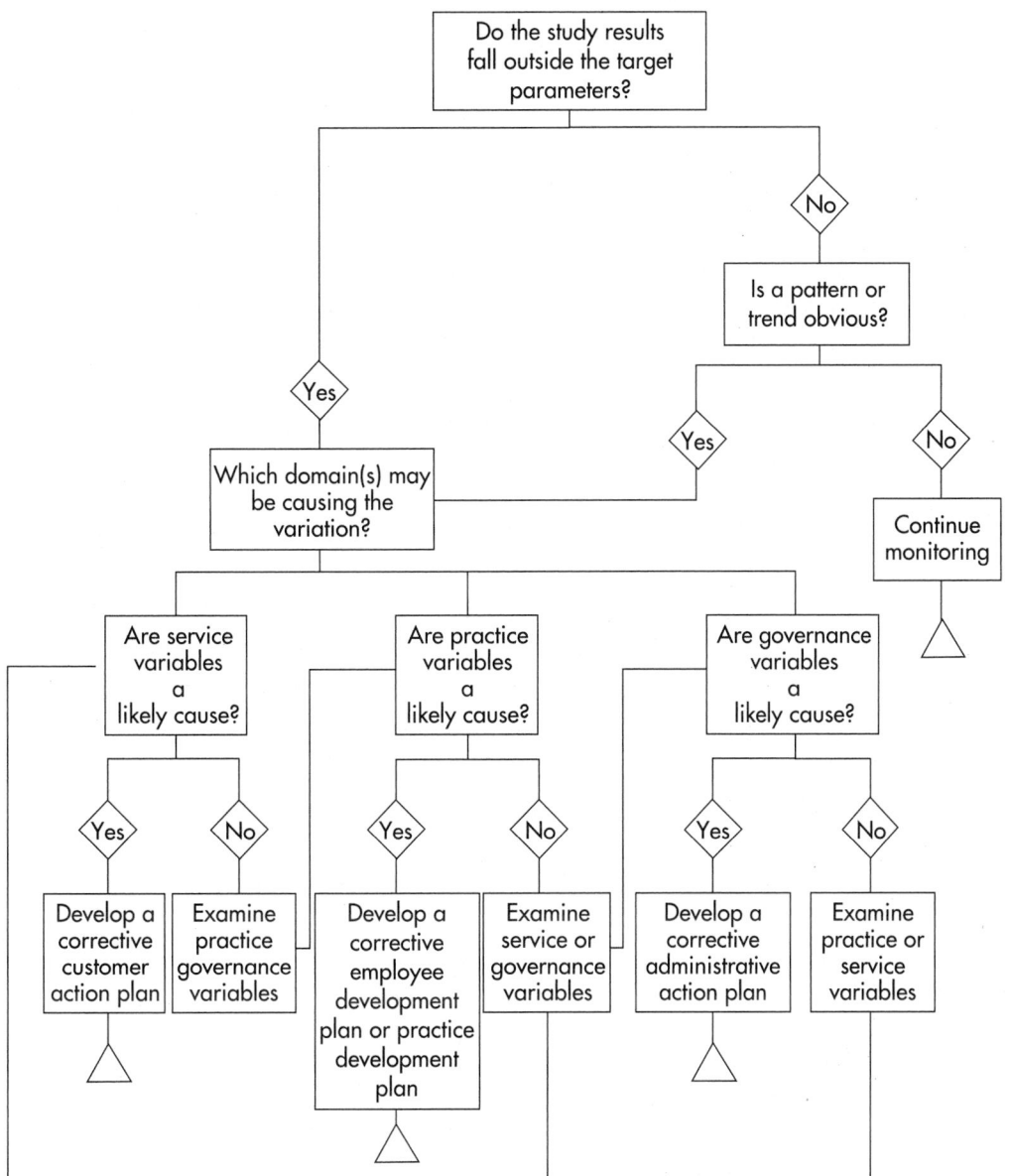

Figure 12-10   Variance decision-making tree.

in the study results obvious?" The control chart is reviewed to note any trends in the study results. If the answer to this question is no, the variation is probably common cause and the system is probably in statistical control with a variation due to chance. Because corrective action might result in tampering, it is probably best to wait until the next scheduled study period and compare the results to see if a trend is forming. If, however, a trend or pattern does exist, this may indicate a special cause variation, which requires analysis of the service, practice, or governance variables that are causing the variance and the initiation of appropriate action planning.

The variance decision-making tree creates a trifocus for problem solving that helps to isolate the likely causes of variation in measurement results. The more quickly sources of problems can be pinpointed, the more quickly solutions can be designed and implemented. Swift solutions to problems result in cost savings and improved performance.

Rafael Aguayo says, "The companies that rely on inspection to improve quality believe that quality is expensive (because of the way they believe improvements are made). The Deming companies, on the other hand, are constantly improving the process and the product without justifying every improvement, confident that higher productivity, lower costs, and higher profits will result."[1]

"Ignorance is the most expensive commodity in the world."[1] In today's health care environment, health care workers can no longer ignore the resource-saving, cost-effective statistical methods of performance measurements.

REFERENCES

1. Aguayo R: *Dr. Deming: the American who taught the Japanese about quality,* New York, 1990, Carol Publishing Co.
2. Deming WE: *Out of the crisis,* Cambridge, Mass, 1986, Massachusetts Institute of Technology Center for Advanced Engineering Study.
3. Eskildson L, Yates GR: Lessons from industry: reusing organizational structure to improve health care quality assurance, *Quality Rev Bull,* 17(2): 38-41, 1991.
4. Green E: Taking control of control charts, *Nursing Quality Connection,* May/June 1995, pp 4-5.
5. Ishikawa K: *Guide to quality control,* Tokyo, 1982, Asian Productivity Organization.
6. Joint Commission of Accreditation of Healthcare Organizations: 1995 accreditation manual for hospitals, Chicago, 1995, The Association.
7. O'Leary DS: President's column, *Joint Commission Perspectives,* 10:2, Nov/Dec 1990.
8. Scholtes PR: *The team handbook,* Madison, Wis, 1990, Joiner Associates, Inc.
9. Sines B: Personal communication, April 21, 1991.
10. Walton M: *The Deming management method,* New York, 1986, The Putnam Publishing Co.
11. Walton M: *Deming management at work,* New York, 1990, G.P. Putnam's Sons.

Part Five

CREATING AN ORGANIZATION-WIDE PERFORMANCE IMPROVEMENT PROGRAM

Chapter 13

Developing and Implementing a Performance Improvement Plan

It was a manufacturer's worst nightmare come true. On September 29, 1982, the first of seven Chicagoans died after ingesting cyanide-laced Extra Strength Tylenol capsules. This incident panicked the public and rocked the very foundation of Johnson & Johnson, the parent company of McNeil Laboratories, the maker of Tylenol.

Something needed to be done and quickly. However, the wrong move could worsen rather than correct the problem. Within hours of the incident, the switchboards at Johnson & Johnson were overloaded with calls from pharmacies, doctors, hospitals, poison control centers, and consumers, not to mention news reporters.

Recognizing the need for swift and decisive action, Johnson & Johnson executives mobilized a three-phase plan of action. Phase one involved problem identification and containment. By the end of the first day, the executives were convinced the poisonings did not originate at the plant, either accidentally or intentionally. This was confirmed the next morning, when the capsules taken by the sixth victim were identified to have been from a lot that had been produced at another location. Containment required the recall of all Tylenol capsules—over 31 million packages nationwide. The company also halted all further production of the capsules and suspended advertising of the product.

The second phase involved communication between the company, the police, the health authorities, and the public. Clarification of the incident was made in advertisements, letters to the trade, and statements to the media. Emergency phone lines were installed to answer questions.

By the second weekend, the company had moved into the third phase: rebuilding the brand name. (The idea of ending all further production of Tylenol was never a consideration, although industry experts suggested reintroducing the product under a new name.) The rebuilding phase involved a strategic plan that included reestablishing public trust in the product. A triple-seal, tamper-resistant package was designed. Coupons were distributed to the public offering free packages of Tylenol, and higher than normal discounts were given to retailers so that shelf space for Tylenol would be regained. Johnson & Johnson offered a $100,000 reward to anyone who provided information leading to the arrest and conviction of those responsible for the tragedy.

As a result of this incident, the Food and Drug Administration (FDA) and the over-the-counter pharmaceuticals organization formed a committee to develop standards for tamper-resistant packages. Previously, Tylenol had commanded about 35% of the $1.3 billion analgesic market, outselling the next four leading analgesics combined, but during the crisis, sales of Tylenol dropped 80%. By February 1983, however, Tylenol had regained almost 70% of its former market share.

The tragedy could have meant the end of Tylenol production and a significant blow to Johnson & Johnson. Success was achieved because swift and decisive action was taken.[1,8,11]

The story illustrates a critical point. To solve problems effectively or seize opportunities for quality improvement, a plan is necessary. The key to effective action is to act, not to react. Successful action requires a strategy. "Strategy is not about adaptability in behavior, but about regularity, not about discontinuity but about consistency. Organizations adopt strategies to reduce uncertainties, to set direction, focus effort, reduce risks, and define the organization."[5]

A performance improvement plan requires a proactive approach, not haphazard attempts or quick fixes.

PERFORMANCE IMPROVEMENT

Performance improvement involves the resolution of performance problems and the exploitation of performance opportunities. Performance problems are either unsatisfactory or undesired outcomes or those obstacles within the service that interfere with achievement of desired customer outcomes. These problems may deal with service, practice, or governance. A service problem might be an increase in the number of injury-related falls. A practice problem might be a deficit in documentation of patient care. A governance problem might be inadequate staffing to meet customer needs.

Performance opportunities consist of those occasions when, although the performance target is adequate, an opportunity exists to improve the outcome of the service or the process by which the service is delivered. These situations provide the opportunity to "work smarter," not harder, to add value to the service while controlling costs. They may be service, practice, or governance related. For example, although the surgical wound infection rate falls to within the desired target parameters, staff may identify an opportunity to decrease costs without compromising patient outcomes by replacing sterile dressings with clean ones in dressing changes or environmental services may find a more cost-efficient way to dispose of hazardous waste. Thus, while the target parameters are maintained, cost of service may be considerably reduced.

Inherent in performance improvement is change. In 500 BC Heraclitus said that nothing endures but change. More recently, both Waterman[13] and Peters[12] have discussed change as a necessary factor in today's corporate environment. Waterman defines change as a dynamic imbalance. "There is a kind of rhythm to the process: first, a constant search for standard ways of doing things that makes life easier. Then, the deliberate breaking of old rules, familiar patterns, past practice. . . ."[13]

Change is indicated whenever there is a discrepancy between what is actual and what is desired. The discrepancy can involve either the outcomes, the process, or the structure of the service, practice, or governance. Improvements in the nosocomial infection rate or in patient compliance are examples of a change in desired customer outcomes. A change in practice, such as the discontinuation of bedside-based laboratory monitoring, is an example of a process change. A structure change might involve expanding the type of personnel who can perform certain processes.

Change is a complex, continuous process. Brooten describes it as a process that leads to alterations in individual or institutional patterns of behavior.[3] It may occur haphazardly or in an organized manner. Haphazard change simply happens. Brooten calls it "change by drift" and suggests that it is caused by benign neglect. It is marked by failure to consider the consequences of a series of actions. The spiralling costs of health care are an example of this type of change. The parties involved are carried along by the change much like a boat adrift in a sea. The process is undirected and the results are unpredictable.

A second type of change is reactive change. Spurred by an unmanageable situation (the proverbial straw that broke the camel's back), what happens can be described as a "knee-jerk" reaction. For example, the mother of the chairman of the board received cold meals during a recent hospital stay. Memos and directives are issued and policies and procedures are immediately changed. Reactive change can have positive or negative results; however, the greatest problem with this type of change is that it is situational.

Planned change, on the other hand, is a deliberate, conscious, controlled process. It is proactive, involving collaborative goal setting and active participation by the parties involved. Activity is directed toward improving processes to achieve predefined outcomes.

Change requires movement. In haphazard change, the movement is uncontrolled. Reactive change is controlled, but the results may not be optimal because of lack of forethought. During planned change, there is a deliberate attempt to control the change process by predetermining outcomes and adjusting the operating processes to achieve the desired results.

PLANNING FOR CHANGE

Planned change necessitates a strategy for change. Resolution of performance problems or exploitation of performance opportunities requires strategic planning.

Strategic planning is the vehicle for responding to and shaping change by developing and implementing outcome-directed processes to manage that change.

"Strategic planning is a continuous, systematic process of making risk-taking decisions today with the greatest knowledge of their effects on the future; organizing efforts necessary to carry out these decisions; and evaluating results of those decisions against expected outcomes through reliable feedback mechanisms."[7] It is the process of making decisions about the design and delivery of the service, practice, and governance of the organization. Strategic planning turns desired results into a plan of action.

NEED FOR PLANNING

In the midst of constant change, planning provides stability. In today's health care economy, organizations *cannot* afford *not* to plan. Garner suggests, however, that the same factors that necessitate planning are also the acknowledged reasons given for not planning.[9] These pressures include service diversification, competition, changing consumer preferences, accelerated technology, economic constraints, changing professional expectations, and organizational complexity.

The benefits of planning are numerous. Planning establishes standards by which performance can be evaluated. It provides a sense of direction. It determines limits by building in controls that focus full attention on the task at hand. It assigns responsibility and accountability for structure, process, and outcomes. A strategic plan provides a barometer to measure variance from the intended path while affording an organized approach to complex projects or problems. It reduces the costs of human and material resources by focusing on their effective and efficient use. It is a lifesaver when a crisis strikes, because it provides the necessary redirection in the midst of chaos. Had Johnson & Johnson failed to plan, Tylenol may have been lost forever.

Planning facilitates collaboration and creativity, because it focuses on a critical issue and fosters the exchange and development of new ideas and solutions. Planning, however, is a skill in which many individuals lack expertise. This may account for some reluctance to plan. Other reasons for not planning relate to the problems inherent in the traditional approach to strategic planning.

REDEFINING THE STRATEGIC PLAN

The traditional strategic plan set the overall goals and direction for the organization. It was global in scope, dealing with ways to maximize market position and financial outcomes. It was generally considered to be an executive function and often remained exclusively in the board room. The focus was projecting a 5-year plan to move the institution toward its vision.

Today's organizational visions have a much shorter range, because the economic and technologic stability of health care is constantly changing. Thus the entire approach to strategic planning needs to be rethought. Today's plans need to focus on the short term. One-year plans now replace the replanning syndrome of the past, wherein much time was spent generating 3- to 5-year plans that had to be redesigned within a year because of unpredicted change. This also contributed to a reluctance to participate in the planning process and reinforced the perception of planning as an academic exercise.

No longer is planning an executive function. Today strategic planning is an essential tool for the entire organization. It is a critical element whenever and wherever change is needed at the divisional, unit, or individual level. Councils and task forces need to use strategic planning also to manage change. Garner suggests, "Not only do health care organizations need a vibrant and results oriented planning process but planning is crucial at all organizational levels."[9] The 3M Company develops a new strategic plan each year. Each of its businesses outlines its strategy for the year and submits it to headquarters, where a corporate plan is developed.

The traditional view of strategic planning is changing. Peters suggests that flexibility in planning is the watchword of the future.[12] The planning process and therefore the plan itself is dynamic. To be responsive, flexible, and customer-driven, the process must be "bottom-up," i.e., it must start at the front line and include those staff members who will implement the change. Decisions regarding the plan must be made by the councils expected to carry out the plan.

DECISIONS, DECISIONS, DECISIONS

Decision making is a critical skill in the planning process. Unlike routine or operational decision making, which focuses on day-to-day situations, strategic decision making involves new ways to do things or to solve problems on a large scale. Decisions are made in all three phases of planning.

In the first phase, priority setting, decisions are made regarding which critical issues will be addressed and whether those issues are service, practice, or governance in nature. Decisions are also made regarding priorities for action based on which issues have the greatest influence on customer outcomes. The tools and techniques outlined in Chapter 7 are helpful in making these decisions.

In the next phase, outcome setting, decision making focuses on the results to be achieved for each of the defined priorities. Questions to be asked include, "What are the desired outcomes for this critical issue?"

and "What will the results of this planned change in service be?" If, for example, the critical issue is documentation, the desired outcomes of a high performance documentation system must be defined before any attempt is made to change the current system. One outcome might be that there will be a legally sound record of patient care activities in each department of the organization and patient responses to those activities. Another might be the elimination of redundancy or a decrease in documentation time. This is the phase that clearly separates planned change from reactive change.

Many organizations omit this phase of the planning process. They plan activities, implement them, and wait to see the results. Determining outcomes before changing a process is critical to ensuring that the planned processes focus on achieving desired results. No resources are wasted on extraneous or nonessential, nonproductive activities. All processes are directed and purposeful.

The third phase, intervention planning, involves deciding how to achieve the predetermined outcomes. Decisions include who will do what by when. Deciding who will act delegates the responsibility, awards the authority, and establishes accountability for completing specific activities. The specified activities must include only those actions essential to accomplish the desired results. Actions must be resource driven and sequential. Being resource driven means that the constraints of people, equipment, operating systems, money, and other resources are considered when making activity choices. The time line portion of this phase defines the completion date for specific activities and ensures achieving the outcome by the target date.

DEVELOPING AN EFFECTIVE PLAN

Curtin states "the most successful strategies for action or change capitalize on existing value structures."[5] These value structures are evident in written standards. The box at the top of the page lists the policies that must be in effect for successful planning. These policies or rules for plans must be adhered to diligently.

Deep and Sussman describe four inhibitions that prevent good planning.[6] The first is that many people consider planning a luxury. They are so busy "putting out fires" that they cannot free themselves from their immediate duties to focus on tomorrow. Second, because planning is a future-oriented activity, many feel that it constitutes little more than an educated guess. A third obstacle is society's emphasis on *doing* rather than *thinking*. "We erect statues and name streets after people who successfully execute the plan, not those who devise it."[6] Finally, Deep and Sussman believe that many people lack planning skills. They

POLICIES FOR PLANS

1. Plans must be written.
2. Plans must be developed with input from staff responsible for implementation.
3. Plans must be specific to the defined critical issue.
4. Plans must be realistic.
5. Plans must be flexible.
6. Plans must define outcomes, actions, and responsible parties.
7. Plans must be reviewed and/or revised periodically.
8. People affected by the plan must be kept informed.
9. Planned actions and outcomes must be timed.
10. The timespan of a plan must be no longer than 1 year.

ELEVEN CHARACTERISTICS OF AN EFFECTIVE PLAN

These features must all be in place before the plan is implemented:

1. It is stated clearly in terms of the desired end results.
2. It is put into writing.
3. It has been drafted by people who will also be responsible for its implementation.
4. It has been communicated to all those it affects for their comments.
5. One person is ultimately accountable for its implementation.
6. A specific date is established for its completion; earlier dates are established for intermediate milestones as appropriate.
7. Criteria for success of the plan and how to apply those criteria are determined.
8. Intermediate review steps for "go/no go" decisions or revisions of the plan are laced throughout the implementation period.
9. Potential problems that may arise during implementation are identified and anticipated with preventive action.
10. Potential opportunities that may arise during implementation are identified so as to take advantage of them.
11. The supervisor of the plan is held accountable for reporting progress and revisions to the plan on a regular basis to superiors and to all those involved with implementation.

From Deep S, Sussman L: *Smart moves,* Reading, Mass, 1990, Addison-Wesley.

suggest that firefighters, uncertainty avoiders, doers, and skill-deficient individuals can benefit from simple, straightforward planning advice. They offer the 11 characteristics of an effective plan listed in the box above.

PLANNING

OUTCOME ➡ PROCESS

IMPLEMENTATION

PROCESS ➡ OUTCOME

Figure 13-1   Relationship of process and outcome during planning and implementation.

Responsible party	Who	5 West staff
Outcome verb	Will Do	will increase
Conditions	What	their compliance to the alteration in skin integrity protocol
Criteria	By how much, When	by 10% in one year

Figure 13-2   Anatomy of an outcome.

WRITING EFFECTIVE OUTCOMES

Probably the most difficult part of planning for most health care professionals is writing outcomes. This may be because they are accustomed to carrying out actions and waiting to see the results. In the implementation phase, this is exactly what happens. However, in the planning phase, the desired outcomes must be devised *first*, then the activities required to achieve those outcomes are designed. It is only after the action plan has been developed that the implementation phase begins. It is during this phase that the planned activities are carried out and it is noted whether these activities produce the desired results. Figure 13-1 depicts the relationship of process and outcome during planning and implemenation.

Without well-written outcomes, the planning process is doomed to fail. Outcomes provide the foundation for all actions that follow. They represent the difference between motion and direction. Without them, activities have no focus. The effective planner writes SMART outcomes:

Specific: *Define only one intention/result per outcome.*
Measurable: *Quantify the intention/result.*
Appropriate: *Ensure the intention/result is suitable for the identified critical issue.*
Realistic: *Set challenging but achievable results given the available resources.*
Timed: *State when the result is to be achieved.*

Outcomes must be written in terms of the results to be achieved—not how to get there. For example, say, "The staff will reduce the number of level IV falls in geriatric patients to less than 5% within 6 months" rather than "The staff will develop a falls prevention program." The first is a result, the second is an action designed to achieve the result. To facilitate this process, use results-oriented verbs, such as *increase, decrease, reduce, maintain, expand, eliminate,* and *improve,* rather than process verbs, such as *design, develop, identify,* and *evaluate.*

An effective outcome defines who will do what, by how much, and when. Figure 13-2 depicts the anatomy of an outcome. Depending on the type of plan needed, outcomes may be service, practice, or governance in nature.

Action Planning Tools

A number of planning tools have been designed to assist teams in developing action plans. Brassard outlines seven key management and planning tools in his book *The Memory Jogger +*.[2] The tools are not new; rather, most of them have their roots in post-World War II Operations Research work and in the Japanese quality control efforts. These tools include the following:

1. The Affinity Diagram
2. Interrelationship Digraph
3. Tree Diagram
4. Prioritization Matrices
5. Matrix Diagram
6. Process Decision Program Chart (PDPC)
7. Activity Network Diagram

Affinity diagram.   This tool gathers large amounts of language data and organizes it into groups based on natural relationships among the items. For example, when identifying possible solutions to a problem, write each idea from a brainstorming session on an individual adhesive note. After the brainstorming session, group the ideas according to major classifications. This tool helps to sort a large volume of information into manageable chunks. It is helpful in providing structure after brainstorming.

Interrelationship digraph.   This tool graphically maps out the cause and effect links among all items generated during brainstorming and organized into an affinity diagram. For each adhesive note, ask, "Does this cause or influence any of the other notes displayed?" If the answer is yes, draw an arrow from that note to the one(s) it causes. Repeat the procedure for all the notes. Prioritize the notes from highest to lowest number of arrows. This tool helps to provide direction on which are priority topics for action. It is especially helpful when resources for improvement are scarce.

Tree diagram.   This tool systematically maps out the actions needed to be accomplished to correct a problem or to meet an improvement goal. Place the goal or problem statement in a box on the left of the page. Then ask, "What needs to happen to resolve this problem or achieve this goal?" It is useful once a problem has been identified or a goal established. The Tree Diagram provides specific action steps that need to occur to resolve the problem or achieve the goal. It is helpful when broad objectives need to be broken down into specific implementation detail and when assignments need to be made.

Prioritization matrices.   This tool helps to prioritize tasks based on weighted criteria. It is a combination of the Tree Diagram and the Matrix Diagram. It helps to eliminate undesirable or ineffective options. Again, this tool is most useful when resources are scarce.

Matrix diagram.   This tool shows the relationship between each idea in one group of items and each idea in one or more of the other groups. It is helpful when you need to show the logical connecting points between items in each set. There are a number of different matrix formats depending on the number of sets of items being evaluated. This tool helps to identify the strength of the relationships among items of different sets.

Process decision program chart.   This tool maps out every conceivable event and contingency that might occur in moving from a problem or goal statement to action. It is used when the cost of failure is high and/or the implementation phase must be kept to a tight time frame. Often a Tree Diagram is used, and at each step the question asked is, "What could go wrong?" Solutions to the potential problems are brainstormed and countermeasures are built into the plan.

Activity network diagram.   This tool is used to plan the most appropriate schedule for any complex tasks. It is helpful when simultaneous improvement plans must be coordinated and when the time frames for completion are critical.

Figure 13-3 depicts each tool, its relationships with the others, and diagrams the typical flow of its use.

DEVELOPING CLINICAL PLANS

When the critical issue for change deals with service, the written plan is directed toward the customer. In the first phase of service planning, the critical issue to be decided is the type of service plan to be used. If the service is patient-oriented, the plans will be clinical in nature. Clinical action plans include clinical paths, algorithms, practice guidelines, and patient teaching plans. Depending on the clinical situation and the health care delivery system, the type of plan utilized may vary. Nevertheless, in a resource-driven environment, decisions must be made regarding appropriate priorities of care relative to the patient's phase of acuity, projected length of stay, and available resources. For example, given a length of stay of 3.5 days for a mastectomy patient, resolution of body image disturbance is not a realistic outcome. A more appropriate result might be that the patient is able to use existing coping mechanisms to manage the emotional trauma associated with breast removal. An example of a customer service plan in the medical records department might relate to information sharing between the hospital and the home health service.

The decisions in the second phase relate to defining customer outcomes. Customer outcomes may be desired or expected. Desired outcomes are those results you wish to obtain as a result of specific interventions. Expected outcomes are those you can anticipate as a result of a process. For example, fever, nausea, and vomiting are expected outcomes of chemotherapy. The desired outcome in this situation might be that the patient maintains his or her current weight during the treatment period or that the patient's fluid and electrolyte balance is maintained within plus or minus 10% during the treatment period. Certain things happen as a result of medical and nursing processes; it is important to recognize these expected results and take them into consideration when writing outcomes. Controlling the fever, nausea, and vomiting is a means to an end. These processes are necessary to achieve the desired results whether the results are maintaining weight, fluid and electrolyte balance, or comfort.

All departments are responsible for certain customer-related processes and their resultant outcomes. For example, the biomedical department is responsible for electrical safety and its safety outcomes.

Clinical outcomes are patient focused, not practitioner focused. For example, use "The patient's fluid and electrolyte balance is maintained within plus or minus 10% during the treatment period," rather than "The practitioner will monitor the patient's fluid and electrolytes."

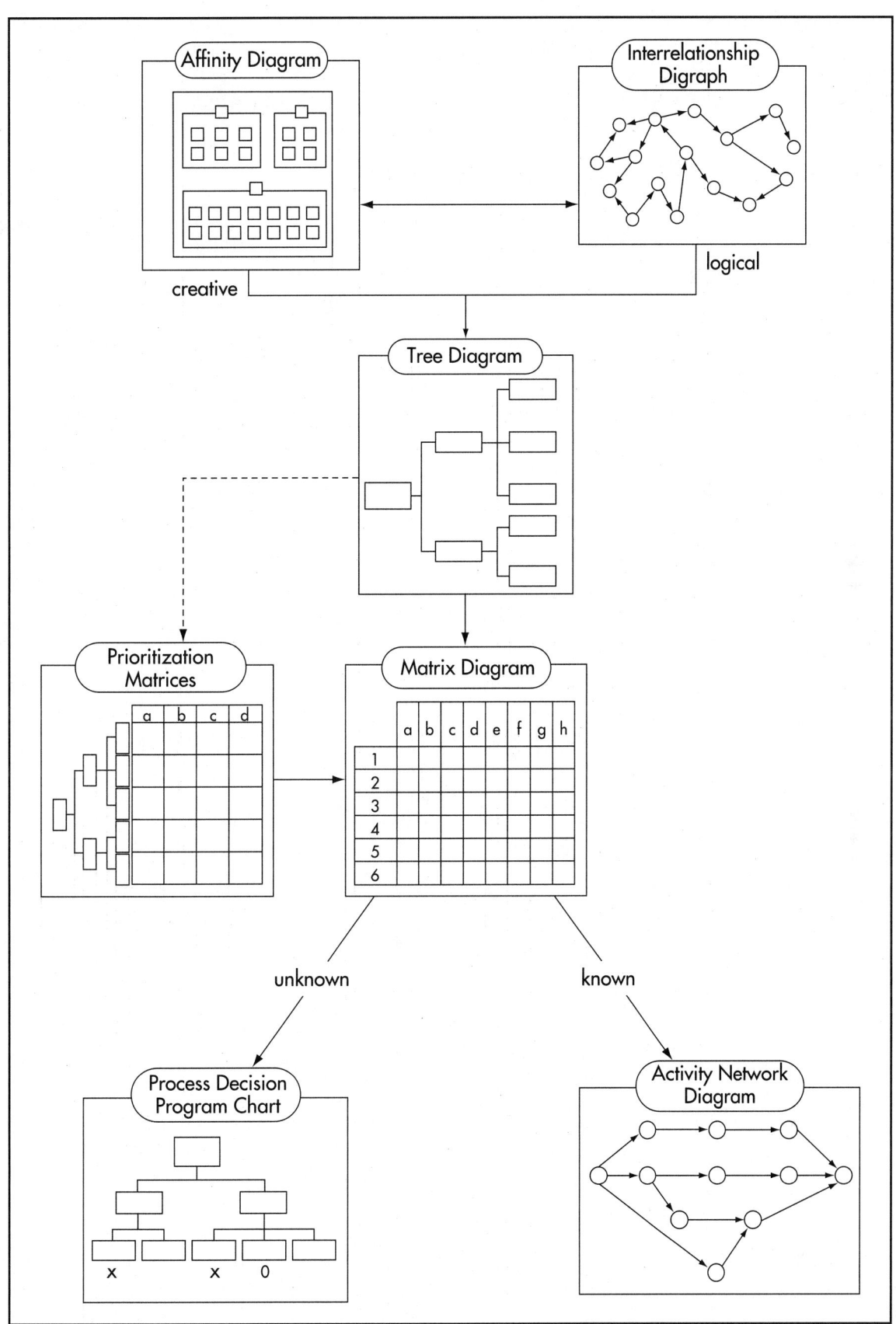

Figure 13-3   Seven management and planning tools—typical flow. (From *The memory jogger plus +: featuring the seven management and planning tools pocket cards,* Methuen, Mass, 1989, GOAL/QPC.

In the third phase of customer planning, the decisions revolve around which processes are essential to assist the customer in achieving the predetermined outcomes. Those activities may be referred to as interventions or orders. Interventions are delineated for each of the defined customer outcomes. Each of the orders then identifies who will do what by when. The "who" may be a physician, a nurse, another health care worker, the patient, or a significant other. Although the outcomes are customer centered, the processes carried out to achieve those outcomes are practice centered and may be performed by any number of individuals. The "what" defines the action or task to be performed and the "when" defines the deadline for completion.

The traditional nursing-specific care plans have given way to interdisciplinary clinical paths. These new plans attempt to reduce length of stay and cost while maintaining quality service and positive patient outcomes. They are typically written for a patient population with a specific medical diagnosis, such as an uncomplicated myocardial infarction or for a population who are undergoing a specific surgery or procedure such as coronary artery bypass or uncomplicated vaginal delivery. Figure 13-4 is an example of a clinical path.

Although the format for these plans vary, there are some critical factors to be considered in the development of these paths:

1. They must manage the patient's priority symptomatology, not the tasks to be performed.
2. They must consider phases of acuity, not days of treatment.
3. They must be outcome driven with outcomes written in each domain for each phase of acuity.

Practice guidelines are another fairly new form of patient care plan. They also occur in many different formats. The AHCPR has written guidelines, as have many professional associations. Managed care organizations are developing organization-specific practice guidelines to standardize care among practitioners. To differentiate practice guidelines from clinical paths, we have defined clinical paths as plans that address the care of medical diagnoses. Practice guidelines outline the care and outcomes for specific patient symptoms, such as decreased cardiac output or impaired gas exchange. Both of these symptoms may be present in a patient with an acute myocardial infarction. Thus the symptoms make up the medical diagnosis. Because practice guidelines outline the care of symptoms, they are the building blocks of clinical paths. Appendix 13-1 is an example of a practice guideline.[10]

Regardless of the format adopted for clinical paths or practice guidelines, it is clear that these new types of plans are going to play a major role in standardizing services in a managed care environment.

DEVELOPING A PROFESSIONAL PRACTICE PLAN

When the performance issue to be addressed involves the health care workers who provide the service, the improvement plan must focus on the practitioner. Two types of plans are commonly used: the employee development plan and the staff development plan.

The Employee Development Plan

The employee development plan is used when a staff performance problem occurs or when there is an opportunity to facilitate the growth and development of an individual. In the first phase of planning for performance correction the nature of the performance problem must be determined. Figure 13-5 depicts a performance problem decision tree. The problem may relate to competency or productivity, the two components of performance. Competency is the ability to do something at some level of proficiency. It is composed of some combination of knowledge, skills, attitudes, and values. Productivity is the application of knowledge, skills, attitudes, or values to yield favorable or useful results.

An employee development plan can be helpful regardless of the nature of the performance problem. Achieving an individual's potential is also facilitated by the use of this plan. In the first phase, the critical areas for development or improvement are identified. In the second phase, outcomes are defined for each critical issue. These outcomes focus on the individual staff member and define the results necessary to demonstrate an improvement in performance or an achievement of potential. Next, activities necessary to fulfill the outcomes are specified. A sample format for an employee development plan is shown in Figure 13-6. The benefits of an employee development plan include the following:

- Increasing staff members' control over their own jobs through a self-administered improvement plan
- Increasing staff members' accountability for their own performance
- Shifting focus of control from a conventional manager-imposed system to self-control
- Providing staff members with a personal benchmark against which to measure growth

The employee development plan is self-directed and self-administered. The employee, with the assistance of the manager, develops the plan. Together they identify critical elements for development or improvement. Then, outcomes are determined and specific activities outlined with a timeline for each element.

Total hip DRG: 209/210	Date: Day:	Date: Day:	Date: Day:	Date: Day:	Date: Day:
	Admission	Intraoperative	Post Op Day 1	Post Op Day 2	Post Op Day 3
Initiation of practice guidelines and applicable stages	☐ Anxiety 0 1 2 3 4 ☐ Admission 0 1 2 3 4 **Pre-operative** ☐ Anxiety 0 1 2 3 4 ☐ Falls prevention 0 1 2 3 4 ☐ Sleep pattern disturbance 0 1 2 3 4 ☐ Preparation for surgery 0 1 2 3 4 ☐ Transfer 0 1 2 3 4	☐ Alterations in skin integrity 0 1 2 3 4 ☐ Fluid volume deficit 0 1 2 3 4 ☐ Hyper-thermia 0 1 2 3 4 ☐ Impaired gas exchange 0 1 2 3 4 ☐ Infection prevention 0 1 2 3 4 ☐ Surgical wound 0 1 2 3 4 ☐ Transfer 0 1 2 3 4 **Post-anesthesia recovery period** ☐ Acute pain 0 1 2 3 4 ☐ Alterations in skin integrity 0 1 2 3 4 ☐ Alterations in peripheral vascular perfusion 0 1 2 3 4 ☐ Hypo-thermia 0 1 2 3 4 ☐ Surgical wound 0 1 2 3 4 ☐ Impaired gas exchange 0 1 2 3 4 ☐ Transfer 0 1 2 3 4	☐ Acute pain 0 1 2 3 4 ☐ Alterations in skin integrity 0 1 2 3 4 ☐ Alterations in cerebral perfusion 0 1 2 3 4 ☐ Falls prevention 0 1 2 3 4 ☐ Fluid volume deficit 0 1 2 3 4 ☐ Impaired mobility 0 1 2 3 4 ☐ Impaired gas exchange 0 1 2 3 4 ☐ Infection prevention 0 1 2 3 4 ☐ Nausea and vomiting 0 1 2 3 4 ☐ Self-care deficit 0 1 2 3 4 ☐ Surgical wound 0 1 2 3 4 ☐ Alterations in peripheral vascular perfusion 0 1 2 3 4	☐ Anxiety 0 1 2 3 4 ☐ Acute pain 0 1 2 3 4 ☐ Falls prevention 0 1 2 3 4 ☐ Fluid volume deficit 0 1 2 3 4 ☐ Hyper-thermia 0 1 2 3 4 ☐ Impaired mobility 0 1 2 3 4 ☐ Impaired gas exchange 0 1 2 3 4 ☐ Infection prevention 0 1 2 3 4 ☐ Sleep pattern disturbance 0 1 2 3 4 ☐ Surgical wound 0 1 2 3 4 ☐ Alterations in peripheral vascular perfusion 0 1 2 3 4	☐ Anxiety 0 1 2 3 4 ☐ Acute pain 0 1 2 3 4 ☐ Consti-pation 0 1 2 3 4 ☐ Falls prevention 0 1 2 3 4 ☐ Fluid volume deficit 0 1 2 3 4 ☐ Hyper-thermia 0 1 2 3 4 ☐ Impaired mobility 0 1 2 3 4 ☐ Impaired gas exchange 0 1 2 3 4 ☐ Infection prevention 0 1 2 3 4 ☐ Sleep pattern disturbance 0 1 2 3 4 ☐ Surgical wound 0 1 2 3 4 ☐ Alterations in peripheral vascular perfusion 0 1 2 3 4
Standing Orders		☐ NPO	☐ 20 lbs weight bearing ☐ OOB w/hip precautions ☐ Ambulate w/walker/crutches ☐ Clear liquids p̄ OR	☐ 20 lbs weight bearing ☐ OOB w/hip precautions ☐ Ambulate w/walker/crutches ☐ Regular diet	☐ Weight bearing to tolerance ☐ Stair climbing ☐ Exercise (PT) BID ☐ Regular diet
Medications	☐ Pre-op medications	☐ ? Transfuse blood ☐ Antibiotic protocol ☐ Pain med protocol ☐ Antiemetic protocol ☐ Coumadin protocol ☐ Renew routine med orders	☐ ? Transfuse blood ☐ Antibiotic protocol ☐ Pain med protocol ☐ Antiemetic protocol ☐ Coumadin protocol	☐ ? Transfuse blood ☐ Antibiotic protocol ☐ Pain med protocol ☐ Coumadin protocol	☐ ? Transfuse blood ☐ Antibiotic protocol ☐ Pain med protocol ☐ Coumadin protocol

Initials	Signature	Initials	Signature	Initials	Signature

Figure 13-4 Example of a clinical path. (Copyright 1997 Eleanor Green and Jacqueline Katz. Reprinted with permission.)

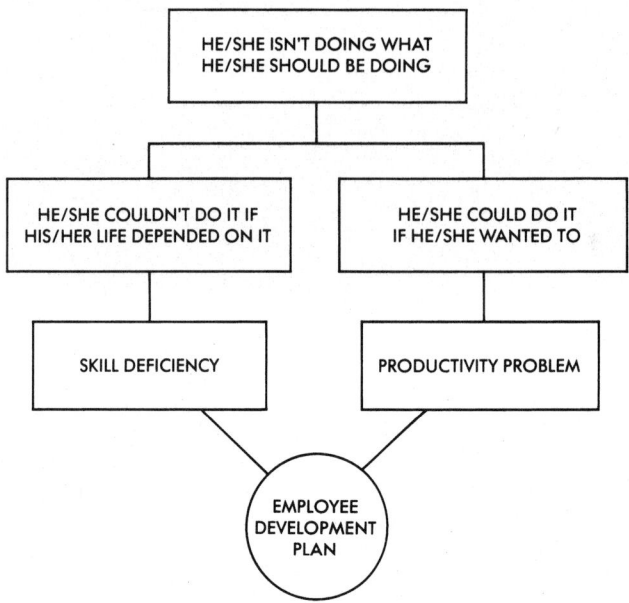

Figure 13-5   Performance problem decision tree.

The employee and the manager negotiate an incentive package for successful plan completion. The employee then implements the plan and periodically reviews and documents progress with the manager, who acts as a facilitator in this process. In a peer review system, the employee would present documentation of successful completion to the peer review body, who would then decide upon promotion.

The Staff Development Plan

When there is a competency deficit in more than one staff member or when an opportunity exists to expand the potential of more than one individual, the staff development plan is used. Issues that require a staff development plan might include preparation of staff to implement a new procedure, such as PICC line insertion, or the development of computer literacy skills. Another example might be a plan to certify all the health care workers in basic life support. The process of planning is similar to that used for the employee development plan. A sample format for a staff development plan is shown in Figure 13-7.

The benefits of staff development planning include the following:

- Timely and appropriate education of all health care workers
- Establishment of a link between performance improvement and staff development
- Improved consistency in organization-wide educational planning

The human resource department is ultimately responsible for the development, implementation, and evaluation of the staff development plan. These three areas of responsibility may be carried out solely by the educators in the human resources department or by designated educators in each department.

DEVELOPING AN ADMINISTRATIVE ACTION PLAN

In the governance domain, an administrative action plan is the tool of choice. It is used when a performance problem or an opportunity related to the system is to be addressed. Examples of governance issues include implementation of a new system, e.g., care delivery; use of a new subcontractor for laboratory services; a merger or acquisition; reorganization of the organization or division; and development of a yearly performance plan. Any time that systems must change, an administrative action plan is needed. In the first phase of planning, decision making focuses on which priorities must be addressed first. Being resource driven, priority is given to those changes that will have the greatest effect on customer outcomes. In the second phase, outcomes are developed to specify the desired results of administrative change and its anticipated impact on the system. Governance outcomes deal with ways in which the organization must change to effect performance improvement. Reducing overtime hours as a percentage of total hours worked is one example of a governance outcome. Another might involve reducing the salary cost per patient day, or reducing the absentee rate. Finally, specific actions are outlined that will facilitate the achievement of the defined outcomes. Figure 13-8 provides a sample format for an administrative action plan.

EMPLOYEE'S NAME _____

DATE OF PLAN _____

Area for Development	Expected Outcome	Target Date/ Monitor(s)	Actions	Responsible Persons	Completion Date		Incentive
					Projected	Actual	

_____ _____
Employee Signature   Date

_____ _____
Nurse Manager   Date

Figure 13-6   Employee development plan.

Critical Issue	Learner Objectives	Learning Activities	Responsible Person(s)	Completion Date		Evaluation Methodology	Threshold		Remarks
				Projected	Actual		Projected	Actual	

Figure 13-7   Staff development plan.

Critical Issue	Desired Outcome	Target Date	Actions	Completion Date		Responsible Person(s)
				Projected	Actual	

Figure 13-8 Administrative action plan.

Administrative action planning may be used by all managers and every department or work group. For example, administration develops a strategic plan, and a task force/team may develop a plan to implement clinical paths or a new recordkeeping system. A manager uses the administrative action plan to outline the achievement of annual department objectives, and the performance improvement council may use an administrative action plan to computerize the data collection and analysis system.

The benefits of administrative action planning include the following:

- the integration of service at all levels within the department or organization
- coordination of managerial activities
- improved utilization of resources

These benefits are realized because the process of planning focuses attention on the councils or teams involved in and affected by a change and the resources necessary to effect that change. The mere act of planning means that attention is given to what results are needed and what is the most efficient way of obtaining those results. Managerial responsibilities then revolve around providing the environment in which those planned activities can happen.

Following the example of pain management in terminally ill cancer patients, analysis of the variance may lead to the development of a number of different plans. A patient teaching plan might be indicated if analysis reveals that patients are uncomfortable because they are not using the equipment correctly. An employee development plan might be indicated if a particular worker is having difficulty passing a required credentialing examination. A staff development plan may be designed if analysis indicates an overall need for health care workers to reassess their values related to customer service. Finally, an administrative action plan and budget modifications may be needed if analysis of variance defines the lack of equipment to be a factor in achieving satisfactory levels of customer satisfaction.

TURNING PLANS INTO ACTION

It is not enough to create good plans; they must be enacted. A plan is no better than the paper on which it is written, if it is not implemented. Without action, the plan is simply rhetorical, a statement of intended performance.

According to Clemmer, our performance results are determined by what we finish, not what we start. Planning is the start of the improvement process but it is the implementation of that plan that makes the difference. "It's ultimately your improvement action that determines your performance results. The effectiveness of that action hinges on your follow through and stick-to-it-iveness."[4]

Moving the plan from paper to practice is facilitated by establishing timetables for completion of specific activities and assigning responsibility for accomplishment of those tasks. Each responsible party must act in accordance with the plan and complete the assigned activities in the time allotted, if the plan is to succeed.

The key to successful action is planning. The traditional view of planning must change from that of an academic exercise to that of a dynamic tool used at every level of the organization.

Decision making is the heart of planning and occurs in each of the three phases of the process. In the initial phase of planning, the decisions relate to identification of the critical issues and establishment of priorities for action. In the second phase, decision making focuses on the desired outcomes to be achieved, and in the final phase, decisions are made regarding the actions needed to accomplish the outcomes.

Plans take many forms and may address service, practice, or governance priorities. Regardless of the type of plan, however, as one anonymous sage put it, one must

Plan purposefully
Prepare prayerfully
Proceed positively
and
Pursue persistently.

REFERENCES

1. A death blow for Tylenol? *Business Week,* p 151, Oct 18, 1982.
2. Brassard M: *The memory jogger +,* Meuthen, Mass, 1989, GOAL/QPC.
3. Brooten D, Hayman L, Naylor M: *Leadership for change,* ed 2, Philadelphia, 1988, JB Lippincott.
4. Clemmer J: *Pathways to performance,* Rocklin, Cal, 1995, Prima Publishing.
5. Curtin L: Creating a culture of competence, *Nurs Manage,* 21(9): 7-8, 1990.
6. Deep S, Sussman L: *Smart moves,* Reading, Mass, 1990, Addison-Wesley.
7. Drucker PE: *Management: tasks, responsibilities, policies,* New York, 1974, Harper & Row.
8. Fannin R: Diary of an amazing comeback, *Market Media Decis,* special ed, pp 129-133, Spring 1982.
9. Garner JF, Smith HL, Piland NF: *Strategic nursing management,* Rockville, Md.,1990, Aspen Publishers.
10. Green E, Katz JM: *Clinical practice guidelines for the adult patient,* St Louis, 1995, Mosby.
11. Moore T: The fight to save Tylenol, *Fortune,* pp 45-49, Nov 29, 1982.
12. Peters T: *Thriving on chaos,* New York, 1988, Alfred A. Knopf.
13. Waterman RH Jr: *The renewal factor,* New York, 1987, Bantam Books.

Appendix 13-1   Practice Guideline for Management of Alterations in Skin Integrity Related to Pressure Ulcers

Severity Index

Stage 0:

At risk, but no visible evidence of alterations in skin integrity

Stage 1:

Nonblanchable erythema of intact skin

Stage 2:

Partial thickness skin loss involving epidermis and/or dermis. The ulcer is superficial and presents clinically as an abrasion, blister, or shallow crater.

Stage 3:

Full thickness skin loss involving damage or necrosis of subcutaneous tissue that may extend down to, but not through, underlying fascia. The ulcer presents clinically as a deep crater with or without undermining of adjacent tissue.

Stage 4:

Full thickness skin loss with extensive destruction, tissue necrosis, or damage to muscle, bone, or supporting structures (for example, tendon or joint capsule). Note: undermining and sinus tracts may also be present.

INDICATIONS:

1. Loss of pain/pressure sensations
2. Malnutrition
3. Anemia
4. Infection: bacterial, viral, fungal
5. Immobility (bed-bound, body cast, chair-bound)
6. Spinal cord injuries: quadriplegia, paraplegia
7. Oversedation (anesthesia)
8. Metabolic and endocrine disorders (diabetes, cirrhosis)
9. Peripheral vascular disease
10. Subcutaneous edema
11. Immunologic deficiencies
12. Excessive uncontrolled excretions/secretions (e.g., diarrhea, urinary/fecal incontinence, sweating)
13. Aged, elderly
14. Obesity
15. Preexisting history of pressure ulcers
16. Orthopedic patients
17. Critically ill patients
18. Impaired nutritional status
19. Altered level of consciousness
20. Radiation therapy

DEFINITION OF TERMS:

1. **Sinus tract:** pathway that can extend in any direction from the wound surface; results in dead space with potential for abscess formation
2. **Undermine:** tissue destruction underlying intact skin along wound margins

REFERENCES:

Bryant R et al: *Pressure ulcers in acute and chronic wounds nursing management,* Bryant R, editor, St Louis, 1992, Mosby.

U.S. Department of Health and Human Services: *Pressure ulcers in adults: prediction and prevention clinical practice guideline number 3,* Rockville, Md, 1992, Public Health Service, Agency for Health Care Policy and Research.

AUTHORS:

Jacqueline Katz, MS, RN
Eleanor Green, BSN, RN

APPROVAL BY:

DATE:

REVIEW DATE:

REVISE DATE:

DISTRIBUTION:

Alterations in Skin Integrity Related to Pressure Ulcers

STAGE 0:

At risk, but no visible evidence of pressure ulcer

Competencies:

In order to manage patients in this stage the individual must be able to:

1. Identify the signs and symptoms of stage 0 of alterations in skin integrity
2. Perform the processes outlined in this stage
3. Achieve the outcomes outlined in this stage
4. Identify the complications associated with this stage
5. Identify the causative factors that produce alterations in skin integrity
6. Describe the dangers associated with fixation devices such as tape, skeletal pins, casts, splints, and braces and their contribution to alterations in skin integrity
7. Select appropriate support devices
8. Position patient according to procedure

Credentialing:

None

ASSESSMENT:

1. Perform a baseline head-to-toe skin inspection and monitor at least once a day, with particular attention to bony prominences.
   Observe for:
   - delayed blanching
   - paleness
   - tissue sponginess
   - maceration
   - flakiness
   - scaling
   - skin temperature changes, either increased or decreased
   - induration (hardness)
   - skin turgor
   - capillary refill
   - loss of hair
   - color
   - edema
2. Monitor peripheral pulses q day
3. Observe patient's hygiene routine
4. Collect information regarding patient's/significant others' knowledge about alterations in skin integrity

Diagnosis:

1. Stage level of alteration in skin integrity
2. Identify the impact of external mechanical forces: pressure, friction, and shear
3. Determine patient's and significant others':
   - involvement in care
   - communication and support needs
   - knowledge base and readiness to learn

Outcomes Identification:

Patient

1. Absence of nonblanchable erythema; skin integrity is maintained
2. Identifies early signs and symptoms of alterations in skin integrity and reports them as they occur

Staff

1. Identifies and stages patient at risk for alterations in skin integrity
2. Utilizes processes outlined in this stage
3. Identifies signs and symptoms of worsening condition and restages patient status
4. Maintains communication regarding the patient's clinical condition and treatment plan with all involved persons

System

1. A qualified staff member is available to care for this patient
2. Equipment necessary to stage 0 processes is available as needed:
   - egg crate mattress

Planning:

In-house

1. Design a movement/turning schedule for bed-bound patients
2. Design a repositioning schedule for chair-bound patients
3. Modify the interventions outlined in this stage as indicated by patient condition or physician order
4. Modify patient education outlined in this stage based on patient's and/or significant others' knowledge of altered skin integrity
5. Modify the outcomes outlined in this stage based on assessment data

Discharge

1. Identify resources for obtaining support devices needed for home care
2. Continue positioning schedule

Education:

1. Demonstrate preventive care of skin
2. Teach factors that enhance skin integrity, such as adequate nutrition and fluid intake
3. Provide instruction in proper use of preventive aids
4. Teach patient to shift position every 15 minutes
5. Provide patient with all information to make informed health care decisions

Interventions:

1. Keep all skin clean, dry, free of body excretion. Avoid hot water and use a mild cleansing agent that minimizes irritation and dryness of skin. During cleansing minimize the force and friction applied to the skin
2. Keep bed clothing dry, free from crumbs, and other irritating material
3. Use lifting devices (such as pull sheets or trapeze) to avoid shearing and friction in lifting patient
4. Provide foot and nail care to avoid abrasions by scratching adjacent skin areas
5. Use moisturizer to treat dry skin; avoid massage over bony prominences
6. Maintain environmental humidity greater than 40%
7. Avoid exposure to cold
8. Use a lubricant such as:
   - corn starch or creams
   - protective films (such as transparent film dressings, skin sealant)
   - protective dressings (such as hydrocolloids)
   - protective padding to reduce friction injuries from moisture between skin folds, tape irritation
9. Use positioning devices such as pillows or foam wedges to pad bony prominences
10. Keep patient's heels off the bed. Do not use donut-type devices
11. When in side-lying position, avoid positioning directly on trochanter
12. Maintain head of bed at lowest degree elevation consistent with medical conditions or other restrictions. Limit amount of time the head of the bed is elevated.
13. Use an egg crate foam mattress
14. Avoid prolonged sitting; reposition every hour

15. Implement turning and/or repositioning schedules. Turn at least every 2 to 3 hours
16. Initiate indicated stage of altered nutrition: less than body requirements practice guideline

Complications

1. Nonblanchable erythema of intact skin
   - initiate stage 1 of alterations in skin integrity practice guideline

Evaluation:

1. Analyze patient progress toward outcomes
2. Analyze response to interventions, treatments, and medications
3. Evaluate effectiveness of teaching
4. Analyze the degree of understanding and cooperation with plan of care

Communication:

Verbal

1. Report:
   - any alteration in skin integrity

Written

1. Record initiation and specific stage of the practice guideline on the Careprint
2. Note any modifications to the stage on the Careprint and rationale for each modification as it occurs
3. Chart all baseline data, ongoing monitoring data, interventions taken, and the patient's responses on the patient care flowsheet
4. Record the evaluation of patient outcomes on the progress record
5. Record all patient teaching

STAGE 1:

Nonblanchable erythema of intact skin

Competencies:

In order to manage patients in this stage the individual must be able to:

1. Identify the signs and symptoms of stage 1 of alterations in skin integrity
2. Perform the processes outlined in this stage
3. Achieve the outcomes outlined in this stage
4. Identify the complications associated with this stage
5. Identify causative factors that produce alterations in skin integrity
6. Describe the dangers associated with fixation devices such as tape, skeletal pins, casts, splints, and braces and their contribution to alterations in skin integrity
7. Select appropriate support devices
8. Position patient according to procedure
9. Describe signs and symptoms of infection

Credentialing:

None

Assessment:

1. Perform a baseline head-to-toe skin inspection and monitor at least once a day, with particular attention to bony prominences.
   Observe for:
   - delayed blanching
   - paleness
   - tissue sponginess
   - maceration
   - flakiness
   - scaling
   - skin temperature changes, either increased or decreased
   - induration (hardness)
   - skin turgor
   - capillary refill
   - loss of hair
   - color
   - edema
2. Monitor peripheral pulses every day
3. Observe patient's hygiene routine
4. Collect information regarding patient's/significant others' knowledge about alterations in skin integrity

Diagnosis:

1. Stage level of alteration in skin integrity
2. Identify the impact of external mechanical forces: pressure, friction, and shear
3. Determine patient's and significant others':
   - involvement in care
   - communication and support needs
   - knowledge base and readiness to learn

Outcomes Identification:

Patient

1. Absence of nonblanchable erythema; skin integrity is maintained
2. Identifies early signs and symptoms of alterations in skin integrity and reports them as they occur

Staff

1. Identifies and stages patient with stage 1 alterations in skin integrity
2. Utilizes processes outlined in this stage
3. Identifies signs and symptoms of worsening condition and restages patient status
4. Maintains communication regarding the patient's clinical condition and treatment plan with all involved persons

System

1. A qualified staff member is available to care for this patient
2. Equipment necessary to stage 1 processes is available as needed:
   - egg crate mattress

Planning:

In-house

1. Design a movement/turning schedule for bed-bound patients
2. Design a repositioning schedule for chair-bound patients
3. Modify the interventions outlined in this stage as indicated by patient condition or physician order
4. Modify patient education outlined in this stage based on patient's and/or significant others' knowledge of altered skin integrity
5. Modify the outcomes outlined in this stage based on assessment data

Discharge

1. Identify resources for obtaining support devices needed for home care
2. Continue positioning schedule
3. Validate that turning and repositioning schedules can be maintained at home. If not, make referral to home health agency

Education:

1. Provide patient with all information to make informed health care decisions
2. Demonstrate treatment measures for broken skin surfaces
3. Teach factors that enhance skin integrity, such as adequate nutrition and fluid intake, reduced smoking
4. Provide instruction in proper use of preventive aids
5. Teach patient to shift position q 15 minutes
6. Teach how to decrease pressure points and promote optimal circulation

Interventions:

For Unaffected Areas

1. Maintain stage 0 of this practice guideline

For Affected Stage 1 Areas

1. Avoid use of soap or lotion
2. Cleanse area with clear water only; pat, do not rub, skin dry
3. Protect area with a protective film (such as transparent film dressings or skin sealant)
4. Never massage affected area
5. Protect area with positioning devices such as pillows or foam wedges. Do not use donut-type devices
6. Use an egg crate foam mattress
7. Keep patient off affected area
8. Implement turning and/or repositioning schedules: turn at least q 2 to 3 hours
9. Initiate indicated stage of altered nutrition: less than body requirements practice guideline

Complications

1. Partial thickness skin loss evidenced as abrasion, blister, or shallow crater
   - initiate stage 2 of alterations in skin integrity practice guideline
2. Infection:
   - initiate prescribed therapy

Evaluation:

1. Analyze patient progress toward outcomes
2. Analyze response to interventions, treatment, and medications
3. Evaluate effectiveness of teaching
4. Analyze the degree of understanding and cooperation with plan of care

Communication:

Verbal

1. Report:
   - nonblanchable erythema of intact skin
   - fixation devices that could contribute to alterations in skin integrity
   - specific difficulties with positioning patient
   - signs/symptoms of infection

Written

1. Record initiation and specific stage of the practice guideline on the Careprint
2. Note any modifications to the stage on the Careprint and rationale for each modification as it occurs
3. Chart all baseline data, ongoing monitoring data, interventions taken, and the patient's responses on the patient care flowsheet
4. Record the evaluation of patient outcomes on the progress record
5. Record all patient teaching

STAGE 2:

Partial thickness skin loss involving epidermis and/or dermis. The ulcer is superficial and presents clinically as an abrasion, blister, or shallow crater.

Competencies:

In order to manage patients in this stage the individual must be able to:

1. Identify the signs and symptoms of stage 2 of alterations in skin integrity
2. Perform the processes outlined in this stage
3. Achieve the outcomes outlined in this stage
4. Identify the complications associated with this stage
5. Identify the causative factors that produce alterations in skin integrity
6. Describe the dangers associated with fixation devices such as tape, skeletal pins, casts, splints, and braces and their contribution to alterations in skin integrity
7. Select appropriate support devices
8. Position patient according to procedure
9. Describe signs and symptoms of infection

Credentialing:

None

Assessment:

1. Perform a baseline head-to-toe skin inspection and monitor at least once a day, with particular attention to bony prominences.
   Observe for:
   - delayed blanching
   - paleness
   - tissue sponginess
   - maceration
   - flakiness
   - scaling
   - skin temperature changes, either increased or decreased
   - induration (hardness)
   - skin turgor
   - capillary refill
   - loss of hair
   - color
   - edema
2. Observe affected area when changing dressing for:
   - odor
   - color
   - drainage
   - necrotic tissue
   - eschar
   - wound margins
   - size and depth of affected area
   - localized pain
   - granulation (beefy-red shiny tissue)
   - itching
3. Monitor peripheral pulses q day
4. Observe affected area for evidence of infection
5. Collect information regarding patient's/significant others' knowledge about alterations in skin integrity

Diagnosis:

1. Stage level of alteration in skin integrity
2. Identify the impact of external mechanical forces: pressure, friction, and shear

3. Determine patient's and significant others':
   - involvement in care
   - communication and support needs
   - knowledge base and readiness to learn
4. Identify causative factors related to abrasion, blister, or shallow crater, such as acne, eczema, parasites, insect bites, psoriasis, tape allergies

Outcomes Identification:

Patient

1. Resolution of abrasions, blisters of craters
2. Identifies early signs and symptoms of alterations in skin integrity and reports them as they occur
3. Absence of infection
4. All peripheral pulses are present
5. Affected areas do not deteriorate to a more advanced stage

Staff

1. Identifies and stages patient at risk for stage 2 alterations in skin integrity
2. Utilizes processes outlined in this stage
3. Identifies signs and symptoms of improving or worsening condition and restages patient status
4. Maintains communication regarding the patient's clinical condition and treatment plan with all involved persons

System

1. A qualified staff member is available to care for this patient
2. Equipment necessary to stage 2 processes is available as needed:
   - egg crate mattress

Planning:

In-house

1. Design a movement/turning schedule for bed-bound patients
2. Design a repositioning schedule for chair-bound patients
3. Modify the interventions outlined in this stage as indicated by patient condition or physician order
4. Modify patient education outlined in this stage based on patient's and/or significant others' knowledge of altered skin integrity
5. Modify the outcomes outlined in this stage based on assessment data

Discharge

1. Identify resources for obtaining support devices needed for home care
2. Continue positioning schedules
3. Validate that turning and repositioning schedules can be maintained at home
4. Refer to home health agency

Education:

1. Provide patient with all information to make informed health care decisions
2. Demonstrate treatment measures for broken skin surfaces
3. Teach factors that enhance skin integrity, such as adequate nutrition and fluid intake, reduced smoking
4. Provide instruction in proper use of preventive aids
5. Teach patient to shift position q 15 minutes
6. Teach how to decrease pressure points and promote optimal circulation
7. Explain signs and symptoms of infection and need to notify RN or physician

Interventions:

For Unaffected Areas

1. Maintain stage 0 of this practice guideline

For Affected Stage 2 Areas

1. Avoid use of soap, lotion, or topical antiseptics
2. Cleanse area with clear water only; pat, do not rub skin dry
3. Protect area with protective dressing
4. Partial thickness wounds:
   - hydrocolloid dressings
   - transparent adhesive dressings
   - sheet form of gel dressings
   - synthetic barrier dressings
   - emollient dressings with nonadherent secondary dressing
5. Protect area with positioning devices such as pillows or foam wedges. Do not use donut-type devices.
6. Use a pressure-reducing mattress such as static air, alternating air, or gel or water mattress or use a double egg crate mattress without tucking in sheets
7. Keep patient off affected area
8. Use a bed cradle over affected area
9. Place pouching devices on sources of uncontrolled excretions such as drains, stomas, anus (if bowel incontinent)
10. Implement turning and/or repositioning schedules; for bed-bound patients reposition every 2 to 3 hours
11. Avoid prolonged sitting. Reposition q hour
12. Administer daily stool softeners
13. Change dressings every 5 days or as necessary when contaminated or accidentally removed
14. Avoid elevating the head of the bed more than 30 degrees for longer than 30 minutes at a time
15. Initiate indicated stage of altered nutrition: less than body requirements practice guideline

Complications:

1. Full thickness skin loss
   - initiate stage 3 of alterations in skin integrity practice guideline
2. Infection
   - initiate prescribed therapy

Evaluation:

1. Analyze patient progress toward outcomes
2. Analyze response to interventions, treatments, and medications
3. Evaluate the effectiveness of teaching
4. Analyze the degree of understanding and cooperation with the plan of care

Communication:

Verbal

1. Report:
   - abrasion, blister or shallow crater:
     - size
     - thickness
   - fixation devices that could cause/contribute to alterations in skin integrity
   - specific difficulties with positioning patient
   - signs/symptoms of infection
   - specific problems or conditions that could cause/contribute to alterations in skin integrity

Written

1. Record initiation and specific stage of the practice guideline on the Careprint
2. Note any modifications to the stage on the Careprint and the rationale for each modification as it occurs
3. Chart baseline data/ongoing monitoring data and interventions taken and the patient's response on "Alteration in Skin Integrity Flow Sheet"
4. Record patient outcomes evaluation on the progress record

STAGE 3:

Full thickness skin loss involving damage or necrosis of subcutaneous tissue that may extend down to, but not through, underlying fascia. The ulcer presents clinically as a deep crater with or without undermining of adjacent tissue.

Competencies:

In order to manage patients in this stage the individual must be able to:

1. Identify the signs and symptoms of stage 3 alterations in skin integrity
2. Perform the processes outlined in this stage
3. Achieve the outcomes outlined in this stage
4. Identify the complications associated with this stage
5. Identify the causative factors that produce alterations in skin integrity
6. Describe the dangers associated with fixation devices such as tape, skeletal pins, casts, splints, and braces and their contribution to alterations in skin integrity
7. Select appropriate support devices
8. Position patient according to procedure
9. Describe signs and symptoms of infection

Credentialing:

Mechanical debridement

Assessment:

1. Perform a baseline head-to-toe skin inspection and monitor at least once a day, with particular attention to bony prominences.
   Observe for:
   - delayed blanching
   - paleness
   - tissue sponginess
   - maceration
   - flakiness
   - scaling
   - skin temperature, either increased or decreased
   - induration (hardness)
   - skin turgor
   - capillary refill
   - loss of hair
   - color
   - edema
2. Observe affected area when changing dressing for:
   - odor
   - color
   - drainage
   - necrotic tissue
   - eschar
   - wound margins
   - size and depth of affected area
   - localized pain
   - granulation (beefy-red shiny tissue)
   - itching
3. Observe condition of skin adjacent to wound for:
   - discoloration, e.g., erythema or paleness
   - hematoma formation
   - interruptions in integrity, e.g., denudation, erosion, papules, pustules
   - maceration
   - desiccation
4. Palpate surrounding skin for presence of induration

5. Observe affected area for evidence of infection
6. Collect information regarding patient's/significant others' knowledge about alterations in skin integrity

Diagnosis:

1. Stage level of alteration in skin integrity
2. Identify the impact of external mechanical forces: pressure, friction, and shear
3. Determine patient's and significant others':
   - involvement in care
   - communication and support needs
   - knowledge base and readiness to learn
4. Identify causative factors related to abrasion, blister, or shallow crater, such as acne, eczema, parasites, insect bites, psoriasis, tape allergies

Outcomes Identification:

Patient

1. Reduction in size of crater
2. Identifies early signs and symptoms of alterations in skin integrity and reports them as they occur
3. Absence of infection
4. All peripheral pulses are present
5. Affected areas do not deteriorate to a more advanced stage

Staff

1. Identifies and stages patient with stage 3 alterations in skin integrity
2. Utilizes processes outlined in this stage
3. Identifies signs and symptoms of improving or worsening condition and restages patient status
4. Maintains communication regarding the patient's clinical condition and treatment plan with all involved persons

System

1. A qualified staff member is available to care for this patient
2. Equipment necessary to stage 3 processes is available as needed:
   - egg crate mattress

Planning:

In-house

1. Design a movement/turning schedule for bed-bound patients
2. Design a repositioning schedule for chair-bound patients
3. Modify the interventions outlined in this stage as indicated by patient condition or physician order
4. Modify patient education outlined in this stage based on patient's and/or significant others' knowledge of altered skin integrity
5. Modify the outcomes outlined in this stage based on assessment data
6. Follow one treatment methodology for at least 5 days before altering plan
7. Prepare for mechanical debridement

Discharge

1. Home care is not feasible with this level of skin destruction

Education:

1. Provide patient with all information to make informed health care decisions
2. Demonstrate treatment measures for broken skin surfaces
3. Teach factors that enhance skin integrity, such as adequate nutrition and fluid intake, reduced smoking

4. Provide instruction in proper use of preventive aids
5. Teach patient to shift position q 15 minutes
6. Teach how to decrease pressure points and promote optimal circulation
7. Explain signs and symptoms of infection and need to notify RN or physician

Interventions:

For Unaffected Areas

1. Maintain stage 0 of this practice guideline

For Affected Stage 3 Areas

1. Avoid use of soap, lotion, or topical antiseptics
2. Clean wound with normal saline
3. Protect area with a protective dressing
4. Full-thickness wounds that are clean and proliferating:
   - absorption dressing, that is, synthetic absorption dressing or gauze dressings with noncytotoxic solutions or gels
   - as exudate decreases, only moist absorption dressings should be used to prevent desiccation and trauma
   - hydrocolloid dressings, with the addition of pastes, granules, or powders if additional absorption is needed
   - semipermeable polyurethane foam dressings, with the addition of pastes, granules, or powders if additional absorption is needed
   - granulate gel dressings
   - synthetic barrier dressing
5. Full-thickness wounds with exudate or dead space:
   - synthetic absorption dressings (copolymer starch dressings, dextranomer beads, calcium alginate dressings, and absorptive pastes, powders, or granules)
   - gauze moistened with appropriate solution or gel and lightly packed into the wound
   - clean wounds should be managed with noncytotoxic solutions; if antiseptics are used for infected wounds, they should be discontinued as soon as the wound is clean
   - secondary dressing based on amount of protection needed
6. Change dressings every 5 days or as necessary when contaminated or accidentally removed
7. Dress ulcers on all body surfaces EXCEPT coccyx and hip using thin film, transparent dressings: (some examples include but are not limited to: Op-site, Tegaderm, Accuderm). May use moist, saline gauze dressings
8. Dress ulcers on coccyx or hip using hydroactive wafers: (some examples include but are not limited to: Duoderm, CGF, Restore). May use moist, saline gauze dressings
9. Protect area with positioning devices such as pillows or foam wedges. Do not use donut-type devices
10. Use a pressure-reducing mattress such as static air, alternating air, gel or water mattress or use a double egg crate mattress without tucking in sheets
11. Keep patient off affected area
    - use a bed cradle over affected area
    - place pouching devices on sources of uncontrolled excretions such as drains, stomas, anus (if bowel incontinent)
12. Implement turning and/or repositioning schedules; for bed-bound patients reposition every 2-3 hours
13. Avoid prolonged sitting. Reposition q hour
14. Administer daily stool softeners
15. Avoid elevating the head of the bed more than 30 degrees for longer than 30 minutes at a time
16. Perform mechanical debridement as ordered (refer to debridement procedure)
17. Oral medications only, no injections
18. Initiate indicated stage of altered nutrition: less than body requirements practice guideline

Complications

1. Full thickness skin loss with extensive destruction, tissue necrosis, or damage to muscle, bone, or supporting structures:
   - initiate stage 4 of alterations in skin integrity practice guideline
2. Infection:
   - initiate prescribed therapy

Evaluation:

1. Analyze patient progress toward outcomes
2. Analyze response to treatments and medications
3. Evaluate effectiveness of teaching unless teaching has been deferred due to patient condition
4. Analyze the degree of understanding and cooperation with plan of care

Communication:

Verbal

1. Report:
   - amount of damage or skin necrosis of subcutaneous tissue
     size
     thickness
   - fixation devices that could cause/contribute to alterations in skin integrity
   - specific difficulties with positioning patient
   - signs/symptoms of infection
   - specific problems or conditions that could cause/contribute to alterations in skin integrity
   - specific treatments/dressings being used

Written

1. Record initiation and specific stage of the practice guideline on the Careprint
2. Note any modifications to the stage on the Careprint and rationale for each modification as it occurs
3. Chart all baseline data, ongoing monitoring data, and interventions taken and the patient's responses on the patient care flowsheet
4. Record the evaluation of patient outcomes on the progress record
5. Record all patient teaching

STAGE 4:

Full thickness skin loss with extensive destruction, tissue necrosis, or damage to muscle, bone, or supporting structures (for example, tendon or joint capsule). *Note:* Undermining and sinus tracts may also be present.

Competencies:

In order to manage patients in this stage the individual must be able to:

1. Identify the signs and symptoms of stage 4 alterations in skin integrity
2. Perform the processes outlined in this stage
3. Achieve the outcomes outlined in this stage
4. Identify the complications associated with this stage
5. Identify the causative factors that produce alterations in skin integrity
6. Describe the dangers associated with fixation devices such as tape, skeletal pins, casts, splints, and braces and their contribution to alterations in skin integrity
7. Select appropriate support devices
8. Position patient according to procedure
9. Describe signs and symptoms of infection

Credentialing:

Mechanical debridement
Enzymatic debridement

Assessment:

1. Perform a baseline head-to-toe skin inspection and monitor at least once a day, with particular attention to bony prominences.
   Observe for:
   - delayed blanching
   - paleness
   - tissue sponginess
   - maceration
   - flakiness
   - scaling
   - skin temperature, either increased or decreased
   - induration (hardness)
   - skin turgor
   - capillary refill
   - loss of hair
   - color
   - edema
2. Observe affected area when changing dressing for:
   - odor
   - color
   - drainage
   - necrotic tissue
   - eschar
   - wound margins
   - size and depth of affected area
   - localized pain
   - granulation (beefy-red shiny tissue)
   - itching
3. Observe condition of skin adjacent to wound for:
   - discoloration, e.g., erythema or paleness
   - hematoma formation
   - interruptions in integrity, e.g., denudation, erosion, papules, pustules
   - maceration
   - desiccation

4. Palpate surrounding skin for presence of induration
5. Observe affected area for evidence of infection
6. Check peripheral pulses q shift
7. Assess affected area for the presence of undermining or sinus tracts, including the location and extent
8. Monitor hemoglobin, hematocrit, and blood sugar levels as ordered values

Diagnosis:

1. Stage level of alteration in skin integrity
2. Identify the impact of external mechanical forces: pressure, friction, and shear
3. Determine patient's and significant others':
   - involvement in care
   - communication and support needs
   - knowledge base and readiness to learn
4. Identify causative factors related to abrasion, blister, or shallow crater, such as acne, eczema, parasites, insect bites, psoriasis, tape allergies
5. Estimate extent of undermining or sinus tracts

Outcomes Identification:

Patient

1. Reduction in size of wound
2. Absence of osteomyelitis
3. Absence of infection
4. All peripheral pulses are present

Staff

1. Identifies and stages patient with stage 4 alterations in skin integrity
2. Utilizes processes outlined in this stage
3. Identifies signs and symptoms of improving condition and restages patient status
4. Maintains communication regarding the patient's clinical condition and treatment plan with all involved persons

System

1. A qualified staff member is available to care for this patient
2. Equipment necessary to stage 4 processes is available as needed:
   - egg crate mattress
   - debridement equipment
   - dressings
3. Reimbursement for special bed therapy will not be denied

Planning:

In-house

1. Modify the interventions outlined in this stage as indicated by patient condition or physician order
2. Modify the outcomes outlined in this stage based on assessment data
3. Follow one treatment methodology for at least 5 days before altering plan

Discharge

1. Due to likelihood of surgical interventions, discharge is not considered during this stage

Education:

1. Provide patient with all information to make informed health care decisions
2. Teach patient to shift position every 15 minutes
3. Explain signs and symptoms of infection and need to notify RN or physician
4. Initiate preoperative education

5. Inform patient of treatments as they occur
6. No formal skin care education occurs during this stage

Interventions:

For Unaffected Areas

1. Maintain stage 0 of this practice guideline

For Affected Stage 4 Areas

1. Avoid use of soap, lotion, or topical antiseptics
2. Clean wound with normal saline
3. Protect area with a protective dressing
4. Full-thickness wounds that are clean and proliferating:
   - absorption dressing, that is, synthetic absorption dressing or gauze dressings with noncytotoxic solutions or gels. As exudate decreases, only moist absorption dressings should be used to prevent desiccation and trauma
   - hydrocolloid dressings, with the addition of pastes, granules, or powders if additional absorption is needed
   - semipermeable polyurethane foam dressings, with the addition of pastes, granules, or powders if additional absorption is needed
   - granulate gel dressings
   - synthetic barrier dressing
5. Full-thickness wounds with exudate or dead space:
   - synthetic absorption dressings (copolymer starch dressings, dextranomer beads, calcium alginate dressings, and absorptive pastes, powders, or granules)
   - gauze moistened with appropriate solution or gel and lightly packed into the wound
   - clean wounds should be managed with noncytotoxic solutions; if antiseptics are used for infected wounds, they should be discontinued as soon as the wound is clean
   - secondary dressing based on amount of protection needed
6. Change dressings every 5 days or as necessary when contaminated or accidentally removed
7. Dress ulcers on all body surfaces EXCEPT coccyx and hip, using thin film, transparent dressings (some examples include but are not limited to: Op-site, Tegaderm, Accuderm). May use moist, saline gauze dressings
8. Dress ulcers on coccyx or hip using hydroactive wafers (some examples include but are not limited to: Duoderm, CGF, Restore). May use moist, saline gauze dressings
9. Protect area with positioning devices such as pillows or foam wedges. Do not use donut-type devices
10. Use a pressure-reducing mattress such as static air, alternating air, gel or water mattress or use a double egg crate mattress without tucking in sheets
11. Keep patient off affected area
12. Use a bed cradle over affected area
13. Place pouching devices on sources of uncontrolled excretions such as drains, stomas, anus (if bowel incontinent)
14. Implement turning and/or repositioning schedules; for bed-bound patients reposition every 2-3 hours
15. Avoid prolonged sitting. Reposition every hour
16. Administer daily stool softeners
17. Avoid elevating the head of the bed more than 30 degrees for longer than 30 minutes at a time
18. Perform mechanical debridement as ordered (refer to debridement procedure)
19. Oral medications only, no injections
20. Perform enzymatic debridement as ordered (refer to debridement procedure)
21. Prepare patient for surgical or laser debridement
22. Prepare patient for tissue flap surgery:
   - monitor nutritional status; serum albumin should be greater than 3.0 g/dl
   - administer perioperative prophylactic antibiotics as ordered
   - initiate surgical practice guideline
   - postoperatively place patient in a prone position or on a specialty bed for a minimum of 3 weeks

- monitor drainage in closed drainage system for volume, color, odor
- gradually increase mobility beginning in week 3 postoperatively
23. Initiate indicated stage of altered nutrition: less than body requirements practice guideline

Evaluation:

1. Analyze patient progress toward outcomes
2. Analyze response to interventions, treatments, and medications
3. Evaluate effectiveness of teaching unless teaching has been deferred due to patient condition
4. Postoperatively evaluate effect of progressive mobility on skin flap and suture lines
5. Analyze the degree of understanding and cooperation with the plan of care

Communication:

Verbal

1. Report:
   - amount of skin loss, destruction, necrosis and to which area of the body
     crater size
     undermining
   - fixation devices that could cause/contribute to alterations in skin integrity
   - specific difficulties with positioning patient
   - signs/symptoms of infection
   - specific problems or conditions that could cause/contribute to alterations in skin integrity
   - abnormal lab values
   - specific treatments/dressings being used
   - any surgical interventions

Written

1. Record initiation and specific stage of the practice guideline on the Careprint
2. Note any modifications to the stage on the Careprint and the rationale for each modification as it occurs
3. Chart all baseline data, ongoing monitoring data, interventions taken, and the patient's responses on the patient care flowsheet
4. Record the evaluation of patient outcomes on the progress record
5. Record all patient teaching unless deferred due to patient's condition

Chapter 14

Assessing Activities and Documenting Improvement

Process is not necessarily progress.
Jackie Katz

Perhaps you have heard the story about the patient who went to see his psychiatrist, wearing only a fireman's hat. His entire body was painted purple with red polka dots. He was flapping his arms wildly and clucking like a chicken while he hopped on one foot and then the other. When his doctor asked him what he thought he was doing, the man replied, "I'm keeping the elephants away!" "But we're in the middle of Manhattan," stated the psychiatrist, "there aren't any elephants here." "See how good it works!" exclaimed the patient with a smile.

This chapter is designed to see "how good it works." As with the patient's plan above, performance improvement plans may involve elaborate activities and also may consume valuable resources, but a flurry of activity does not guarantee the desired results. As with the staff nurse, who at the end of a hectic day wonders exactly what has been accomplished, a plan can generate much work with little measurable return. The key to ensuring that the specific actions outlined in a plan are producing what they were intended to produce is periodic review and ongoing documentation of achievement.

This chapter focuses on the process of evaluating and documenting how the implementation of action plans are progressing. It discusses the differences between evaluative and diagnostic judgment, process versus outcome review, and quantitative versus qualitative analysis. It describes the follow-up necessary to validate and record the performance improvement that results from the activities outlined in the action plans.

All plans, whether they are service, practice, or governance in nature, require follow-up analysis. This is the step in the performance improvement process that provides documentation of not only the intent to act but also the outcomes of that intent. In the absence of follow-up, data collection, analysis, and action planning are purely academic exercises. Follow-up evaluation is the grist from the mill of progress. It focuses on the action plan and analyzes both the ends and the means, the outcomes and the process, the results and the interventions. Too frequently, follow-up has focused only on the process of planning and whether or not the activities in the plan were carried out. Little, if any, attention was given to the results of the planned activities. It is imperative to measure the progress made toward the results for which the plan was designed and initiated.

Timing is everything in follow-up. Change takes time. If a change is evaluated too early, the expected results may not yet be apparent. A covert reason for a lack of performance improvement may be hasty remeasurement. Concurrent and retrospective review may help to eliminate this as a cause of less-than-optimal achievement. Concurrent review occurs while the plan is being carried out and focuses on the accomplishment of interim objectives. These interim objectives are benchmarks of progress along the way toward the ultimate desired outcomes. Retrospective review is carried out after all the interventions outlined in the plan have been completed.

> *Performance improvement does not end when actions are taken. Not only must staff continue to assess key processes for future opportunities for improvement, but to determine whether actions taken are successful in improving care or service. The results of continued measurement and evaluation should provide information to make that determination.*[3]

JUDGMENT: A CRITICAL DECISION-MAKING SKILL

Follow-up evaluation relies heavily on decision-making skills. Decision making requires judgment.

Bleich suggests that many experienced professionals are uncomfortable with taking responsibility for making and documenting judgments and therefore are reluctant to do so. Reasons for discomfort in making and documenting judgments might include accountability aversion and lack of understanding, skill, and consistent evaluative terminology.[1] One must understand what a judgment is and be skilled in making judgments so that there is confidence that the judgment is sound. Once a judgment is made and documented, the individual who made the judgment owns it and must be willing and able to defend it. The reluctance of professionals to make judgments is evidenced by the number of recommendations and contingencies cited by the Joint Commission in the area of documentation of the evaluation phase of patient care.

DIAGNOSTIC JUDGMENT

Bleich outlines two types of judgment—diagnostic and evaluative.[1] In general, practitioners tend to be more comfortable with the former.

Diagnostic judgment involves the collection, analysis, and synthesis of data. It is used during the assessment, diagnosis, and planning steps of the problem solving/diagnostic process. There is a heavy emphasis on these steps in all disciplines within the health care arena. Today, physical assessment, history taking, and formulating diagnoses are stressed not only in the basic medical and nursing educational programs but also in other health care professional educational programs. Much time and effort has been spent, therefore, in improving all practitioner's skills in this area across the continuum of care.

Impetus for continual improvement of these skills has come from the Joint Commission's *Assessment of Patients* and *Care of Patients* functional standards.[3] The standards continue to state that the assessment includes biophysical, psychosocial, environmental, self-care, educational, and discharge-planning factors based on identified diagnosis and/or patient care needs across the continuum of care. Thus the need for sophisticated skills in diagnostic judgment in each patient care area across the continuum of care is well documented.

Diagnostic judgment focuses on problem identification, whether the problem is related to service, practice, or governance. However, it can also be used to identify opportunities for improvement where no problem currently exists. This is the preventive aspect of diagnostic judgment, which enables practitioners to identify potential problems or opportunities to intervene to improve the efficiency or the effectiveness of the process. Traditionally, the thrust of diagnostic judgment has been problem finding; consequently, practitioners are less adept at using their diagnostic judgment for prevention. Problem finding may involve identifying the signs and symptoms of digoxin toxicity in a patient, identifying a lack of dietary staff compliance with a new procedure, or the misappropriation of linen on the weekend shifts. Prevention, on the other hand, enables the professional to identify symptoms of a potential problem, e.g., identifying patients at risk for digoxin toxicity, predicting dietary staff's response to a new situation, or anticipating that the volume of linen required on a particular weekend will be heavier than usual.

To diagnose effectively, one must be able to synthesize. Synthesizing is having the ability to combine separate elements to form a coherent whole. For example, identifying that a patient's incision is red, painful, and warm to the touch, and that the sutures are taut requires observation skills. To recognize that those symptoms may signal wound infection requires the ability to synthesize.

"This is a process of working with elements, parts, etc. and combining them in such a way as to constitute a pattern or structure not clearly there before."[2] Combining collected data in ways that form patterns requires sophisticated analysis skills. Mapping trends in measuring results is another example of synthesizing. For instance, data collection from six of eight departments may report a slight increase in the volume of injury-related falls in a specific quarter. Taken individually, each report may not be significant; however, when viewed together, a major safety problem may be apparent. The preventive aspect of diagnostic judgment can also be seen in this example. Prevention of increases in injury-related falls may result from discovering and eliminating significant contributing factors, such as heavily waxed floors or slippers with slick soles.

Using diagnostic judgment is like playing detective. It is the professional's job to identify the various clues to a particular service, practice, or governance problem and to determine the "culprit." Knowing the problem and the cause is only half the battle, however. Once the source of the problem is identified, the professional uses his or her diagnostic judgment to devise a plan that will solve the problem once and for all.

In the previous steps of this process, diagnostic skills have been utilized. At this point, however, a different kind of judgment is required.

EVALUATIVE JUDGMENT

Evaluative judgment frustrates many professionals. Its absence is frequently cited in Joint Commission recommendations. Although many practitioners confuse diagnostic and evaluative judgment, they are very different. Both require critical thinking skills, but diagnosis is not evaluation. Many practitioners erroneously interchange the words "assessment" and "evaluation." These are two distinct processes, and, although assessment receives much attention in basic education, evaluation frequently does not. Being able to differentiate the two is a critical first step in identifying when to use each.

Evaluation involves making judgments about the value of ideas, solutions, methods, or materials. It uses standards for appraising the extent to which actions or results are accurate, effective, economical, or satisfying. Evaluation can be quantitative or qualitative. An example of quantitative evaluation is the statement that the room temperature is 95° F as measured by thermometer. A qualitative corollary is "It's sweltering in here!" Quantitative evaluation involves numbers; qualitative evaluation involves perceptions.

According to Bloom, people evaluate, judge, or appraise almost everything they come in contact with. However, most of those judgments are highly egocentric, i.e., they are quick decisions made without much forethought and based on the individual's frame of reference. They fall more into the realm of opinion rather than judgment and into the subconscious rather than the conscious realm.[2] For example, if an owner is dissatisfied with the service on his or her car, that individual may choose never to purchase a car of that make again. Although a rude or ineffective service representative may have had nothing to do with the quality of the car, an opinion is generalized about the company and its product based on a personal experience that may or may not reflect reality. Patients in hospitals may form similar opinions about the quality of the medical or nursing services based on their reactions to the "hotel" services they do or do not receive.

True evaluation, however, requires a conscious effort and is based on objective criteria.

Internal and External Criteria for Follow-up

Objective criteria are used to follow up on action plans. These criteria may be internal or external. Internal standards relate to the action plan itself. Is the plan consistent in approach? Is it on target? Internal standards are used to determine that there are no major errors in the format of the plan or the planning process, i.e., the plan design.

External standards relate to the appropriateness of the plan to achieve the desired ends. Did the plan produce the intended results? These criteria consider the efficiency, economy, or utility of specific activities to achieve specific results. Do the activities chosen represent the best solution to the problem posed? Are the activities chosen the most appropriate ones in light of the alternatives? Do the activities chosen produce results other than those desired?

In using the external standards, both the process and outcomes of the plan are analyzed. Process review is accomplished using formative evaluation, whereas outcome review requires the use of summative evaluation.

Formative Versus Summative Evaluation

Formative evaluations analyze the response to a specific intervention. Summative evaluations evaluate progress toward established outcomes. Formative evaluations look at the particular pieces of the action plan and the relative importance to the whole, whereas summative evaluations analyze how well (or how poorly) the pieces worked together to achieve the desired results. Formative evaluations therefore tend to focus on the process of carrying out the action plan, and summative evaluations focus on the achievement or lack of achievement of outcomes.

Both formative and summative evaluations are used in the scientific, or problem-solving, process. Figure 14-1 compares the use of diagnostic and evaluative judgments in both the scientific process and the measurement and evaluation process. The dividing line between diagnostic and evaluative judgment is the implementation of the action plan. Whether the plan is a clinical path, a teaching plan, an employee development plan, a staff development plan, or an administrative action plan, once the activities outlined in the plan are initiated, the type of critical thinking skills shifts from diagnostic to evaluative. Evaluative judgment analyzes the efficiency and effectiveness of the plan; therefore, follow-up of the

Type of Judgment	Scientific Process Steps	Measurement and Evaluation Activities
Diagnostic judgment	Assessment Diagnosis Planning	Data collection/analysis Problem/opportunity identification Action planning
Evaluative judgment	Evaluation	Evaluation of variation

Figure 14-1   Relationship of diagnostic and evaluative judgment and the scientific and measurement and evaluation processes.

plan of action must include an efficiency and effectiveness analysis.

EVALUATING EFFICIENCY AND EFFECTIVENESS

Evaluation measures the overall efficiency and effectiveness of any set of activities designed to achieve a desired end. Efficiency is measured by process review. Outcome review measures effectiveness. Efficiency measures the relationship of what an organization gets out of the plan in comparison to what it puts into making the planned activities happen. Efficiency involves doing right things right. It requires working smarter, not harder.

Outcome evaluation deals with effectiveness. Effectiveness is the degree to which the activities outlined in the plan produced the desired results. Did the strategy work? Lancaster defines two major effectiveness criteria or standards. The first is appropriateness or accuracy, i.e., the fit between the problem or opportunity and the chosen strategy. The second criterion is resource allocation. Without proper allocation of resources, even the best strategy will fail.[4]

WHAT TO EVALUATE AND WHEN

First and foremost, the focus of the follow-up should be the effectiveness of the plan. Did the plan do what it was designed to do? Has the action plan achieved the desired results?

Evaluation of the effectiveness of the action plan is usually accomplished by remeasuring the original indicator. If, for example, a teaching plan was developed to teach terminally ill cancer patients how to use patient-controlled analgesia units, success or failure of the plan would be based on the increase in the patient's comfort level because of better understanding of how to use the equipment. Therefore, remeasuring the original process would indicate an improvement if the study results fell within the control limits as a result of implementing the teaching plan, when they did not fall within the limits prior to patient teaching. By using the same study, the initial results can serve as a baseline to track the degree of progress or improvement.

There are three possible results that can be obtained by remeasuring the original study after action plan implementation:

1. *The desired results outlined in the plan were achieved.* The problem has been corrected or the opportunity capitalized upon. The predetermined outcomes have been achieved and the remeasurement data fall within the control limits. In this case, the original measurement schedule is resumed to ensure that performance improvement is sustained.
2. *The desired results have not been met, but there is significant progress toward their achievement.* Remeasurement data fall closer to the control limits than the initial study. The problem seems to be resolving. In this case, a process review or formative evaluation is necessary in addition to the outcome review. In this review, the outcomes, actions, resources, and target dates are reevaluated and revised as necessary to facilitate the achievement of the desired results. Perhaps additional time is necessary to complete the activities, because a crisis created a temporary diversion. Perhaps more resources are necessary to fully execute the plan. Perhaps some of the specified activities or interventions were out of sequence or were not carried out according to the timeline. Adjustment of the plan is necessary to meet the desired outcomes. Questions to ask during a process review include the following:

- Were the outcomes SMART?
- Were the target dates for accomplishment realistic?
- Has enough time elapsed for the desired change to occur?
- Were the actions/interventions carried out as specified?
- Were sufficient resources allocated for the accomplishment of the results?

Once the plan has been revised, it must be implemented and evaluated by remeasuring the original indicator once again to see if the changes have produced the necessary improvement to boost the results into the desired control limits.

3. *The outcomes have not been met and appear to be unlikely to be met given the current state of circumstances.* Remeasurement data are not significantly closer to the control limits than in the initial study and may even be farther away.

In this case, the first step is to reevaluate what you are asking people to do. Whether they are staff, patients, vendors, or other professionals, people generally wish to cooperate. When they are consistently resistant or noncompliant, it may be that what you are asking them to do is unrealistic. Determine if the standard to which you are holding them accountable is reasonable and appropriate. If the standard itself is the source of the problem, revise it. However, if the standard is adequate, then evaluation of the appropriateness of the plan for the identified problem or opportunity should be undertaken.

Next, take another look at the information in Chapter 12 to determine if the etiology of the problem was correctly identified. A new analysis of the variance must be done to determine if a contributing variable might be responsible that may not have been identified during the indicator selection process, or if one of the identified contributing variables may be playing a more significant role than was previously thought. If so, an alternative plan may need to be developed. If not, all contributing variables must be identified and a new plan developed that addresses all of the contributing factors. For example, if a staff development plan to improve the nurses' compliance to documentation using nursing diagnosis fails to achieve its purpose, a staffing problem rather than ineffectiveness of the plan may be the cause. Questions to ask include the following:

- Is the standard a good one?
- Was the cause of the problem properly identified?
- Was the plan appropriate for the problem or opportunity?
- Did the plan address all of the contributing variables?
- If not, what other factors need to be addressed to resolve the problem or to take advantage of the opportunity?
- Should the plan be abandoned or merely revised?

If the plan must be abandoned, a new plan must be devised utilizing the strategies outlined in Chapter 13. If the plan simply needs revision, then a process review as outlined in step 2 above should be carried out and the necessary revisions made. The diagram in Figure 14-2 shows the relationship among the three results and their subsequent options.

WHAT TO DOCUMENT

Documentation is frequently the benchmark by which performance is measured. It is an accreditation requirement and a legal necessity. Once written, the plan becomes evidence of the intent to act on an identified problem or opportunity. The process of implementation must also be documented. Process documentation involves recording what was done and when. Outcome documentation involves documenting progress.

Documentation may be broken down into three parts: data collection and analysis, planning, and evaluation. Data collection involves recording the collection of information. That information may be data regarding initial assessment or ongoing measurement. Data may be service, practice, or governance in nature. For example, recording radiation levels over time is data collection, as is recording the number of radiology technicians attending a continuing education event or the number of admissions, transfers, discharges, and deaths in a particular department for a particular shift. Data collection documentation also involves recording the implementation of routine activities such as turning patients every 4 hours or carrying out the essential activities listed in an action plan. Tools used to collect data usually take the form of flowsheets or checksheets, which provide a quick summary of such things as numbers, activities, or symptoms over time. The data collection tool (see Figure 11-1) is an example of a data collection flowsheet. Data collection is process documentation. The collected data must support the need for a plan of action. The analysis of the data provides that support.

Another form of process documentation is a plan. As mentioned earlier, it is the written record of the intent to act on a problem or opportunity. The tools used to record planning are the plans themselves. Plans are the second integral component of a comprehensive documentation system. Examples of plans are given in Chapter 13. The plan must delineate the results expected to be obtained once the plan has been implemented.

The third component of a good documentation system is evaluation. Documentation of evaluation is accomplished by keeping progress records, which serve as a diary of movement toward predetermined outcomes. Those outcomes are defined in the action plan. The tool most commonly used to document

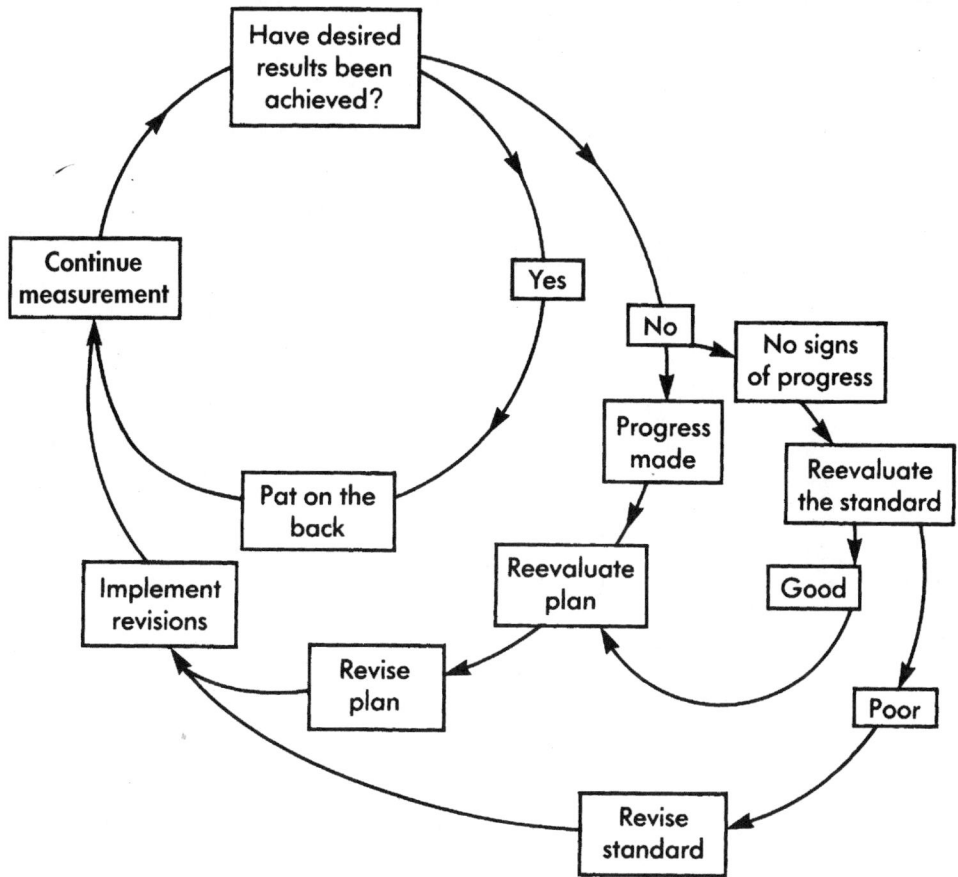

Figure 14-2   Critical path of effectiveness analysis.

evaluation is the progress record. If the issue is service oriented and involves patient care, progress toward patient outcomes is recorded. If the issue is practice oriented, a staff progress record is required. A governance progress record is required to follow the progress toward governance outcomes as defined in the administrative action plan. Figure 14-3 is an example of a generic progress record. The critical issue may be a customer problem if the plan is service in nature. It may also be an area for development if the plan relates to the staff, or a system's issue if the plan relates to governance.

Data collection is used to diagnose the problem or opportunity. A plan of action is designed and implemented. Data regarding the effects of the action plan are gathered through remeasuring of the initial indicator so that an evaluation of change or progress toward the outcomes designated in the plan can be made. At each of these points, documentation is required. This documentation provides a record of:

- Performance problem or opportunity identification
- Planned strategy to address the performance improvement opportunity
- Implementation of the plan for improvement
- Effectiveness of implementation

Whether the underlying problem or opportunity is service, practice, or governance in nature, both process and outcome documentation are essential. Process documentation defines the performance improvement opportunity and what is to be done about it; outcome documentation records the results achieved when the plan is implemented.

In conclusion, follow-up of the action plan requires evaluative judgment, i.e., the ability to evaluate the efficiency and effectiveness of the plan. The efficiency of the plan can be evaluated by using techniques such as cost-benefit analysis, whereas the effectiveness is analyzed by remeasuring the original indicator to identify performance improvement.

CRITICAL ISSUE	DATE	PROGRESS ENTRY	SIGNATURE

Figure 14-3   Progress record example.

Documentation of data collection, action planning, and follow-up provides written proof of the performance improvement efforts and their results.

REFERENCES

1. Bleich M: Clinical judgments: essential elements of the nursing process, *J Nurs Qual Assurance*, 4(4): 1-6, 1990.

2. Bloom B et al: *Taxonomy of educational objectives, handbook 1, cognitive domain*, New York, 1956, David McKay.

3. *Comprehensive accreditation manual for hospitals*, Chicago, 1996, Joint Commission on Accreditation of Health Care Organizations.

4. Lancaster J, Lancaster W: *Concepts for advanced nursing practice: the nurse as a change agent*, St. Louis, 1982, Mosby.

Chapter 15

Communicating Results

*Everyone talks about communicating
but no one does anything about it.*
Mark Twain

And they said: Come let us build us a city, and a tower, with its top in heaven, and let us make us a name; lest we be scattered abroad upon the face of the whole earth. And the Lord came down to see the city and the tower, which the children of men builded. And the Lord said: Behold, they are one people, and they have all one language; and this is what they begin to do; and now nothing will be withholden from them, which they purpose to do. Come let us go down, and there confound their language, that they may not understand one another's speech. So the Lord scattered them abroad from thence upon the face of all the earth; and they left off to build the city. Therefore was the name of it called Babel; because the Lord did there confound the language of all the earth; and from thence did the Lord scatter them abroad upon the face of all the earth.

Genesis 11:1-9

Nothing is more powerful than communication. Poorly planned and/or executed communication is like a tower of Babel—a hodgepodge in which the right hand does not know what the left hand is doing.

Communication is the transfer of information from one person to another. Hamilton defines communication as the process of sharing thoughts, ideas, and feelings with others in commonly understandable ways.[4] Business communication refers to all of the oral and written information that is directly or indirectly applicable to the organization. Rosenblatt defines business communication as "purposive interchanges of ideas, opinions, instructions, and the like, presented personally or impersonally by symbol or signal as to attain the goals of the organization."[8] It is part of the internal operational communication, i.e., the structured communication that relates to achieving organizational work goals. *Structured* means it is built into the plan of operations—part of the routine communication that oils the organizational wheels. Typically, this type of communication is carried out through specific activities. For example, data collection reports, annual program evaluation reports, and quarterly trending reports may all be required communication.

CHARACTERISTICS OF BUSINESS COMMUNICATION

Communication is the lifeline of any business. Its significance cannot be overestimated. Communication can be upward, downward, or lateral. It facilitates decision making at all levels, promotes understanding, and fosters organization and coordination. It is the culmination of hours of activity. Often the effects of work time are lost because its impact was poorly communicated. Frequently the reporting phase is viewed as anticlimactic and treated as an afterthought. Data are hurriedly slapped together and a brief summary of activity is generated. Communication, the most powerful tool available to influence decision making, is being used inappropriately and/or is underutilized.

Regardless of whether the communication is informal or formal, verbal or nonverbal, there are some common factors that bear on its success.

1. All communication must be receiver centered. In every communication, there is a sender and a receiver. The sender must understand the needs of the receiver and target the essence of the message to meet those needs. The receiver must understand the utility of the message if it is to be effective. For example, the possibility of contracting AIDS from an accidental needle stick makes the information regarding needle precautions extremely relevant to the practitioner.

2. Communication should be brief. The operant adage here is "Cut to the chase." What one has to say is only effective if it is heard/read and understood. Time is of the essence, so the quicker the point can be made, the more likely the receiver is to listen/read about the issue. Convey the main idea in as few words as possible.

3. Simple is better than complex. This goes hand-in-hand with brevity. *KISS* means "keep it simple and short." Choose the simple and straightforward over the complex and abstract.

PLANNING TO COMMUNICATE

Although much communication happens spontaneously, truly effective communication requires planning. Everyone at some point has been misunderstood or misinterpreted with unfavorable results. The key to success in outcome-driven communication is to focus on the desired results and plan the communication to achieve those ends.

Just as the lead paragraph in a newspaper article explains the five Ws (Who, What, Where, When, and Why), effective communication requires four Ws and one H. Before communicating, the sender must define the following:

1. Who needs to know about this?
2. Why do they need to know about it?
3. *How* is the message communicated most effectively?
4. What is appropriate to communicate?
5. When should the communication occur?

Each of the components translates into a distinct planning step.

Step 1: Who Needs to Know About This?

In this step you define your audience(s). There may be more than one individual or group who needs to receive your message. The question to ask is, Who needs to know about the results of this study? Is it the staff? The Quality Management Board? Other departments?

The audience is determined by three factors. First, those individuals or groups who are affected by the results should know about them. Second, administrative policy may outline who routinely receives communication regarding performance issues. Third, specific information may be generated that a particular group, which does not routinely receive this information, needs to act on. In this case, a special audience may be defined, such as the board of directors, a department, and/or a patient group.

Once the audience is determined, you can tailor the communication to your audience. Each individual or group approaches communication according to the individual's or group's current frame of reference. You should consider questions such as "Does this group have 'the big picture' or is it more concerned with a small piece of the pie?" According to Hamilton, since no two people have the same frame of reference, difficulty in communication is likely.[4] To avoid communication breakdown, it is necessary for the sender to understand the receiver's frame of reference. For instance, administrators frequently think in terms of cost and productivity and tend to have a broader frame of reference than staff. Staff members often perceive matters personally, i.e., how will this information affect daily practice or individual responsibilities? Departments often view messages from the perspective of their own service, practice, or governance.

No two groups are alike, and it is the sender's challenge to identify the differences. What makes a particular group or individual unique? Do not overlook demographic variables such as age, sex, and academic preparation, or personality variables or styles such as commitment, authoritarianism, flexibility, and openness. The individual's or group's role or position in the organization may have a profound bearing on how communication is perceived. A vice president brings a different perspective than a new orientee. A group of patients may perceive information differently than a vendor group would. Tailoring communication to its intended audience is discussed more fully in step 4.

Audience analysis also includes a determination of how much the audience already knows about the subject presented and whether the receiver may have any preconceived opinions about the presenter. The credibility of the presenter can do much to facilitate or impede communication. An audience will listen to or read the words of a credible presenter and ignore a message presented by someone they do not respect.

Hunt suggests using a worksheet to list important audience variables.[5] Figure 15-1 presents an example of an audience analysis worksheet.

Step 2: Why Do They Need to Know About It?

Typically, we communicate to inform, persuade, or recognize. Informational communication conveys data. It is the transmittal of facts and figures only. People in organizations need information to do their jobs. Dissemination empowers individuals and groups and enables them to make decisions and act on them. Rosenblatt suggests that business today "depends on a continuous supply of information, and a dependable distribution or communication system for both the receiving and delivering of the information messages to those responsible for making decisions and controlling operations."[8] An informational performance report is generated for specific individuals or groups who need to keep abreast of the data generated on a routine basis; such groups might include the Quality Management Board or the pharmacy and therapeutics committee.

Directional communication is a type of informational communication. It provides instruction on how to perform specific activities or tasks. It enables people to learn how to accomplish desired outcomes.

Although all reporting has an informational component, an informational report is generated for the data alone. Other types of communication use information to achieve specific ends. For example, the information in persuasive communication is used to influence, to motivate, or to control behavior in a predetermined way.

Persuasive communication is routinely used in health care. Convincing a staff member to work a double shift or a pediatric patient to take an unpleasant-tasting medication requires persuasive skills. The objective of this type of communication is attitude change ultimately leading to behavior change.[7] Persuasive communication is a critical tool in reporting results. It is the key to promoting the value of performance and may be the objective in reporting to the staff, administration, other departments, or any individual or group representing a barrier to performance improvement. Negotiation is a type of persuasive communication. The participants establish a common ground. Both sender and receiver may need to modify their attitudes/behaviors to achieve "a meeting of the minds." Ideally, the outcome is a win-win situation that is acceptable to all. Negotiation is a vital skill in communicating about performance improvement. However, many people are not comfortable negotiating or lack the necessary skills. There are many excellent references available to assist in developing or refining the requisite skills.

Recognition communication is essential to meet the social and psychological needs of workers. It motivates individuals to strive for continued growth. A pat on the back is only inches from a kick in the seat of the pants but miles apart in its effects. Unfortunately, performance measurement has traditionally been viewed as a mechanism for identifying problems and placing blame. However, recognition reporting is a particularly useful tool for acknowledging an individual's or group's achievement of or improvement in meeting performance goals.

A progress report may be generated to inform, persuade, or recognize achievements. It is a status update. A progress report provides a comparison of how things were and how they have changed. Are they better, worse, or the same? Progress reports may be concurrent, reporting how things are going, or retrospective, describing past performance. Fellows and Ikeda suggest that progress reports are worthless unless they address *why* something has changed. Without such an explanation, the report merely cites trends.[2] They advocate reporting the issue, the cause, the response, and the results. Performance reporting therefore must go beyond tracking and discerning trends. To be comprehensive, it must address the gamut of improvement efforts. Progress reports are part of the routine reporting within an organization.

As part of defining the purpose of the communication, you must also delineate the expected effect of your communication on the receiver. What are the desired outcomes of the communication? What impact will the communication have? Will knowledge improve? Will the receiver feel empowered? Will he, she, or they take action? What actions will be taken? Will attitudes and behaviors change? Which behaviors or attitudes will change? Will the receiver feel rewarded and appreciated? Defining the expected outcomes is critical because the content of the message will change based on the results to be achieved.

A cardinal error made by many professionals is providing the same report to different groups having different frames of reference. Typically, one report is generated and circulated to everyone on the routing list. Step 4 in the planning process targets the content to the receiver.

Step 3: How Is the Message Communicated Most Effectively?

This step deals with the channel through which the message is communicated. The two major channels are verbal and written, and both channels are either informal or formal. A "one on one" conversation about the results of a study between a manager and the department representative may describe informal verbal

DEMOGRAPHIC CHARACTERISTICS

    Age: Economic Status:

    Educational Level: Political Status:

    Occupational Type: Other Influences:

GENERAL AUDIENCE ATTITUDES

    What are their political orientations?

    What are their social orientations?

    Where do they get their information?

    What constituencies do they serve?

SPECIFIC AUDIENCE ATTITUDES TOWARD PROPOSAL

    What do they think of your proposal?

    Sources of their attitudes?

    What attitudes can be changed?

    What strategies may work?

SPECIFIC AUDIENCE ATTITUDES TOWARD COMMUNICATOR

    What do they think of you?

    What are your strengths (with listeners)?

    What are your weaknesses (with listeners)?

    Possible sources of credibility?

Figure 15-1   Audience analysis worksheet. (From Hunt GT: *Communication skills in the organization,* ed 2, Englewood Cliffs, NJ, 1989, Prentice-Hall.)

communication, whereas a verbal presentation to the board of directors about the status of performance improvement efforts requires a formal approach. A written communication to one department regarding a particular study may be handled through a memo, whereas the annual departmental performance report is a formal document.

There are advantages and disadvantages to both modes of communication. Verbal communication provides an opportunity for immediate feedback, whereas written does not. The written mode, however, enables the receiver to pace himself or herself for maximum comprehension, whereas the verbal mode does not. Written communication is more likely to be carefully thought out; verbal communication is typically more spontaneous.

Hamilton suggests six factors to consider in deciding which mode to use[4]:

1. The importance of the message
2. The needs and abilities of the receiver
3. How much and how soon feedback is needed
4. Whether a permanent record is required
5. The cost of the mode
6. Whether formality or informality is required

Sometimes the situation requires a combination of oral and written communication. For example, written handouts usually enhance a verbal presentation. Vardaman lists the key situations in which oral, written, or combined communication is most desirable[10] (Figure 15-2).

Once you determine the medium, turn your attention to what is to be communicated and how it is to be presented.

Step 4: What Is Appropriate to Communicate?

When you have completed the above steps, you are ready to tackle the mountain of data, analyses, and quality improvement results you need to communicate. The challenge is to develop order within the information. First you must determine the appropriate content for each receiver. Not everyone who requires information needs the same information at the same depth. Steps 1 and 2 targeted the audience. Step 3 targets the format. Step 4 targets the message itself. What should be conveyed? Content that is appropriate for one audience may be inappropriate for another. Appropriateness is defined as suitability or fit for a particular use. Assessing appropriateness requires determining how the particular audience will use the information provided. The content should be tailored accordingly. If, for example, the purpose of the communication is to persuade the service improvement council to reevaluate the falls-prevention program and action is the desired result, then the information presented in the communication must convince the council to act on your suggestion. If, on the other hand, the purpose of the message is recognition for meeting the performance targets set for pain management and the desired outcome is maintenance of performance, then the message must reinforce the desired behaviors.

Once the content for each audience has been identified, content must be arranged in the sequence it will assume in the report. A content outline is usually most helpful. Arrange the content outline from most important to least. If time is at a premium, the main points of the message will be delivered to the receiver in the first

ORAL	WRITTEN	COMBINED
1. Confidential matters	1. Impersonalization desired	1. "Carry home" ideas desired
2. Warmth, personal qualities needed	2. Extension in time and space proper	2. Follow-up needed
3. Open atmosphere desired	3. Storage and retrieval needed	3. Optimal understanding needed
4. Stronger feelings needed	4. Reliability/validity important	4. Clarity and impact needed
5. Exactitude/precision not required	5. Idea verification/authentication needed	5. Exploratory communication
6. Immediacy required	6. Objective references needed	6. Audience participation needed
7. Crucial situations	7. Writing more acceptable	7. Abstract/remote ideas
8. Added receiver impact needed	8. Crucial decisions/actions	
9. Personal authentication needed	9. Review/reconsideration needed	
10. Meeting social needs	10. Supplement to speaking	

Figure 15-2   Summary of conditions for communication form. (From Vardaman G: *Effective communication of ideas*, New York, 1970, Van Nostrand Reinhold.)

few minutes. Lesikar describes three types of sequencing: logical, direct, and chronological.[6] Logical sequencing uses inductive order, i.e., it moves from the known to the unknown. The facts are presented and then analyzed, and conclusions are drawn. In direct sequencing, deductive order is used. Conclusions are presented first, then the facts and analysis from which they are drawn. Chronological sequencing presents the findings in the order in which they occurred. It gives a historical perspective.

When constructing a content outline, remember the KISS principle: keep ideas as short and simple as possible without sacrificing the intent of the message. A general rule of thumb is that the length of the report is directly proportional to the severity of the problem it addresses. The more severe the problem, the more formal the report should be. According to Lesikar[6], an outline should do the following:

- Organize information to maximize understanding
- Show relationships among the pieces of information to be included
- Make the information fit together logically in the reader's mind

Keeping it simple also means selecting words that the audience understands. Avoid a long word when a short one will do. Use everyday language that the audience can relate to. Avoid using jargon or unfamiliar words.

When the audience is heterogeneous, with different levels of knowledge about the issue, or when the audience's academic preparation varies, aim the message at the lowest knowledge level to avoid miscommunication.

Once the outline is generated, it provides the skeleton upon which to hang the meat of the report. In constructing the report, use active, rather than passive, verbs. Active verbs show the subject of the sentence doing the action. Passive verbs show the subject being acted upon. For example, "the staff of 4W reduced the incidence of level III medication errors by 10%" is a more powerful message than "the incidence of level III medication errors has been reduced by 10% by the staff of 4W." The first version is not only clearer but also shorter.

Choose precise words that convey an accurate description. A precise message leaves little room for misunderstanding and misinterpretation.

Keep sentences short. Long sentences are more difficult to understand than short ones. They tend to be less clear. Convey one idea per sentence. Lesikar suggests that sentences be bite sized.[6] A chunk of food that is too big is difficult to swallow. Similarly, a sentence that is too long is difficult to understand. Shorter sentences communicate more effectively.

Planning Visual Aids

A picture is worth a thousand words. Graphic displays enhance all reports; however, they rarely can tell the whole story. Irvin S. Cobb stated, "Don't tell me that one picture is worth a thousand words. Sometimes it's not worth one word. If I'm drowning, what do I do—hold up a picture? Hell no, I yell 'Help!'"[2] Do not allow visual aids to detract from the message. Choose them wisely.

Visual aids should clarify, i.e., they should help the audience understand the content. Many people do not like to read numbers, and much information reported in performance reports involves numbers. Graphs and tables are useful tools for presenting quantitative data. They enable the reader to visually compare and contrast data.

There are four principles to keep in mind when using graphics:

1. Use them only when they are needed, i.e., when they clarify data or facilitate presenting a large quantity of data in a limited space.
2. Prepare the reader for the visual aid, i.e., tell the audience members that they are about to view a graphic aid.
3. Explain what it is.
4. KISS: Keep it short and simple.

Charts, graphs, and tables break up the content and can enhance visual interest. People are accustomed to visual depictions. They are pervasive in contemporary life, from the newspaper to the TV. We are bombarded with visual images.

The most common types of graphic aids include graphs and tables. A graph shows how pieces of data are related. It compares different classes of data. There are several types of graphs: the line graph, the bar graph, and the pie graph.

A run chart connects points on a scale to show trends. It depicts a change in some variable over time. Plotting the results of data sets on a run chart and connecting the dots (Figure 15-3) creates a dynamic visual. Typically the bottom line (horizontal axis) represents time and the side line (vertical axis) represents the variable that is expected to change over time.

Bar graphs depict relationships between two variables. Like a run chart, a bar graph may show change over time or it may compare two other variables, such as the relationship of the study results on a particular indicator by unit or by month. The differences within the data are shown by variations in the length of the bars. Figure 15-4 gives two examples of bar graphs. Bars may be horizontal or vertical, but each bar must be labeled. As in the line graph, there is a vertical and a horizontal axis, each representing a distinct variable being compared.

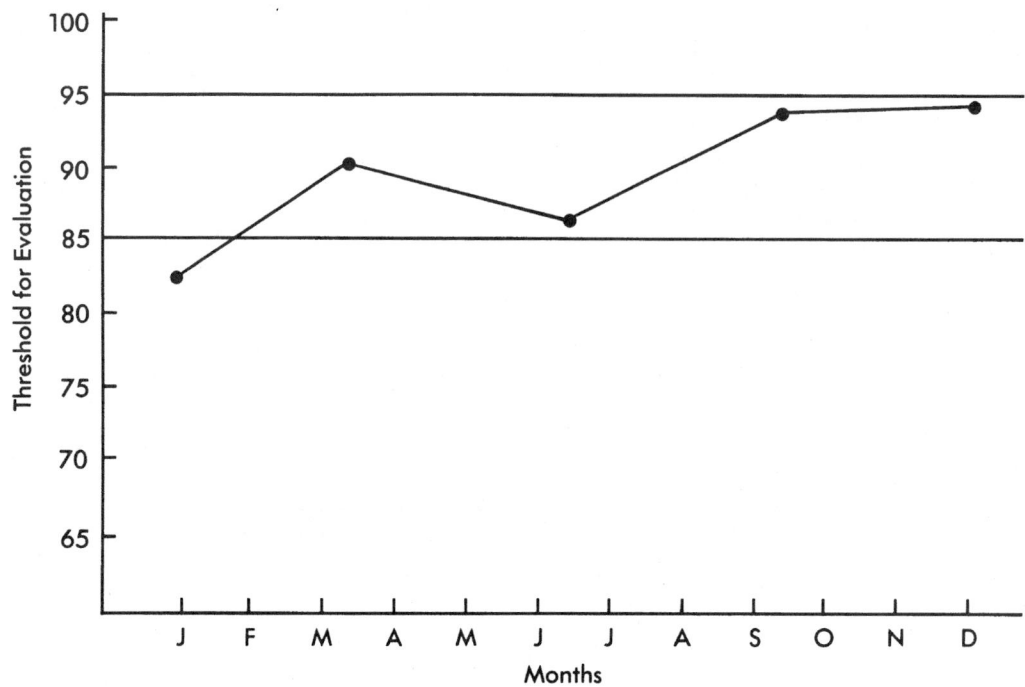

Figure 15-3   Line graph of thresholds for evaluation.

A pie graph depicts proportions. It depicts the phenomenon being analyzed in the form of a pie. A wedge of the pie is assigned to each of the components that make up the pie. Each wedge represents a percentage of the total item being analyzed, and differences are shown by the sizes of the wedges. Figure 15-5 is a pie graph representing the percentages of radiology escort service trips per week.

A table is an orderly arrangement of data. The data are arranged vertically in columns and horizontally in rows. Both columns and rows must be labeled. Tables are often used to clarify the relationships and meaning of the numbers. A table is an excellent mechanism for depicting large amounts of numerical data in a relatively small space. If particular numbers require special explanation, they should carry an asterisk or otherwise be marked, and a footnote should be added at the bottom of the table. The numbers for a rate-based indicator might be represented in tabular form (Figure 15-6).

Lesikar outlines five general rules for effective table construction[6]:

1. If rows are very long, repeat the row heads on the right side.
2. Use a dash or an abbreviation such as "n.a." (not applicable) rather than a zero when data are not available.
3. Key footnote references to numbers in the table with asterisks or other unambiguous, nonnumeric symbols.

4. Include totals and subtotals whenever they enhance the value of the table. Columns and/or rows may be totaled.
5. Make clear the units in which the data were measured (e.g., years, months, dollars, clinical units).

Color is useful to highlight contrasting information. Using different colors for the lines, bars, wedges, or columns helps the reader compare the data.

Step 5: When Should the Communication Occur?

Timing is crucial. The practicability and desirability of acting on the communication depend on appropriate timing. The best planned communication is wasted if it is poorly timed. The likelihood of the receiver attending to what is presented and thinking about the information is determined not only by how but also by when the information is presented.

Vardaman lists four checkpoints to use in assessing communication feasibility: (1) situational conditions, (2) resource availability, (3) data adequacy, and (4) programming with other communications.[10] Situational conditions include timing, significance, credibility, and realism.

Situational conditions. Bad news should never be delivered "cold," nor should an idea for radical change. It is important to time the communication for presentation when the receiver is most likely to be open to and to comprehend its significance. For example,

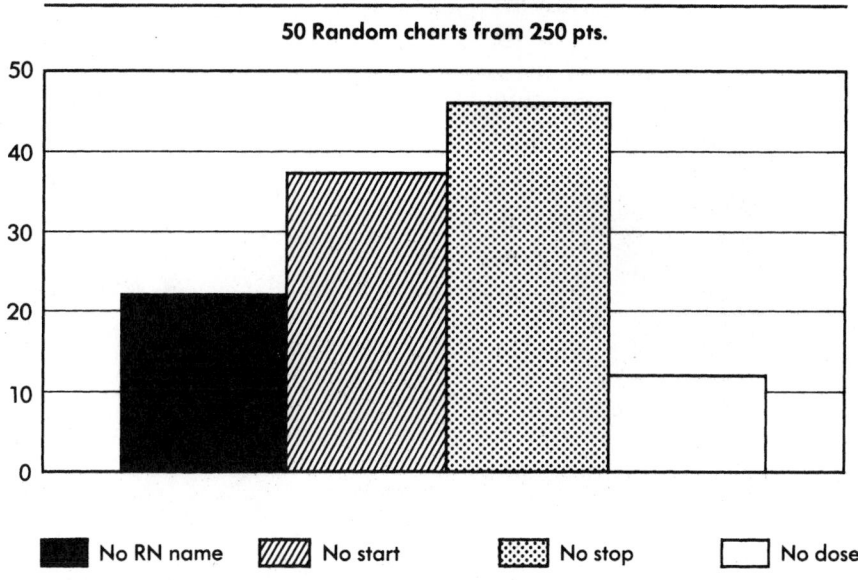

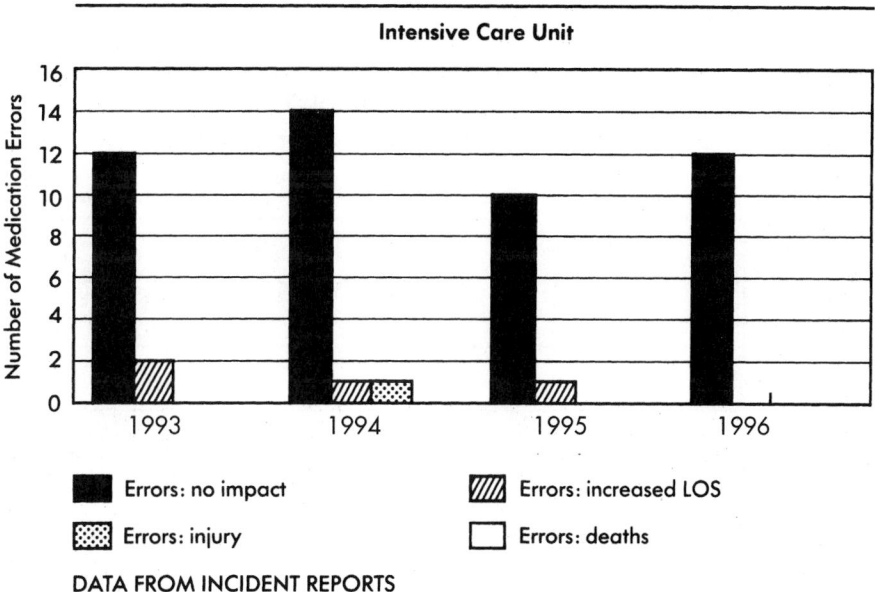

Figure 15-4   Two examples of bar graphs.

administrators often are more receptive to ideas for change immediately before and after an accreditation site visit.

Resource availability. Are sufficient fiscal, human, or material resources available to support the communication? If not, the content of the message would be moot. These resources must be secured before communication can occur.

Data adequacy. Are the data sufficient to build the case? Has the change been in effect long enough to demonstrate the desired results? If not, the message may be premature.

Programming with other communications. Finally, the message must blend with other communications if it is to be successful. Receiving the report when other issues are consuming most of an individual's attention diminishes the force of the communication and decreases the likelihood of its being understood. Timing involves knowing who else in the organization is communicating what and to whom, and how your report is

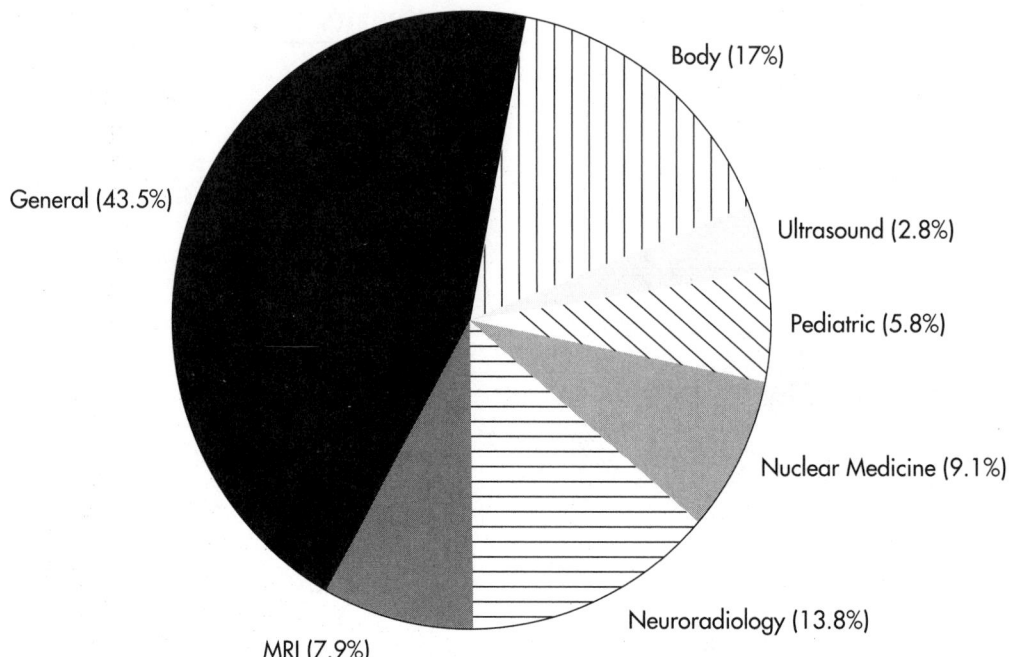

Figure 15-5   Example of a pie graph. (From Schroeder P: *Improving quality and performance: concepts, programs, and techniques,* St. Louis, 1994, Mosby.)

PATIENT FALLS

(Jan. 1, 1996 to December 31, 1996)

	Stage I	Stage II	Stage III	Stage IV
ICU/CCU	1	0	1	0
NICU	0	0	0	0
DETOX	5	2	4	2
OB/GYN	0	0	0	0
ONCOLOGY	2	1	3	2
MED-SURG	7	0	8	3
PEDS	11	2	14	3

Stage I: Witnessed, no injury
Stage II: Witnessed, injury
Stage III: Unwitnessed, no injury
Stage IV: Unwitnessed, injury

Figure 15-6   Example of a table.

enhanced or diminished by these other communications. Sometimes "piggybacking" reports of a similar nature can strengthen the grouped reports, and the synergy among them can increase the likelihood of a positive response to each.

Displaying Data Effectively

Carey and Lloyd suggest three tips for effective display of data from a study:

1. Provide a comparative reference on benchmark data.
2. Provide guidelines for interpreting the statistical significance or organizational importance of the data.
3. Provide graphs of key findings.[1]

An enumerative study is one that is performed on a static population for a given period of time and/or location. It is designed merely to describe outcomes. This type of data is best presented in a pie chart, bar graph, Pareto chart, or histogram.

An analytic study is one done on a dynamic process. It is not restricted to single points in time. It focuses on predicting the future rather than describing the past. Its purpose is to determine why outcomes were observed and how to improve the processes that produced the observed outcomes.

To evaluate this type of study, a control chart is the best form of visual data display.

One method of displaying study data simply and effectively is a storyboard. Producers of multimedia projects use storyboards to visually plot the progress of a story line. A storyboard is a visual depiction of all the steps of a study. This technique enables the observer to get the "whole picture" at a glance, quickly and concisely.

A storyboard can be an effective visual display of the performance improvement story. Figure 15-7 is an example of a storyboard format depicting the various stages in the performance improvement process and the tools used at each stage. Formats for storyboards vary; however, all three programs of the performance management system must be represented.

WRITING EFFECTIVE REPORTS

Written reports are probably the most common form of communication in organizations. Of course, they are effective only when they are read and understood. With the volume of paperwork that each administrator faces, the likelihood of a report being read is inversely proportional to the number of other reports in the administrator's "in" box. The busier a person is, the more likely he or she is to take reading shortcuts. Staff members are now busier than ever. Long, drawn-out reports full of statistical analyses are likely to be scanned rather than read. Never assume that because a report was written and distributed, it was read, even if reading it was requested or required.

Using the techniques suggested earlier in this chapter will yield more effective communication. Below are a few more suggestions to enhance the readability of a written presentation.

Reports have a greater impact when they are organized and presented appropriately. A written report represents the thoughts and work of the writer. It is a visual representation of its creator. When readers judge a report, they are considering not only the content but also the appearance of the work. In fact, the reader's impression of the content may be positively or negatively affected by the look of the report. A sloppy, disorganized report may suggest poorly developed, illogical ideas, whereas a well-organized and carefully formatted report may contribute to the credibility of the content.

Always include a cover sheet that identifies the title of the report, the date submitted, to whom the report is directed, and who prepared the report. Even if the report is merely a brief summary sheet, a cover sheet should be used. If the report is lengthy (e.g., more than 15 pages), include an abstract at the head. The abstract should be no longer than one page and should include the key points of the report. This way, a hurried reader can get the message quickly and return to the full report to digest the particulars as time permits.

Number all pages, figures, and appendices. There is nothing more frustrating to a reader than not being able to find a reference, figure, or chart. When possible, include the chart or figure in the body of the work so that the reader does not have to flip back and forth between the pages.

Doublecheck spelling and grammar. Excellent computer programs are available to check spelling and grammar. If these are not available, consult a dictionary. If your report is important and especially if it is also lengthy, you should consider having someone else read it to identify grammatical or spelling errors before you finalize and distribute the report.

DELIVERING AN EFFECTIVE ORAL PRESENTATION

Most individuals fear public speaking. The mere suggestion of an oral presentation is enough to induce palpitations, sweaty palms, and a dry mouth. Although much communication is written, sometimes an oral report is needed. The presentation may take the form of an informal briefing at a staff meeting or more formally as a report given at a council meeting or to an administrative group.

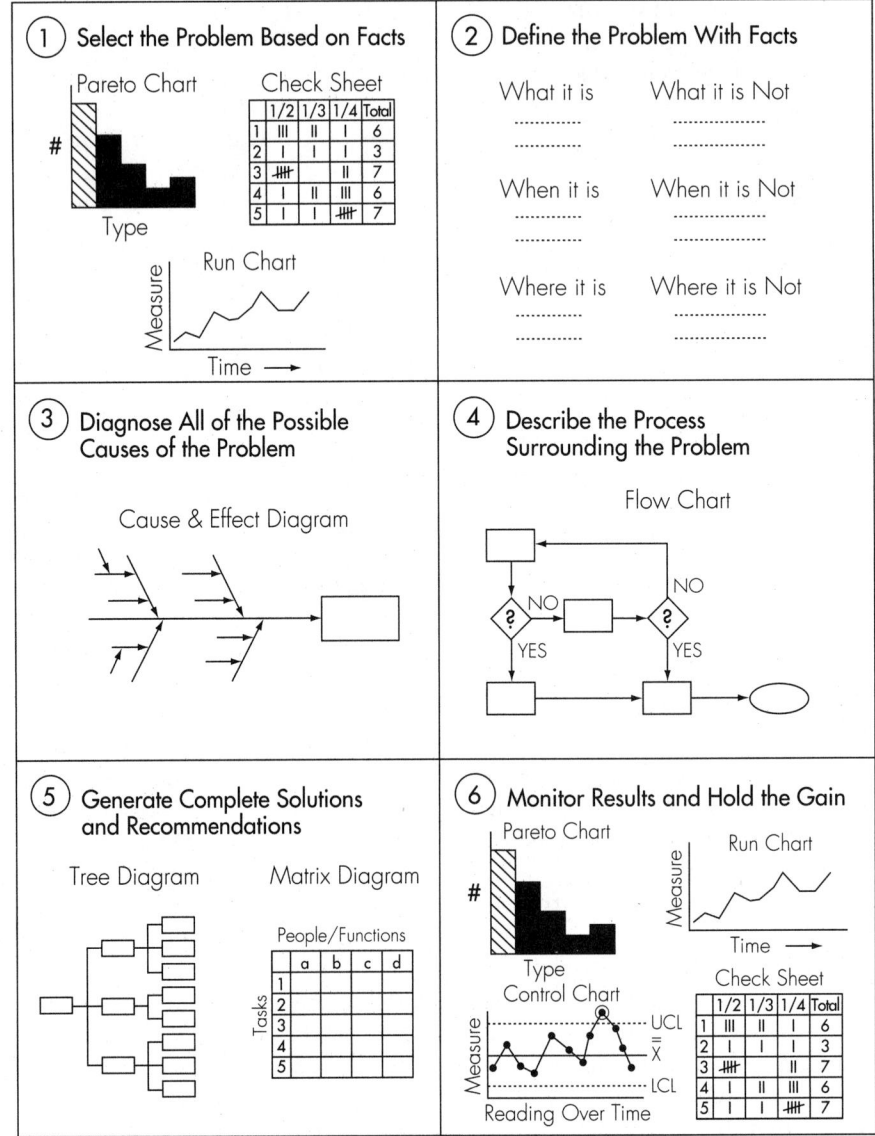

Figure 15-7 Storyboard format. (From Brassard M: *The memory jogger +: featuring the seven management and planning tools, pocket cards*, Meuthen, Mass, 1989, Goal/QPC.)

Many of the techniques described earlier in the chapter are useful in preparing a successful oral presentation. In addition, a few key points are given below.

In a written report, the writer is behind the scenes. In an oral one, the speaker is part of the message. The audience takes in both the message and the speaker's delivery and appearance. How they perceive the speaker can have a tremendous effect on how they relate to the message being conveyed. An anxious, disorganized, or unenthusiastic presenter can negatively affect the audience's perception of the speaker's competence and credibility, thus discrediting the message, too. A confident, enthusiastic, informed speaker can enhance the impact of the message.

There are two ways to deliver a verbal message: speaking one-on-one to an individual or delivering the message to more than one individual. When a message is conveyed one-on-one, it is a conversation. When it is delivered to a group, it may be thought of as an expanded conversation. An expanded conversation is merely an economical way of communicating the same message to many individuals.[8]

To diffuse the panic associated with speaking before a large group, look for ways to reduce the presentation to a conversation. Seek out a friendly face. Initially, talk to that person. After about a minute, make eye contact with someone else and speak to that person for a little while. Move from face to face. Should you encounter an uninterested face, return to a friendly one for a confidence boost.

By and large the biggest mistake most novice presenters make is to read their work. An effective oral presentation is not a recitation. Think back to when you enjoyed being read to. Probably it was when you were a child, just before bedtime. No wonder audiences dislike being read to—it makes them feel childish and sleepy. Even the finest content may be destroyed by being read. If you need help remembering key points, write key phrases on note cards and number them to indicate the proper sequence. Show the major points on an overhead, slide, or flip chart so that you do not lose your train of thought, but *never* read.

Preparation is the key to effective content and practice is the key to effective delivery. Rehearse, rehearse, rehearse. It will free you from clutching a prepared script as a life preserver.

Another important point to remember is that the brain can absorb only what the seat can endure. Many people become fidgety during presentations. Individuals listen more closely if the message relates to them. Relate the utility of the content for the audience early in the presentation, within the first 5 minutes if possible. This helps to set the stage for the information that follows. Another hint to set the stage for your presentation and to increase the likelihood of being heard is to eliminate environmental distractors. It is difficult to be heard in the midst of telephones ringing and beepers beeping. If the presentation is a planned formal one, choosing a site that minimizes disturbances of this kind is crucial. You do not want the VP to be beeped just as you are reaching the climax of the presentation.

Do not take yourself or your content too seriously—and do not forget to smile. Appendix 15-1 provides some additional tips for successful presentations.

ADDITIONAL COMMUNICATION MECHANISMS

Two other mechanisms can be used to enhance communication about quality activities: the performance management bulletin board and the institutional newsletter.

Swindle maintains that nearly everyone reads bulletin boards and almost no one reads newsletters.[9] That is because the information placed on bulletin boards is seen as important to the individual's relationship to the organization. The bulletin board must be strategically placed and properly controlled. Newsletters, however, are often seen as folksy tidbits about individuals within the organization, births, marriages, retirements, and sports scores. Changing that view requires a commitment to include pertinent and relevant information regarding the performance management system activities and the impact of that system on the individual's daily practice.

Both bulletin boards and newsletters are excellent tools to inform and recognize individuals for their performance. We suggest dividing the bulletin board into six sections to help staff find information quickly.[3] These sections include the following:

- general organization information
- department information
- the performance improvement program
- recognition
- required reading
- communication from other departments

To control paper flow, each item should be dated with its posting date and its removal date. One person, typically the department secretary, is designated to post and remove items in a timely manner and to record in the department's notebook the names of those staff members who have not completed required reading.

Organizing an effective newsletter can also promote an important communication link between staff and the organization. A regular column related to performance excellence can be used to educate staff, to foster a culture of performance excellence, to inform staff about significant study findings, and to recognize the staff's performance improvement efforts. One way to ensure that staff members get the message is to make the newsletter required reading on the bulletin board.

Although communicating results is the last piece in a study, it also is the first step in identifying problems or opportunities. Communication of relevant results is only as good as the feedback that the report elicits. What impact did the communication have and what results did it evoke? Mechanisms must be put in place to enable individuals, departments, councils, and administration to respond to the communication.

Everyone within the organization needs to be touched by the performance management communication network. It is the lifeline of organizational growth and development.

REFERENCES

1. Carey R, Lloyd R: *Measuring quality improvement in healthcare,* New York, 1995, Quality Resources.
2. Fellows H, Ikeda F: *Business speaking and writing,* Englewood Cliffs, NJ, 1982, Prentice-Hall.
3. Green E, Katz J: Make your bulletin board a QA tool, *RN,* 53(1): 38-39, 1990.
4. Hamilton C, Parker C, Smith DD: *Communicating for results,* Belmont, Cal, 1982, Wadsworth Publishing.
5. Hunt GT: *Communication skills in the organization,* Englewood Cliffs, NJ, 1980, Prentice-Hall.
6. Lesikar RV: *Business communication: theory and application,* ed 3, Homewood, Ill, 1976, Richard D. Irwin.
7. Rappsilber C: *Persuasion as a mechanism for change.* In Lancaster J, Lancaster W, editors: *The nurse as change agent,* St Louis, 1982, Mosby.
8. Rosenblatt SB, Cheatam TR, Watt JT: *Communication in business,* Englewood Cliffs, NJ, 1977, Prentice-Hall.
9. Swindle R: *The business communicator,* Englewood Cliffs, NJ, 1980, Prentice-Hall.
10. Vardaman G: *Effective communication of ideas,* New York, 1970, Van Nostrand Reinhold.

Appendix 15-1   Presentation Tips

- If you make a mistake, fix it and go on. Participants would prefer to find out the correct information and are very forgiving when you admit an honest mistake.

- If you feel tired and burned out, it will show when you present. Develop personal relaxation methods to relieve your stress and energize yourself before, during, and after your presentations. Exercise, noncaffeinated drinks, foods high in carbohydrates, and classical music work well.

- A good rule of thumb for your handouts: participants hear you say it, they see you display it, and they will need to write it down—so you will want to provide them with the appropriate space to record their thoughts.

- Check to make sure the public address (PA) system and other equipment are set up and working properly! A check of all equipment 1 hour in advance can prevent a lasting negative impression.

- Room temperature in the comfort range promotes learning and understanding! A temperature of 68 to 70 degrees produces better retention than 2 degrees below or above this standard.

- Materials that fall off the wall break concentration! Finding several ways to attach materials will cut down on this distraction. Try using masking tape, straight pins, push pins, sticky tack, or a variety of these.

- Writing on the bottom third of the flipchart makes it tough for your participants to see. Since no one can see that portion of the page, the solution is to write in the flipchart's upper two thirds and print two to three times larger than normal.

- Wear comfortable clothing and shoes. For both men and women, wear shoes that do not pinch or bind your feet; avoid wearing brand-new shoes on session days. Wear clothing that is loose and comfortable and that you feel your best in—avoid wearing new suits or outfits that you are not used to.

- Play your favorite music while setting up your presentation room or preparing for the next day. Some people may prefer soothing classical music; some may prefer rock. Use the kind of music you know you need for that day.

- Drink plenty of water while presenting. If in a hotel facility, have the banquet staff provide fresh lemon slices for your water. Pour several glasses at the back table so the ice will have time to melt down, as ice-cold water will tighten your vocal cords and cause your voice to go up several octaves.

- Select a professional look. Try to dress up one step from the participants. You are the person they look to for the answers. Dress the part!

- When using index cards for your notes:
  (1) Write on only one side and number on the back side the order in the presentation's sequence.
  (2) Rubber band together the whole presentation set of cards.
  (3) Pull out the card after you are finished with it and lay it aside.
  (4) Reassemble the cards according to the numbers on the back *after* the presentation is complete.
  These simple techniques will help your confidence in the presentation and will also indicate the correct order just in case the cards get mixed up.

Modified from Backer L, Deck M, McCallum D: *The presenter's survival kit*, St. Louis, 1995, Mosby.

- If your audience is small, use overhead transparencies, which are easier to change and make it easier for you to monitor your audience's reactions. If your audience is large (50 to 100 or more), consider using the more formal 35-millimeter (35mm) slides.

- Once your slides or transparencies are projected on the screen, do not read from them to your audience. Elaborate on the main points presented.

- Print on your flipcharts in uppercase and lowercase letters. Avoid cursive writing; it is harder to read.

Modified from Backer L, Deck M, McCallum D: *The presenter's survival kit*, St. Louis, 1995, Mosby.

Part Six

MANAGING THE PERFORMANCE OF THE PERFORMANCE MANAGEMENT SYSTEM

Chapter 16

Creating an Awareness of the Performance Management System

*The performance of a health care organization
is in direct proportion to its planned, organized,
systematic commitment to excellence.*
Ellie Green

Santiago, an old fisherman, was ridiculed by his fellow villagers, because he was unable to catch any fish. They attributed his failure to fate. Santiago disagreed with them; he knew he had the ability to catch fish. He taught Manolin, a village boy, how to fish. Manolin was the only one who still believed in him.

One night, Santiago was inspired by a dream to catch a huge fish that would prove his fishing abilities to everyone. Early the next morning, he set off in his old fishing boat. He caught a marlin, which was so huge that it dragged Santiago's boat around for days. Eventually, Santiago was able to harpoon the fish and secure it to his boat. Triumphant about his catch, Santiago headed for shore. However, before he could make it to shore, sharks smelled the marlin's blood and devoured all the meat off of the huge fishbones. Nevertheless, the villagers were awed by the size of the fishbones. They praised Santiago's fishing abilities. Manolin learned an important lesson—never to give up and to believe in internal values, regardless of other people's opinions.[3]

THE PERFORMANCE MANAGEMENT SYSTEM

Implementing a new culture in a health care organization today in which a performance management system

can thrive requires the same commitment and perseverance to internal values as did Santiago in Hemingway's famous novel *The Old Man and the Sea.* Health care organizations today require a new culture, because the former health care culture recommended and rewarded status quo and tenure. The new culture rewards innovation, commitment, and perseverance. In spite of criticism and negative comments, a performance management system is like Santiago's boat. It is the vehicle that can take a health care organization farther than they have ever been before to excellent performance.

The goal of the performance management system is to provide the framework within which the performance awareness, measurement, and improvement programs may be developed (Figure 16-1). Once developed, these three programs, synchronized within the performance management system, provide three great benefits. First, within the performance awareness program, the organization is enabled to create standards in the service, practice, and governance domains as well as develop a culture of excellence. Second, within the performance measurement program the health care organization creates and utilizes valid and reliable data from all departments, subsidiaries, and alliances to make rational predictions of present and future resource

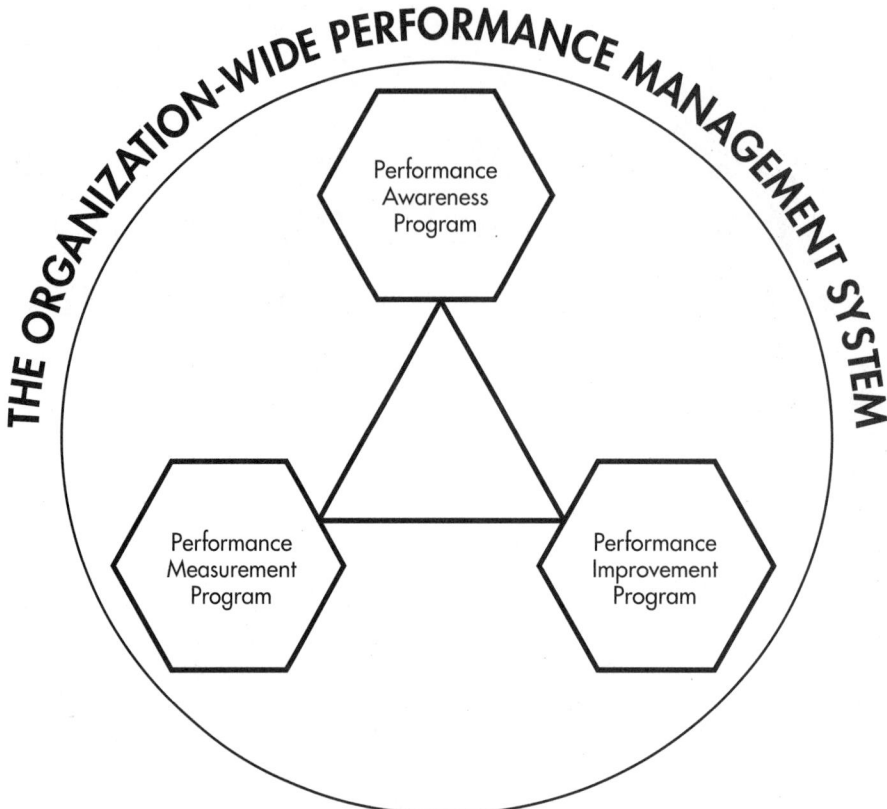

Figure 16-1 Performance management system paradigm.

consumption and performance. Third, within the performance improvement program the organization is enabled to create a systematic method for continual organization-wide performance improvement.

Although most health care organizations attempt to implement some type of performance improvement system to evaluate and improve their efficiency and effectiveness, many are disappointed, because improvement is not always the outcome of their efforts. Furthermore, to many, a performance management system is synonymous with quality assurance (QA) and has come to symbolize time away from patient care, endless audits, and required, excessive—but ignored—paperwork.

This was especially true in the 1960s and 1970s, when quality assurance became associated with audits of details, whether or not there were significant concerns at stake. During the 1980s, the traditional approaches to QA began to change. Some of the driving forces behind those changes included upwardly spiraling health care costs, an older and sicker population, and an explosion of technology that outdistanced research dollars to prove the efficacy and benefit of each new invention. In the 1980s QA was replaced by continuous quality improvement

(CQI). Today, CQI has been replaced by performance management. Unlike the term continuous quality improvement, which became a catch-all phrase for any quality effort, the term performance management is specific. This term encompasses three critical programs: (a) awareness, (b) measurement, and (c) improvement.

An organization-wide performance management system must drive its three critical programs:

1. *awareness*—a program that educates all customers and stakeholders to the standards involved in the organization's three domains of service, practice, and governance
2. *measurement*—a program that delineates exactly how measurement of key functions and critical processes will occur in the three domains and how the data will be used to reduce errors and calculate the cost of nonconformance
3. *improvement*—a program that will delineate expected outcomes in each domain and benchmark success against historical or national indicators. It will use these outcomes as building blocks for performance improvement as well as serve the organization-wide vehicle for innovation.

THE PERFORMANCE MANAGEMENT SYSTEM: A KEY FUNCTION

A key function is defined as a goal-directed, interrelated series of processes.[4] By this definition the performance management system within a health care organization serves as a key function and therefore must be allotted the same scrutiny as other organizational key functions.

Organizations do not, of course, measure and improve the key functions per se. The improvement focus is always on the *critical processes* that lie within each key function.

When performance management is considered a key function, there are three critical processes that lie within it: (a) awareness, (b) measurement, and (c) improvement. Each of these three processes is so encompassing in scope that an organization cannot capture all necessary activities within each process without great thought and systematic planning. Given the limited resources of most health care organizations, the simplest method for implementing the necessary activities required by a thorough performance management system is to create a program for each of the three critical processes of awareness, measurement, and performance. Each program may then be developed so that all necessary activities are performed. Furthermore, you are able to build into each of these programs benchmarks against which to measure your performance. Figure 16-2 illustrates the key function of performance management and its relationship to the three critical processes that have been developed into three programs of awareness, measurement, and improvement. These three programs synergistically create the performance management system for a health care organization.

Once the organization of the performance management system is created, it is necessary to delineate the scope of each program. Figure 16-3 shows how to utilize the matrix discussed in Chapter 6 to accomplish this. As discussed in Chapter 6, this matrix is divided vertically into the domains of service, practice, and governance. It is divided horizontally into three categories: routinely offered, offered by request or as the need arises, and offered in an emergency.

In the first horizontal box consider what is routinely offered by the performance awareness program in the service, practice, and governance domain. For example, we routinely offer service based on an organizational model. In the second horizontal section consider what is offered by the awareness program by request or as the need arises. For example, in the service domain we offer modification of the outcome and/or process standards of the performance awareness program. In the third horizontal box consider what is offered by the awareness program in an emergency. For example, in the service domain we offer emergency performance measures based on predetermined contingency standards.

Utilizing this matrix helps solidify the direction of the performance awareness program. The performance awareness program creates the standards for the entire performance management system. Therefore, standards are the basis for all measurement and improvement. Without standards, the entire performance management system cannot function.

THE PERFORMANCE AWARENESS PROGRAM

Just as the organization itself must be driven by carefully constructed standards, so too, must the performance management system. In a standards-based system that emphasizes performance, the performance awareness program must be developed first. We recognize that writing standards for the performance management system is a new idea to many. However, these standards, developed within the awareness program, provide the "rules of the game" for the entire

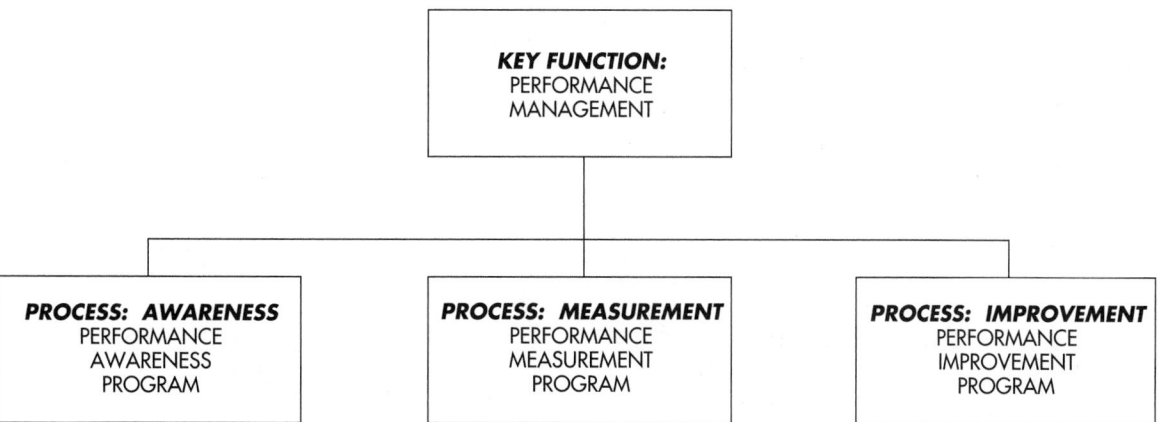

Figure 16-2 Performance management and the relationship of the three critical processes that have been developed into programs.

MATRIX TO DELINEATE SCOPE OF THE PERFORMANCE AWARENESS PROGRAM

IN THE AWARENESS PROGRAM WE OFFER:	SERVICE DOMAIN	PRACTICE DOMAIN	GOVERNANCE DOMAIN
ROUTINELY OFFERED	1. Service based on an organization-wide model 2. Written standards to drive all services 3. Continuous information about performance measurement and improvement results to interested parties 4. The use of performance management information for utilization in the decision making process of care delivery	1. Practice based on an organization-wide model 2. Written standards to drive all practices 3. Information about practices and improvement to practices to interested parties 4. Organization-wide performance management documentation on standardized, designated tools	1. Governance based on an organization-wide model 2. Written standards to drive the governance of the organization 3. Information about governance and system practices to interested parties 4. Organization-wide standardized tools for documentation of the performance management systems information
REQUESTED/AS NEED ARISES	1. Modification of outcome and/or process standards of service of the performance awareness program 2. Readjustments to care delivery that are based on data	1. Modification of outcome and/or process standards of practice of the performance awareness program 2. Adjustments of sample sizes; repeat studies as directed	1. Modification of organization-wide written standards for the performance management system 2. Repeated studies with increased sampling sizes
EMERGENCY	1. Emergency performance measures based on predetermined contingency standards	1. Implementation of contingency standards 2. Education about contingencies	1. Contingency standards addressing sentinel events are developed and available

Figure 16-3   Matrix to delineate scope of the performance awareness program.

performance management system. This is a necessary step within the awareness program, if the measurement and improvement programs are to function correctly. The three programs, then, create an integrated performance management system that results in every employee "singing from the same hymnal."

Because a successful performance management system requires a commitment of considerable resources, thorough advance planning is necessary. Carefully designed systems have not been the traditional method of developing and conducting the various, so-called "quality programs" in most health care organizations. Although health care organizations have developed standards to direct a program of patient care services, they have typically overlooked the development of standards necessary to direct a performance management system. Furthermore, most organizations felt justified in neglecting to develop their performance management system's standards, because there was little in the way of research or written material to guide them, and innovation was not encouraged.

In Chapter 3, THE BLUEPRINT outlines the standards' format for health care organizations. These standards include mission, philosophy, goals, policies, outcomes, procedures, practice guidelines, action planning, documentation, and job descriptions. Using this same format, standards are developed for the performance management system by the organization's top leadership—the CEO and those appointed to the quality management board.

These standards for the performance management system set expectations in writing about how the performance management system will function throughout the organization. Furthermore, these standards should detail responsibility and accountability of all workers, units, departments, and services within the organization for the three programs of awareness, measurement, and improvement. Without written standards, it would be impossible to generate a planned, organized, systematic performance management system. Standards are the yardstick against which we measure compliance to expectations—the basis for determining if the performance management system is doing what it was designed to do.

Develop standards, or written expectations, first when your health care organization is restructuring itself for the competitive managed care environment or developing alliances to meet the continuum of care requirements of today's accreditation agencies. The top leaders of the organization, directed by the CEO, bear the responsibility for creating the organization-wide standards for the performance management system. These standards then act as benchmarks against which the appropriateness, efficiency, and effectiveness of the system is measured and improved. In other words, developing standards for the performance management system is synonymous with the creation of an awareness program.

THE PERFORMANCE MEASUREMENT PROGRAM

The second component of a well-defined and well-planned performance management system is the performance measurement program. This component involves data collection and analysis. How to analyze the performance of your performance measurement program is discussed in Chapter 17.

THE PERFORMANCE IMPROVEMENT PROGRAM

The performance improvement program is the third component of the performance management system. This is the phase in which improvements are made in the process and outcomes of the performance management system itself. How to improve the performance of the performance management system is discussed in Chapter 18.

CREATING AN AWARENESS PROGRAM FOR THE PERFORMANCE MANAGEMENT SYSTEM

A suggested organization of standards for the performance management system is presented in the box on p. 262. We recommend that the performance management system's standards be organized into structure, outcome, and process, just as THE BLUEPRINT organizes the organization-wide standards.

The foundation for an organization-wide, standards-based system that emphasizes performance lies in the development of structure standards. The foundational standards upon which the performance management system is built also begins with structure standards. These include the mission (and vision) statement, the philosophy, the goals, and the policies for the organization-wide performance management system. Outcome standards follow. Outcome standards are the expected results of carrying out the process standards of the performance management system. Process standards of the performance management system include procedures, practice guidelines, action planning, and documentation. The standards for the organization-wide performance management system must be outlined and each standard formatted, using the framework of THE BLUEPRINT. Then the health care organization can create a performance management system manual that contains all necessary information. This ensures uniformity of team management, measurement—including data collection and analysis, statistical reporting, documentation, and improvement of designated outcomes across the continuum of services of the organization.

CREATING AN AWARENESS PROGRAM: ORGANIZATION OF STANDARDS FOR THE PERFORMANCE MANAGEMENT SYSTEM

Structure:

1. Mission (and vision) of the performance management system
2. Philosophy of the performance management system
3. Goals and objectives of the performance management system
4. Policies (and performance descriptions) of the performance management system

Outcome:

1. Service outcomes of the performance management system
2. Practice outcomes of the performance management system
3. Governance outcomes of the performance management system

Process:

1. Procedures for the performance management system
2. Practice guidelines for the performance management system
3. Action planning of the performance management system
4. Documentation of the performance management system

DISSEMINATING THE PERFORMANCE MANAGEMENT SYSTEM'S INFORMATION

The use of an operations manual is important to the dissemination of the organization-wide performance management system's rules, processes, and expected outcomes. An awareness of the performance management system cannot occur without a central reference source that every worker understands, acknowledges, and contributes to as part of his or her daily work experience. If this does not occur, health care organizations will find important information scattered among many memoranda, oral agreements, and minutes. "When there is a central reference source, the information survives despite lapses in memory and employee turnover."[2]

If your organization is totally computerized, the details of a manual may be captured in your database of information and accessed through every department's computer terminals. In the absence of such electronic capabilities, a 3-ring binder may be used. In either case, the goal is to provide the entire health care organization with a well-thought-out, formally approved, easily understandable, and legitimate way of conducting the organization's performance management system.

Hospitals have grown into one of the most complex social institutions within the United States.[1] Many organizations traditionally have become polarized into departments, or units. Today's health care environment calls for all departments and units within the organization, as well as those organizations it associates with, or is allied by contract to, to "sing from the same hymnal." The autonomous and insulated thinking of workers within each department must give way to interdisciplinary sharing, problem solving and data collection. Unless all workers see the overall performance picture of the total organization, view themselves as essential parts of the team, and understand the rules and expectations of the performance management system, that often-used but undefined term, *excellence,* will remain elusive.

The organization of standards for the performance management system presented in the box to the left lists a suggested sequence for the major sections of the performance management system's information manual.

THE MISSION

The mission of the performance management system within an organization is of paramount importance. It is not a repetition of the health care organization's mission, such as "to provide quality care," nor is it a repetition of the division of nursing's philosophy, such as "to foster an environment for continuous quality improvement." It also is not a rewording of ancillary services' mission, such as "to provide high quality services to all customers." It *is,* rather, an explanation of the reason for the existence of the performance management system and why employees should be involved in its operation.

The box below shows a sample mission statement for a performance management system in a health care organization. The mission statement justifies the existence of the performance management system. It

THE MISSION OF THE PERFORMANCE MANAGEMENT SYSTEM

To provide a mechanism to develop, measure, and improve the level of service, practice, and governance provided within the organization.

should blend with and support the organization-wide mission. Just as the mission statement of an organization explains why it exists, so the mission statement of the performance management system explains its purpose. Remember, the mission statement is a structure standard. Place it first in the performance management system's manual.

THE PHILOSOPHY

The philosophy of the performance management system consists of a statement of beliefs, concepts, and principles about this key governance function. These describe the ideas, convictions, and attitudes of the organization about its awareness, measurement, and improvement programs. This philosophy serves as a guide for action and an explanation of action. The beliefs provide a basis for carrying out the mission of the performance management system. Keep in mind that the philosophy of the performance management system should be realistic, understandable, measurable, believable, and achievable.

The philosophy of the performance management system should be written and placed in the next section of the performance management manual. It should be reviewed at least every 3 years. The box on the right shows a sample philosophy of a performance management system. Philosophy is also a structure standard.

THE GOALS

The goals of the performance management system are derived directly from the philosophy. The goals describe how the philosophy will be actualized. Goals express the broad-based desires for the performance management system. They compose the next section of the performance management system's structure standards. If you are using a 3-ring binder to house the performance management system's standards, then make goals the next section. Each month the quality management board should evaluate the goals of the performance management system to alter, update, or record progress toward meeting the goals.

Objectives add specificity to the goals by delineating how the goals will be achieved yearly. The box on p. 264 is a sample of goals with the accompanying objectives. Goals are written to correspond to an organization's philosophy. Realize that philosophy may no longer consist of creative, impressive jargon that has nothing to do with the day-to-day reality of operating the health care organization. In other words, all structure, outcome, and process standards along with the evaluation portion of the framework must "hang together" or exist synergistically rather than exist ran-

THE PHILOSOPHY OF THE PERFORMANCE MANAGEMENT SYSTEM

- Each customer has the right to expect performance excellence.
- Accountability for organizational performance begins at the highest level within the organization.
- Organizational, group, and individual performance is manageable.
- Performance comprises competency and application.
- Performance excellence is each employee's responsibility.
- Performance standards define the performance expectations.
- Awareness of and compliance with performance standards is fundamental to performance excellence.
- Performance excellence can be achieved only through an organized system of awareness, measurement, and improvement.
- Performance excellence cannot be achieved in an environment of fear and blame.
- The system is critical to performance excellence.
- Measurement of performance is ongoing and focuses on key processes within the organization.
- Performance measurement must be statistically based and systematic.
- Improvements must be made in all three domains of performance: service, practice, and governance.
- Improvements can be achieved only as a result of continuous feedback from both internal and external customers.

domly, scattered throughout various manuals of the organization.

Furthermore, goals and objectives are dynamic rather than static. They are written expressions of the activities occurring within the organization. More than one objective may apply to each goal, or several goals may be met through one objective. In any event, formulating goals must not be a paper exercise undertaken solely to get through an accreditation process, but rather the creation of dynamic directives that drive the organization's performance management system. Like the mission and philosophy, goals are also structure standards.

THE POLICIES

Policies, as defined in THE BLUEPRINT, are structure standards and, as such, are nonnegotiable rules. Define those rules governing the performance management system in the next section of the performance management system's manual.

GOALS AND OBJECTIVES OF THE PERFORMANCE MANAGEMENT SYSTEM

Goal 1:

To develop an organization-wide, integrated, interdisciplinary, standards-based performance management system throughout this organization.

Objectives:

- To host a performance management leadership conference for all board members, administrative staff, and managers in October of this year so that they can understand the vision of the organization.
- To schedule employee-manager 4-hour retreats to establish a commitment to performance improvement and design a strategic plan for establishing interdisciplinary priorities of key functions and critical processes for the next 2 years.

Goal 2:

To provide 3% to 5% of the total operating budget to assess and improve service, practice, and governance throughout the organization.

Objectives:

- To redesign the job descriptions of every employee of the organization to include a commitment to excellence of performance in each domain.
- To include the performance management system as a cost center within the organization.

Goal 3:

To utilize statistically derived measurements as the basis for decision making regarding the delivery of service, practice, and governance of the organization.

Objectives:

- To train all workers on the principles of statistics and use of statistical process control tools.

- To develop storyboards to display the results of the performance management system's studies and to display these storyboards in a highly visible area of the organization.

Goal 4:

To foster an environment of open communication, trust, cooperation, and risk-taking that eliminates fear in the workplace.

Objectives:

- To institute a process for anonymous incident-reporting in each domain.
- To institute a process for performance and technology measurement in each domain.
- To implement a program to facilitate work and process redesign and innovation in each domain: service, practice, and governance.

Goal 5:

To make the performance management system a visible part of every employee's daily work experience.

Objectives:

- To install a performance management system bulletin board in each department/unit of the organization.
- To require that 15 minutes of every staff meeting be devoted to the subject of the performance management system and its three programs.
- To create and implement a shared leadership governance model that facilitates a top-down commitment to the organization-wide performance management system.

There are three types of policies that are developed for the performance management system:

- service performance management policies
- practice performance management policies
- governance performance management policies.

Remember that every organization is bound by its policies, so be wary of creating impressive-sounding policies for the performance management system that would be impossible to implement with available resources and/or defend in court.

Service Performance Management Policies

Policies that govern the service domain of the performance management system occupy the next section of the manual. These policies outline the nonnegotiable rules of the performance management system in the customer domain. This includes all services such as patient care, education, and discharge callbacks to check on postdischarge recovery. If the policy is a service one, it must contain the organization's own rules for governing patient care and service. The policies must be realistic, understandable, measurable, believable, and achievable, based on the organization's available resources.

Publication of a complete outline of a performance management system's policies in this book is not feasible. However, examples include statements dictating that performance management studies routinely will be conducted on the top three to five patient populations that are admitted annually into the organization's health care system, and that a trifocus approach will be used in all performance analysis. Rules will be delineated in this section regarding the types of clinical studies to be conducted as well as the rules for conducting clinical trials and patient research, sample size, routine departmental quality control, or frequency of measurement. In short, this section includes any non-negotiable rules of the performance management system directly pertaining to the awareness program, i.e., creating standards for its operation, or rules pertaining to the program of performance measurement, and rules pertaining to the program of performance improvement.

Practice Performance Management Policies

Performance management system's policies in the practice domain include the nonnegotiable rules for measuring the professional practice of all staff members. The second division of the policy section of the performance management system's manual comprises these policies.

The policies in this practice domain section address key issues of employee participation in the three performance management system's programs. For example, participation in the performance awareness program would include such issues as serving in the shared leadership council structure and adhering to the performance management system's standards. Employee participation in the performance measurement program would include such issues as using proper sampling size; employing accurate data-gathering techniques, using the designated information management processes; and figuring the cost of variances. Employee participation in the performance improvement program would include such issues as establishing and meeting expected outcomes and working as members of the process improvement teams.

Governance Performance Management Policies

The policies of the performance management system in the governance domain are the nonnegotiable rules for administering the performance management system itself. These policies provide the "bones" or working skeleton, of the performance management system. The policies in this section specify the responsibility and accountability for organization-wide performance management that drive the total organization-wide thrust for excellence. These rules include those for shared leadership council structure, the performance improvement chain-of-command; for organization-wide measurement, such as who will collect data, how often, and on which processes; for use and responsibility of translation of data into statistics; for creation

and use of storyboards; for creation of teams; for allocating a length of time for improvement of processes; for managing data information, including archive requirements, benchmarking, and the use of national data bank information.

This section should also specify frequency of reviews and updates of all standards. Outline the "rules of the game" for the performance management system in an organized manner and maintain them in the performance management system's manual. Remember, however, that policies are nonnegotiable, so develop them wisely.

Job Descriptions

Within the performance management system there are several key personnel whose job descriptions are an integral component of the success of the performance management system. These include, but are not limited to, the organization-wide performance management coordinator(s), the risk manager(s), the utilization review personnel, and the case or outcomes manager.

Each job description within the organization—from the CEO to the dishwashers—should specify responsibility and accountability for performance management. However, the job descriptions mentioned above are critical to the outcomes of the performance management system, because these employees perform the actual hands-on, behind-the-scenes duties of meeting outcomes; gathering, compiling, and translating data into information; and handling the continual changes inherent in the present health care environment associated with awareness, measurement, and improvement of key functions and critical processes.

The job descriptions for the employees directly associated with the inner workings of the performance management system are critical, because they provide written rules for the scope of responsibility and accountability over the key function of performance management. Furthermore, the job descriptions of today's performance management specialists should reflect the boundaries and obligations along a continuum of care that follows the patient from home and community into the health care system and back into the home and community. No longer will the traditional "in-house" job description for a performance management specialist be adequate.

Today it is necessary to outline the extent of authority of the performance management specialist as he or she functions beyond the organization's walls. This will require a clear understanding of the role of performance management specialists as they function outside the primary organization. They must understand the paraprofessionals' role and the community resources available to the patient; the written rules for the awareness, measurement, and improvement programs that include interaction with a wide variety of people both within and outside the organization; reporting; and information management. It will necessitate creating and establishing an extended performance management system that includes measurements from a variety of outside sources. This is the only way to keep track of patients over extended periods of time. This information has become an expected part of the performance management system's research on outcomes, to prove the effectiveness of an organization's treatments and interventions.

Do not assume these key roles. Articulate them in detail and house them in the performance management system's manual for easy access to all interested workers. These key roles also include the positions of council chair and member. A concise, well-detailed job description will provide the necessary written authority to proceed unhindered in carrying out required duties of the performance management system.

Outcomes

Next, delineate the outcomes that the organization expects from its performance management system. The written outcomes describe what the organization hopes to achieve by implementing a performance management system. Every organization wants to enhance the appropriateness and effectiveness of the delivery of patient care. To do that, the organization must first develop its own standards or performance awareness program, performance measurement program, and performance improvement program and the expected outcomes of each. Together, these three programs contain the organization-wide expected outcomes of the performance management system. The outcomes of this system then become the benchmarks against which all performance is measured. This includes performance within the service, practice, and governance domains of the organization.

Performance management outcomes are incorporated into the process standards of the performance management system. For example, an outcome within the service domain might include a practice guideline for patient discharge that refers to discharging a particular patient population group within a designated hospital length of stay. Within the practice domain the outcome of the practice guideline for conducting a performance improvement study might be obtaining valid and reliable data. This would require using a systematic, ongoing measurement method by the same data collector, using a specific patient population, the same evaluation tool, and the same statistical program to analyze the data—all of which is spelled out in the performance awareness, measurement, and improve-

ment programs. Within the governance domain an outcome (objective) might be to reduce the number of lost patient charges for supplies by 20% for the year.

Always establish outcomes as you develop standards. These outcomes, as stated, can be met only if they are realistic, understandable, measurable, believable, and achievable. Remember that outcomes are standards in their own right and, as such, should be given the same attention and authority as structure and process standards.

Processes

Process standards of the performance management system include procedures, practice guidelines, action plans/pathways/algorithms, and documentation related to performance management.

Procedures. All procedures for the performance management system should follow the same format. The procedures of the performance management system include explanations of how to carry out tasks or calculations, such as standard deviation, data entry into a computer, or the procedure for a post-discharge patient telephone interview. Procedures are process standards. Like all procedures, they describe psychomotor skills involved in meeting the outcomes of the performance management system.

One suggested format that may be used to describe how to carry out the tasks of the performance management system is shown in Figure 16-4. These procedures are maintained in the performance management system's manual for easy access and reference. We recommend that the performance management system's procedures be reviewed and updated every 3 years.

Practice guidelines. Practice guidelines for the performance management system are written to guide staff members in the critical thinking skills necessary to initiate and implement certain performance management processes when predetermined targets have been met.

Practice guidelines for the performance management system provide an organization with tools for standardizing performance awareness, measurement, and improvement program activities. They promote continuity in practice from department to department and across the continuum of care. Unlike policies, practice guidelines are negotiable. In other words, they provide direction while permitting modifications to be made when warranted by professional judgment. Examples of practice guidelines for the performance management system might include management of variance, management of information, or management of process improvement teams.

When practice guidelines are implemented for the performance management system, things happen the

POST-DISCHARGE TELEPHONE INTERVIEW PROCEDURE FOR THE PERFORMANCE MANAGEMENT SYSTEM

Title: Post-discharge Procedure for Patient Telephone Interview

Desired outcome: To provide data about the degree of customer satisfaction with (a) service care, (b) professional practice, and (c) governance of the organization.

Tools, forms, and location: Use form A-2101, entitled "Discharged Patient Telephone Interview". This form is located in the blue manual, Section 4.

Steps:

1. Obtain patient discharge list.	This list is available daily from medical records.
2. Call patients beginning at the top of the list.	If no answer, note on list. Call may be repeated later at the discretion of the interviewer.
3. Request time and charge for each long distance call.	Time and charge must be a verbal request to the operator.
4. Explain purpose of call to the patient as outlined.	If met with resistance, pleasantly terminate the call.
5. Ask interview questions in order.	Do not ad lib. Do not interject personal comments.
6. If a complaint is registered, promise a call back.	Refer to appropriate person to answer complaint.
7. Place completed telephone interview forms in red manual.	Red manual will be picked up and calls evaluated monthly at quality management board meetings.

Documentation: Document interview on form A-2101.
Document patient's name, phone number, time and charges in the telephone log.
Document positive, neutral, and/or negative responses on Performance Management System's Telephone Response Tally Sheet.

References: Katz, Jacqueline, RN, MS, Green, Eleanor, RN, BSN, Managing Quality, Mosby-Year Book, St. Louis, 1996.

Approval:

Review date:

Revision date:

Distribution: Volunteer Office, Same-Day Surgery, Clinic, Emergency Department, Dialysis Department.

Figure 16-4 An example of a performance management system procedure.

way they are planned to happen. This standardization reduces costs, increases employee compliance, and removes the traditional haphazard, frantic activities associated with health care organization's performance management systems. For further information refer to the discussion of practice guidelines in Chapter 8.

Action planning. The importance of action planning in the performance management system has been given much attention not only by accrediting agencies but also by the internationally known W. Edwards Deming, who incorporated planning into his much-touted "Shewhart's Cycle for Quality." Planning is an integral component of this famous "plan-do-check-act" cycle for quality.[5] Note that planning always comes first. An old adage says, "If you fail to plan, you plan to fail." There is much truth in this statement, which is why each health care organization carefully plans and constructs the standards governing its own performance management system.

In addition to these standards, an organization-wide performance management plan should be developed. This plan should do the following:

1. include a visual representation of how the performance management system is structured
2. outline the mission, vision, goals, and philosophy of the performance management system
3. interface with all other organizational plans, such as the information management plan, the infection control plan, and the seven environmental control plans
4. provide a list of tools to be used organization-wide in the performance management system.

Action plans are highly individualized for each organization's performance management system, because each organization will outline its own structure, outcome, and process standards. These will drive the action plans. Action plans are used in each domain when an opportunity for improvement arises. Specific actions to correct the area of concern and names of specific employees to carry out the actions are included on the plan. Traditional phrases such as the following are never included in today's action planning:

- action will be taken
- continue to monitor
- will discuss at the next staff meeting

The anatomy of an action plan should include *who, will do what, by how much,* and *when.*

Ideally, maintain the written organization-wide performance management system plan in the performance management system's manual in the section that follows the practice guidelines. Each organization must develop an individualized performance management system plan that fits its unique situation.

Documentation. Documentation used within the performance management system includes every tool, form, and chart developed for performance management. Standardized documentation ensures consistency. For example, we recommend that one data collection tool be used throughout the organization (see Chapter 11). Furthermore, there should be one method employed to analyze and compile data. The method should be simple enough to enable colleagues from all departments as well as across the continuum of care, to understand the measurement method, interpret the results, draw conclusions, and act to create improvement. These details should be part of the practice guideline for the management of information.

The documentation used in the performance management system is the responsibility of the quality management board, chaired by the CEO. It is always a carefully considered process rather than a haphazard assortment of forms and reports generated randomly by various employees throughout the organization. Because data collection is the backbone of the performance management system, the importance of accurate recording of information cannot be overemphasized.

Some of the pieces of documentation that may be used in the performance management system are the following:

- Shared leadership structure chart that provides details of the performance management system
- Matrix for delineating scope of care and service
- Patient, staff, management profiles
- Matrix for recording important processes of service, practice, and governance
- Indicator development tool
- Data collection tool/data analysis tool
- Threshold parameter tool and control charts
- End-of-shift report tool
- Satisfaction survey tools
- Incident reporting tools
- Quality control tools
- Team worksheets

Although this list may seem to represent a large volume of documentation, remember that the performance management system represents a separate cost center and, as such, it holds the same importance as a department. The operation of a department cannot be accomplished without standardized tools for documentation. The documentation of the performance management system must be carefully considered with one form or tool building upon and complementing another. Remember, documentation is a process standard.

Structure, outcome, and process standards, along with the necessary education to make them operational, results in a performance awareness program.

THE VALUE OF A PERFORMANCE AWARENESS PROGRAM

The value of a performance awareness program may be determined by its ability to identify indicators to be used as barometers to measure the soundness of the performance management system. We have identified five indicators of performance to be used in the performance awareness program as measures of success. They are (1) an organization-wide governance model, (2) a shared leadership framework driving all council and team structures, (3) a CEO that is involved in the decision-making processes of the performance management system, (4) developed and written structure, outcome, and process standards for the performance management system, and (5) a budget earmarked for the operation of the performance management system.

An *organization-wide governance model* provides the framework for the creation of standards within the entire organization as well as the performance management system. A model organizes the system's values into a logical pattern that is understood at a glance by all workers within the organization. THE BLUEPRINT, for example, enables an organization to establish a tri-focus emphasis as the basis for operating its awareness, measurement, and improvement programs (see Chapter 3). This trifocus partitioning permits health care workers to approach opportunities for improvement in small segments without becoming overwhelmed by the complexity of a problem. Furthermore, the tools of statistical process control used to identify, clarify, and improve processes lend themselves quite well to this trifocus approach. A comparison of your organization's governance framework with that of THE BLUEPRINT will serve as an indicator of performance for your performance management system.

A *shared leadership framework* provides the details of the day-to-day operating structure of the organization's performance management system. It provides a visual paradigm of how the organization is structured to accomplish the programs of awareness, measurement, and improvement as well as how workers are assigned to the necessary synergistic roles and activities that form the foundation for productivity of the performance management system. An analysis of the visual paradigm of your performance management system compared with that discussed in Chapter 5 will provide an indicator against which you can benchmark.

A CEO that is involved in the decision-making processes of the performance management system is an absolute necessity. In fact, the entire success of the performance management system of a health care organization is virtually dependent on the performance of the CEO. A health care organization's systems and interdependent interactions of awareness, measurement, and improvement are complex and in most organizations it is the CEO who has the broad overview of the organization's vision combined with a knowledge of the budget. His or her day-to-day interest in and actions relevant to the performance management system will make or break its success. If the CEO provides a positive, enthusiastic role model for the workers of a health care organization, emphasizing the importance of the performance management system to organizational success, all employees will follow suit. Without the influence of such a role model the potential of the performance management system will never be realized. An indicator of your organization's potential for success lies in your CEO. Compare your CEO's potential leadership with the one discussed in Chapter 5 and use it as your benchmark.

Fully developed structure, outcome, and process standards for the performance management system are crucial to its implementation and success. Once developed, these standards become the basis for all decisions regarding the performance awareness, measurement, and improvement programs. The standards of the performance management system provide the "rules of the game" for health care professionals assigned to roles within its three programs of performance awareness, measurement, and improvement and all performance outcomes proceed from the standards that direct these three programs.

Standards form the basis of the performance measurement system and provide the crucial baseline "yard stick" by which we measure performance. Well-defined standards conserve resources by reducing confusion, duplication, and errors. Benchmark the standards for your performance management system against those described throughout this book.

A *budget earmarked for the operation of the performance management system* is crucial to its success. It is impossible to stay abreast of accreditation requirements, increase productivity, and contain costs without planned, systematic, organized methodology backed by a sound budget.

Many CEOs attempt to conserve resources by integrating a haphazard performance management system into the daily work of an already overworked staff by requiring "QA" as part of each employee's daily job. These CEOs are noted for delegating all performance responsibilities as well as for refusing to consider the financial aspects of a performance management system as a necessary and critical component of their organization's operation. These actions by a CEO devalue the pursuit of excellence and show disdain for the conscientious workers who have been assigned the impossible responsibility for accomplishing the organization's performance management.

To remain financially viable and survive the present health care crisis requires that organizations develop a performance management system to capture and maintain a competitive lead in their performance awareness, measurement, and improvement programs. Maintaining the competitive lead means that the CEO will position the organization strategically through its three integrated performance programs of awareness, measurement, and improvement to compete in the national health care arena not only on the basis of costs but also on the basis of performance excellence evidenced by the data obtained by the performance measurement program. The present involvement of the CEO in the performance management system of your health care organization is a predictor of success and his or her involvement may be benchmarked against the requirements of the CEO discussed in Chapter 4.

Creation of a sound performance awareness program provides a solid foundation upon which to build the next two components of the performance management system—the performance measurement program and the performance improvement program. Although many health care organizations are struggling to define performance management relative to clinical care, few have identified the need to create an organization-wide performance management system subdivided into three programs. Our experiences of designing performance management systems for health care organizations have led us to see the importance of creating and implementing a standards-based performance awareness program *first* before initiating any work on the development of the performance measurement program or the performance improvement program.

Once the performance awareness program is in place, the performance measurement program may begin. This program is discussed in Chapter 17.

REFERENCES

1. Drucker PF: *Innovation and entrepreneurship*, New York, 1985, Harper & Row.
2. Finch K: *Quality assurance: the open road to excellence in psychiatric nursing*. Speech presented at the Fourth National Conference-Canadian Foundation for the Advancement of Psychiatric Nursing, May, 1990.
3. Hemingway E: *The old man and the sea*, New York, 1952, Simon & Schuster.
4. *Joint Commission accreditation manual for hospitals*, Chicago, 1996, Joint Commission.
5. Scholtes PR: *The team handbook*, Madison, Wis, 1990, Joiner Associates, Inc.

Chapter 17

Measuring the Performance Management System

Long ago in the kingdom called Phrygia in the country of Turkey, there lived a very foolish king. One day the king's servants brought to him a drunken satyr. Since satyrs spent all of their time with Bacchus, the god of wine, it was not unusual for a satyr to be intoxicated. After many days of partying with the satyr, the king decided to send him back to Bacchus. In appreciation for the return of the errant satyr, Bacchus agreed to give the king anything he wanted. Being greedy, the king asked for the power to turn anything to gold simply by touching it. Bacchus knew the implications of this request, but he could not deter the king. "So be it. You have what you want."

The king was ecstatic for, in fact, everything he touched did indeed turn to gold. Flowers, rocks, his cloak, his shoes—everything he touched became gold. He would be the richest man in the world. By the time he returned to the palace he was tired and hungry; however, the bread turned to gold when he tried to take a bite. The wine turned to liquid gold when he tried to drink it. Unable to eat or drink and so heavily weighted with golden clothes and jewelry, the king returned to Bacchus and asked him to undo the gift.

The king in this story is Midas, and variations on the story abound. Two prominent morals exist in any version of Ovid's famous tale: too much of a good thing can be too much, and the cost of something may far outweigh its benefits.

When enough is enough. When is enough enough? The answer to that question is, *"Nobody knows."* There simply have been no logical standards for performance measurements in health care. Currently, government, third-party payers, and health care organizations themselves are struggling to develop indicators as performance measurements of "enough." To date, an individual organization is unable to state unequivocally, "That's as good as this process is going to get, so I am turning to another more critical process for the rest of this year." As sensible and as easy as this approach might sound, organizations are wary of deviating from the few performance standards set by accreditation authorities. Traditionally the 12-month tracking of a process was sancrosanct, and failure to comply would result in a deduction of points from the final accreditation score card.

For example, we consulted with a mid-size hospital that spent almost 3 years implementing an organization-wide performance management system. The hospital developed a new culture by reengineering a shared leadership model and educating every worker to the new performance climate. They educated, at great expense, the entire staff to the tools of statistical process control and importance of accuracy in measuring of outcomes in service, practice, and governance. The data they gathered, under the new system, for 9 months just prior to the accreditation survey was the most complete and accurate ever accumulated in their history. The survey team complimented them on their excellent program and apologized for having to deduct points from their score card, because the measurement data did not show a 12-month track record. Fortunately the requirement for 12-month tracking has been eliminated. Today, the program, not the measurement data, must be in place for 12 months. Additionally, the American health care system is struggling to determine "when is enough enough" not only in the measurement process but also in the reimbursement and treatment processes.

In the reimbursement process, what is enough inaccurate billing claims for reimbursement from Medicare, Medicaid, and the prospective payment system? When will fraudulent claims and willful, inaccurate coding that bilks our government of desperately needed dollars be enough? When have third-party payers reimbursed a patient enough? In the treatment process when are enough medical tests enough on a moribund patient? When are enough medical treatments enough? When should lifesaving heroics cease? How aggressively should neonatal resuscitation be administered to babies that will be blind, cognitively challenged, hearing impaired, and have cerebral palsy? How will these events be measured in our performance measurement programs? So far, there are no answers because nobody knows!

Costs outweigh benefits. Consider the current nation-wide dilemma of health care costs outweighing health care benefits. Because there are few tested performance measurement standards associated with third-party cost reimbursement, many people face heartbreaking dilemmas that sometimes end in patient death followed by litigation attempts from the bereaved, frustrated survivors. When cost of care and treatment become the predominant performance measurement of a third-party payer, patients and their families become incensed. Should costs be the basis for treatment decisions? How can a dollar amount be weighed against a patient's life? On the other hand, how much should be spent on treatments, medications, and other therapies, when all medical tests confirm a patient's imminent death? The King Midas moral of costs outweighing benefits, although practical, does not address some of these ethical and legal problems facing today's health care organizations.

The case of Evelyn Harper vividly demonstrates one example of the dilemma. Evelyn, 47 years old, with two children, learned in the fall of 1990 that her breast cancer had invaded her eyes and liver. Her doctor suggested a marrow transplant to extend her life

for a few months to a few years, but her insurer refused to cover this expensive therapy, reasoning that the cancer was too advanced for any additional therapy to alter the outcome. The following February of 1991 she appealed her insurer's ruling. It was denied and she died a few weeks later.[2]

Tragic? Yes. Her case is typical of the current practice of a third-party payer using costs as a decision-making measurement. Believing that costs outweighed the benefits to Evelyn, the insurance company denied payment for recommended treatment. This case illustrates the pathos involved in using "costs versus probable outcome" as one of the driving forces behind treatment decisions.

"Is there an answer to 'when does the cost outweigh the benefit' that will make everybody happy? Probably not. Who will decide the definition of 'effective' and 'chance for recovery'? How good does a treatment have to be to make it worth the price? Is a few weeks to months extended life to a patient worth the exorbitant costs of treatment?"[8]

How to resolve these everyday, heartrending situations has created a national perplexity with ethical and legal implications for the entire health care industry. Roberts states, "There is just no way to give Americans everything they want from their health care system. What we apparently desire is unlimited access to the world's best care, with no organizational or bureaucratic barriers, and without imposing real costs on either ourselves, our government, or the economy. Such a promised land is not attainable."[17] This being the case, those within a health care organization charged with the necessity of a performance management system should see the importance of (a) carefully formulating and articulating their values within the performance awareness program (as discussed in Chapter 16) and (b) conscientiously constructing a realistic, understandable, believable, and achievable performance measurement program.

THE PURPOSE OF A PERFORMANCE MEASUREMENT PROGRAM

The purpose of examining the performance *measurement* program within the performance management system is the following: (a) to determine when enough is enough within the health care organization—that is, to measure outcomes in each domain to create statistically derived targets as end-points for benchmarking and comparing performance data for use in decision making and (b) to measure the costs of service, practice, and governance to determine if costs outweigh benefits not only of patient care and treatment in the service domain but also of all other activities in the practice and governance domains.

Health care organizations must provide the most cost-effective, timely, and appropriate means for measuring the costs of critical processes and variations from the organization's standards. David Burda, in a cover story in *Modern Health Care,* states that "total [performance] management has become an umbrella term for strategies that identify and meet customer expectations, reduce the cost of non-compliance with standards, strive for 'zero' defects, reduce outcome variability, eliminate the cost of poor [performance], use statistical methods to identify and measure processes and continually work [toward organizational excellence.]"[4] He adds that, although performance improvement has become big business in health care, it may actually be adding substantially to operating costs, "the precise ailment that it is supposed to cure."[4]

To understand operating costs, nonconformance costs, and treatment costs and avoid adding substantially to operating costs, the performance measurement program must function in a planned, organized manner. This means that every health care organization must understand how to cost out its service, practice, and governance processes. We view the performance measurement program as the key to the questions of when is enough enough, and when do the costs outweigh the benefits in a health care organization? In the present environment it is one way to ensure performance excellence while controlling costs.

Not only is the health care industry striving to gather generic national benchmarking data but also individual health care organizations are striving through their performance measurement programs to gather organizational outcomes' measurements of service, practice, and governance. These outcomes should be established on process standards and should be written for each domain (see Chapter 8). One aspect, then, of the performance measurement program consists of comparing the desired outcomes with the actual outcomes and analyzing the variances. In this way, expected outcomes may continually be measured and adjusted until reasonable, achievable outcomes for specific patient populations are verified. Then critical decisions such as the one involving Evelyn Harper will be made—not by "gut feeling" of someone in an insurance office—but by *facts* gathered from accurate performance measurements derived from accurate statistics.

THE ROLE OF A PERFORMANCE MEASUREMENT PROGRAM

The role of the performance measurement program is to provide consistent measurements of service, practice, and governance of a health care organization. Measurements will produce solid, statistically based measurement information of critical processes that in turn will permit the organization to make solid decisions about improvements.

In the past, performance management systems were perceived as luxuries, which could be afforded when things were going well and the institution was operating "in the black," or else were used as a method to corroborate staff testimony in a crisis. No longer is a performance management system considered an optional approach or a crisis management strategy. Today, performance management systems with the three programs of awareness, measurement, and improvement are viewed as a competitive advantage, or an economic life jacket that will provide accurate measurements to prove that things happened the way the organization designed them to happen and predetermined outcomes were, indeed, met.

Many health care organizations cannot see a business advantage to the implementation of a performance management system. "What do we receive in exchange for an outlay of resources for performance management?" they ask. It is difficult to answer, because it must involve the theory of "what if." "It is impossible to project what an organization might do 'if'—if there were an outstanding performance management system we'd gain more market share; if we gained more market share, we'd earn more money. However, research indicates that businesses with *higher performance* gain larger market share and earn margins about five times greater than businesses with lower performance and smaller share."[16] This seems to indicate a definite business advantage, because there is a direct correlation between a health care organization's financial performance and the productivity of its performance management system. Correctly operated performance management systems will improve their processes, which will decrease the costs of nonconformance, which will increase market share, which will increase profits (Figure 17-1).

Recognizing this cycle as true, health care organizations are no longer nonchalant about the caliber of their data. They are, rather, planning their performance management systems with all the skill of generals planning a strategic battle and data serves as their artillery. No longer is a performance management system thought of as a data collection center whose purpose is to satisfy accreditors. Nor is performance management a crisis management strategy or an optional approach. Performance management systems have become a defensive bulwark against haphazard, traditional "QA." In particular, the employees charged with oversight of the performance measurement program have become protectors of the dollars and landlords of the outcomes and their performance measurements drive all organizational decisions.

Productivity Cycle

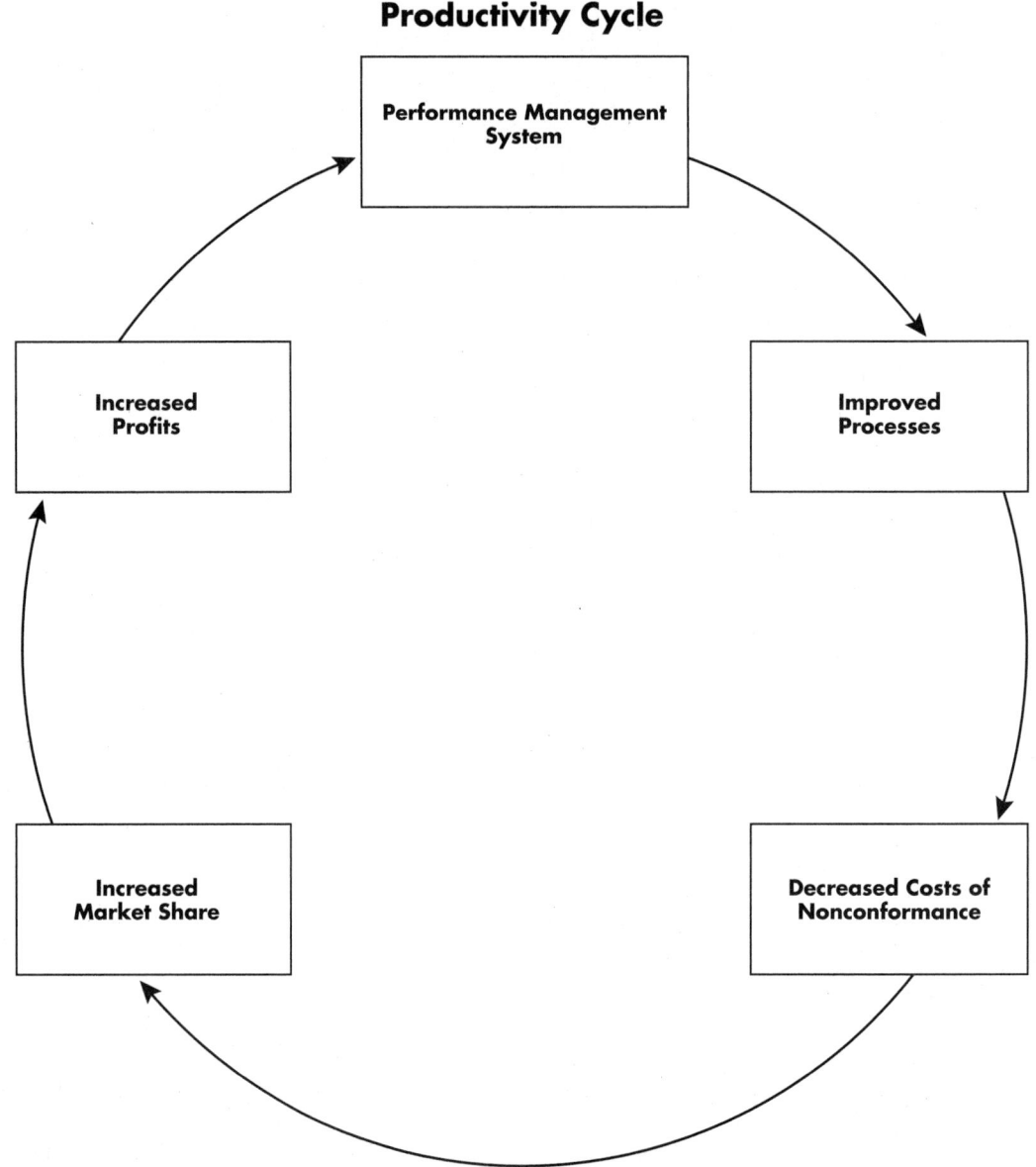

Figure 17-1   Productivity cycle.

For example, one Indiana hospital replaced 11 heart surgeons who had an 8.2% death rate from coronary bypass surgery in 1994. This was more than twice the national average of 4 out of every 100. The team of five surgeons from Chicago that took their place had a 3.6% mortality rate for their coronary bypass procedures.[18]

Although using internal measurements of performance to control practice behaviors is one of the health care industry's stickiest debates, advocates say that it is necessary to provide consumers factual information so that they can make better health care choices. As illustrated by this Indiana hospital, decision making, based on sound data is becoming the backbone of the entire performance initiative across the country.

In the future, this strategy will drive health care organizations to compete on the basis of comparative measurements of performance. These measurements, obtained through the efforts of the performance management system, will serve not only as the organization's *defensive structure*, shielding it against inaccurate allegations, but also as its *offensive structure*, showcasing a fusillade of statistically reliable data used to take decisive action.

Rather than the traditional method of having a QA coordinator identify opportunities for improvement and work toward a single resolution, interdisciplinary employees will function as a process improvement team working toward an organization-wide resolution. This necessitates not only an organized awareness and improvement program but also a measurement program that continually measures outcomes of critical processes, which systematically provide data that identify those processes that fail to conform to identified standards. As in the case of the Indiana hospital data drive the improvement program.

This new focus makes obsolete the traditional, narrow philosophy of volume indicators, i.e., how much or how many. Garvin states, "In my view, most traditional principles of [performance management] were narrow in scope; they were designed as purely defensive measures to pre-empt failures or eliminate defects. What managers need now is a strategy to gain and hold markets with [measures of performance] as competitive linchpins."[10] Deming backs up this opinion. He states, "Inspection with the aim of finding the bad ones and throwing them out is too late, ineffective and costly . . . Quality comes not from inspection but from improvement of the process."[21]

The health care industry today has adopted a new philosophy: measurement decisions cannot depend on emotion or gut feelings but must be made from data. To do this necessitates a program of measurement that understands (a) outcome standards, (b) variances, (c) how to collect data, (d) how to figure the cost of nonconformance of service, practice, and governance, and (e) the value of information management and its relationship to accuracy of data reporting.

THE VALUE OF A PERFORMANCE MEASUREMENT PROGRAM

The value of a performance measurement program lies in its ability to identify indicators to be used as barometers to measure the soundness of the performance management system. We have identified four indicators of performance to be used in the performance measurement program. They are measurement of the following:

1. performance analysis
2. satisfaction analysis
3. research/innovation
4. product analysis

These four indicators fall into two categories of measurement: performance measurement and technology measurement (see box below).

Performance measurement includes measurement of outcomes, productivity, and costs in each domain: service, practice, and governance. Measurement of satisfaction of service, practice, and governance follow. Analysis of these two indicators of performance measurement provides insight into processes that are impaired or nonexistent in the organization, allowing plans to be formulated to initiate corrective action. To facilitate performance measurement, outcomes are written in each domain detailing expected results of processes. Productivity measures include measurement of such things as cost savings, cash flow, elimination of unnecessary workers, market share, employee performance, turnover rates, work processes, teamwork, and morale.[20] Measurement of costs includes measuring the costs of nonconformance and attaching dollar values to service, practice, and governance processes. Satisfaction measurement is usually accomplished by creating questionnaires to poll the organization's internal and external customers, seeking their responses to service, practice, and governance issues of the organization.

Technology measurement includes research/innovation and product analysis. *Research* includes comparative measurements of performance from national databases; measurements of the organization's technology in each domain of service, practice, and governance; and

ORGANIZATION OF PERFORMANCE AND TECHNOLOGY INDICATORS

Performance Measurement

Performance analysis:

1. Outcomes in each domain
2. Productivity in each domain
3. Costs of nonconformance in each domain

Satisfaction analysis:

1. Service satisfaction
2. Practice satisfaction
3. Governance satisfaction

Technology Measurement

Research/innovation:

1. Research/innovative service
2. Research/innovative practice
3. Research/innovative governance

Product analysis:

1. Service products
2. Practice products
3. Governance products

innovations in technology in each domain. Innovation includes improving what already exists or improving on the current methodology of delivering service, practice, and governance. Product analysis measures the performance characteristics of products used to deliver the service.

Technology in the service domain might include such items as modern hospital beds, oxygen and suction apparatus constructed within the hospital's walls, or state-of-the-art hemodynamic monitoring equipment available for all patients.

Technology in the practice domain might include such items as modernized documentation systems and CPR training.

Technology in the governance domain might include fax machines in every department, computerized information management systems, use of national data bank information for organization-wide comparative indicators, and improved medication delivery equipment.

Product analysis includes creating a method for measuring all products used within the organization for effectiveness and comparing these outcomes to the other evaluation indicators. For example, in the service domain, do the intravenous tubes and plastic bags of fluid leak while being infused into a patient? If so, what percent leak? How many times does the patient receive a new needle stick as the result of this faulty product? Would it be more cost-effective to buy more expensive tubing? How much time is the staff devoting to restarting IVs? In other words, it is necessary to compare each product with the other measurement indicators, such as outcome, productivity, costs, and satisfaction, to understand the product's worth.

In the practice domain the process of documentation is an example. Are the tools such as flow charts and physician order forms conducive to consolidating information and saving the employee time? In the governance domain an example would be the cost of handwritten documentation. Is it really less expensive than computerized documentation? Using the research/innovation component along with the costs associated with documenting by hand not only will help an organization come to a satisfying decision based on fact but also will encourage research and innovation, i.e., seeking a quicker, better, smarter method for doing routine jobs.

These four indicators of the measurement program: performance analysis, satisfaction analysis, research/innovation, and product analysis are the last section of the standards described in THE BLUEPRINT model in Chapter 3. They complete the full circle of a standards-based system that emphasizes performance.

Evaluation consisting of performance and technology measurement is an extremely valuable component of the overall performance management system, because it provides the foundation for a health care organization's measurement program. Evaluation may not be ignored because it ensures uniformity of performance and technology across the continuum of service, practice, and governance and provides the organization with systematic measurement data for accurate decision making.

THE PERMANENCY OF THE PERFORMANCE MEASUREMENT PROGRAM

Although many innovative performance methods are being explored, all that *endure* will require a new way of thinking. New creative methodologies, one of which is the carefully constructed performance management system described in this book will, no doubt, provide the present and future direction of the health care industry's performance management techniques. Thus the permanency of the performance measurement program is ensured. It is further ensured because of the planned paradigm of four indicators that are used to measure the success of a performance management system. Performance and technology measurements serve as the guidelines for measurement of a health care organization's performance management success.

Because none of these four indicators can be measured without the cooperation of all workers within a health care organization, success depends on teamwork using an interdisciplinary approach. No process associated with measurement of the four indicators is independent. Each indicator is interdependent and involves many workers to achieve the desired positive results. Surveys show that "a . . . number of health care organizations have proven that process improvement yields dramatic results."[3] Health care organizations may build on this research and implement meaningful performance management systems that include a performance measurement program. Brown and Moore state that, "The health care industry is way behind in realizing the benefits of correctly using [performance management strategies] to improve results."[3]

Once the performance measurement program is underway, and you have begun to gather data, the four indicators—performance analysis, satisfaction analysis, research/innovation, and product analysis—may be tracked and measured. The performance management system's accuracy is verified by data from the measurement of each of these four indicators.

For a performance management system to thrive in a health care organization there will, of necessity, be some trial and error, risk-taking, innovation, experimenting, reengineering, and so on. "For those readers who are the most risk averse, all the common failings of process improvement programs in industry and health care have been analyzed and identified and therefore can easily be prevented because they are easy to recognize."[3] Some of the most common failings are the following:

- A hierarchical form of management is maintained.
- There is no road map or guide, such as THE BLUEPRINT, outlining organizational direction based on the mission and vision.
- There is a lack of a planned, organized, systematic performance management system.
- The performance awareness program is not implemented first.
- The performance measurement program is not organized, planned, and interdisciplinary across the continuum of care.
- The performance measurement system is not statistically based.
- The performance improvement program is haphazard and not directed from the top.
- The organization lacks an information management system to actualize the performance management system.
- The voice of the customer is not heard or considered.
- Knee-jerk reactions to process breakdowns result in tampering, thereby increasing variation and costs.
- Capital investment is used as a substitute for a performance management system.
- Management demands quick, significant financial results.
- The PM system has not been adequately funded or expanded after an initial success, because its implementation is viewed as a short-term accreditation requirement.

The permanency of the performance management system as well as its three programs—awareness, measurement, and improvement—is ensured as its importance becomes more apparent to health care organizations in the midst of upheaval and crisis. "Process improvement is not a fad. It is here to stay because it has a solid theoretical basis of measurement provided by statistics."[3]

COSTS—THE GOLDEN TOUCH?

Many astute health care organizations value their performance management systems as much as King Midas valued gold. In fact, the results that can be realized by initiating such a system may be just short of miraculous. However, rushing out and jumping on the latest bandwagon of managing performance costs is not the answer. The cost of the miraculous results must be carefully and thoughtfully considered, because:

1. A performance management system costs money.
2. Money does not necessarily buy a good performance management system.
3. Some positive outcomes of a performance management system are not worth the added costs.

A performance management system is desirable and essential. But a performance management system with no concern for cost is foolish. Juran identified that performance management could be understood in terms of avoidable and unavoidable costs. Avoidable costs result from defects in products or service failures. Unavoidable costs are associated with prevention, i.e., inspection, sampling, sorting, and other *quality-control* initiatives. To Juran, the failure costs were "gold in the mine" because they could be retrieved with performance [management] efforts.[14]

Crosby defines the expenses associated with a performance management system as the costs of nonconformance. "The cost of nonconformance is the price organizations pay for failing to do things right the first time. This includes the efforts to correct the processes associated with procedural breakdowns and to correct the service as it goes along, to do work over, and to pay for warranty and other nonconformance claims. When you add all these together it is an enormous amount of money. Repetition of failed processes by an employee is very expensive and involves about thirty-five percent of the cost of doing business in a service delivery company."[6] The role of the performance measurement program is, therefore, to measure and cost-out outcomes in each domain and to figure the cost of nonconformance when outcomes in each domain are not met.

Crosby views appraisal costs as those incurred during the problem assessment phase, prevention costs as those incurred in determining "requirements," and failure costs as those incurred because workers failed to follow requirements and the work had to be repeated. This pioneer concept is one of several that has synergistically resulted in the development of the performance management system with three distinct, interactive programs of performance awareness, performance measurement, and performance improvement. Furthermore, figuring the cost of nonconformance as discussed in this chapter is based on Crosby's work.

CALCULATING THE COST OF NONCONFORMANCE

Computing costs for operating the performance management system of a health care organization is not very useful without the ability to use the information in a practical way. For that reason we are including a practical method for calculating the cost of nonconformance (CONC) in a health care organization.

The cost of nonconformance refers to process errors. Process errors are those that occur during the normal activities associated with carrying out your job. Many interrelated processes contribute to increased or decreased productivity. Increased productivity occurs when the process works right the first time exactly as planned. Decreased productivity occurs as the result of breakdowns of the individual steps of activities within a process.

In other words, work errors or failures are due to breakdowns in the steps of the activities that together compose a process. Processes, by design, coordinate several activities to produce one result. There are usually several steps within each activity required to produce one result, which we refer to as a process. Rather than detailing each step, we simply refer to the group of activities as a process and each step is implied. Some examples of this concept include the processes of (a) administering medications, (b) admitting a patient, (c) taking an x-ray, and (d) transferring patients. Note that there are many steps within each of the activities in each of these processes. What happens when some of the steps within an activity are missed or performed incorrectly? Nonconformance to the total process occurs.

The CONC is extremely high in health care organizations. The information provided in this chapter presents one method of determining the cost of nonconformance. What is the value of tracking and computing the cost of nonconformance? When you track process errors and compute their value in lost revenue, prioritization of processes allows you to improve the most costly processes *first!*

Figure 17-2 provides you with two examples of a step-by-step approach to calculating the cost of nonconformance. The first example deals with the pharmacy. The first column, *A,* identifies the process error being considered in this study. In this example it is defined as "errors involved in the process of dispensing medications organization wide to patients."

Column A, identifying the process error, is critical to calculating costs. The error to be considered as a candidate for process improvement must be identified as understandable, measurable, and specific, because in column B it is necessary to delineate not only how the error will be tracked but also the mechanism created to track it. In example 1 the tracking mechanism is a red notebook. Specificity for the errors also has been included: wrong patient name, wrong dose, wrong route, wrong label, wrong time, wrong unit, wrong packaging, or failure to cue an alert such as, "Alert, there are two patients in this unit by the name of Betty Smith."

Once the errors have been tracked over a period of time (usually 3 to 6 months), column C is created. First, calculate the errors per day. Then multiply this number by the number of days in a year. The total yields the annual activity rate. In the case of example 1, the annual activity rate equals 2,190 pharmacy errors per year. Next, materials or waste costs must be computed. As stated earlier, included in these costs are the materials required for the initial work and rework as well as all waste that occurs as a result of process breakdown. In example 1, materials may include the cost of labels, containers, or other associated medication packaging costs. Perhaps some of these costs are salvageable. However, an error made in the process of dispensing medications in the pharmacy often involves use of materials that cannot be salvaged and must be wasted. An example of waste in example 1 is a medication that was prepared in the pharmacy—packaged, labeled, and distributed. The staff RN opens it, handles it, and then discovers the dose is incorrect. The medication may not be repackaged for resale to another patient. It is therefore wasted by the pharmacy and the correct dose must be sent to the staff RN to be dispensed to the patient. In figuring the cost of nonconformance related to process errors such as the one above, the price for the waste of a single dose of the medication must be calculated and recorded. The cost of the wasted medication should be computed at the hospital's cost of resale to the patient, not at the bulk cost of the medication to the hospital. This is referred to as an "opportunity cost" and must be calculated as waste in the cost of nonconformance. In example 1, column C, the materials/waste cost is estimated by the pharmacy department to average $20 per day. Twenty dollars per day for 365 days each year amounts to $7,300 in waste per year in the pharmacy. They did not calculate materials costs, believing most to be salvageable.

Column D is provided for calculation of direct labor costs. It is necessary for the employee, when redoing old work—work that wasn't done right the first time—to time him- or herself to estimate the percent of the workday devoted to redoing work that should have been done right the first time. In this case, the pharmacist reported an average of 40 minutes necessary to fix each error. Forty minutes divided by 60 minutes in an hour equals 0.67 of an hour. Using the generic estimated $30 per hour wage and benefits times the computed 0.67 of an hour, the health care organization will pay $20.10 for each medication error. For accuracy of computation in your organization it will be necessary to obtain the *average* wage and benefits for your employees from your chief financial officer. Workers' salaries are variable. It is the computed *average* that you are seeking in order to calculate the *average* cost of errors. Top management salaries may be included in the computed organization wage and benefits' average or they may be captured in adjusted, estimated overhead costs. If top management salaries are to be

CALCULATING TOTAL COST OF NONCONFORMANCE WORKSHEET

EXAMPLE 1

A. Nonconformance factor	B. Tracking Mechanism	C. Annual Activity Rate	D. Direct Labor Costs	E. Total Direct Labor Costs
Errors involved in the process of dispensing medications organization-wide to patients	Document all medication errors *that left the department.* Use the red designated notebook: Wrong: name, dose, route, label, time, unit, packaging, failure to cue an alert, etc.	6 errors/day 6 x 365 days/yr. Total: 2,190 errors/yr. Materials or waste costs: $ 20/day $ 20 x 365 days/yr. Total: $ 7,300/yr.	Labor time = 40 min/error 40 minutes = .67 of an hour Labor costs = $ 30/hour .67 x $ 30 = $ 20.10/error 2,190 x $ 20.10 = $ 44,019 per year *direct* salary costs spent to fix errors	Must double labor costs because your employer is paying *twice* to get the job done once! Labor costs: first time: $ 44,019 second time: $ 44,019 Total: $ 88,038

Total cost of nonconformance: $ 88,038 + $ 7,300 + $ 44,019 = $ 139,357 per yr. for pharmacy CONCs

Total direct labor   Materials/waste   Overhead*

* Overhead conservative estimate: 50% of total labor costs

EXAMPLE 2

A. Nonconformance factor	B. Tracking Mechanism	C. Annual Activity Rate	D. Direct Labor Costs	E. Total Direct Labor Costs
Nursing data entry errors into the computer: diet orders only	Omission or incorrect patient diet entered into the computer; Highlighted in yellow in computer's recall system	75 errors/day 75 x 365 days/yr. Total: 27,375 errors/yr. Materials/waste costs: 20 meals/day wasted at $ 5/meal (not every meal was wasted) 20 x 365 = 7,300 meals/yr. $ 5 x 7,300 = $ 36,500/yr.	Labor time = 5 min/error 5 minutes = .08 of an hour Labor costs = $ 30/hour .08 x $ 30 = $ 2.40/error 27,375 x $ 2.40 = $ 65,700 per year *direct* salary costs spent to fix errors	Must double labor costs because your employer is paying *twice* to get the job done once! Labor costs: first time: $ 65,700 second time: $ 65,700 Total: $ 131,400

Total cost of nonconformance: $ 131,400 + $ 36,500 + $ 65,700 = $ 233,600 per yr. for data entry CONCs

Total direct labor   Materials/waste   Overhead*

* Overhead conservative estimate: 50% of total labor costs

Figure 17-2   Calculating the cost of nonconformance.

computed in overhead costs, it will be necessary to calculate a greater margin than 50% as used in Figure 17-2. The chief financial officer, along with the CEO, will make this decision.

Since, in column C, there were 2,190 errors per year, and in column D we computed that each error costs the organization $20.10, a simple multiplication of $2,190 \times \$20.10$ will show that approximately $44,019 per year in direct salary costs are spent by the organization to "fix" pharmacy errors.

In column E the total labor costs are computed. Because the organization is paying the pharmacist to "do it right the first time," it is necessary to double the labor costs. The labor costs must be doubled because the employer is paying the employee *twice* to get the correct job done *once!* As you can see in column E, this computes to $88,038 per year.

Now it is time to compute the total cost of nonconformance related to outgoing medication errors in the pharmacy:

$$\text{Total cost: } \underset{\substack{\text{Total labor} \\ \text{cost}}}{\$88,038} + \underset{\substack{\text{Material/} \\ \text{waste}}}{\$7,300} + \underset{\text{Overhead*}}{\$44,019}$$

$$= \$139,357 \text{ per year for Pharmacy CONCs}$$

Example 2 in Figure 17-2 is computed just as the one in example 1. This example of a different type of error is provided to reinforce the concept and help you to remember how to calculate the cost of nonconformance. Every penny associated with the cost of nonconformance cannot be captured; nevertheless, using this simple worksheet provides one method for calculating a ballpark figure. These simple calculations can then be used to assist in making decisions about which processes to improve first. Begin with the ones that are costing the organization the most money. Case managers and outcomes managers should note that this same method is used to calculate the cost of variances within critical pathways.

Track the revenue saved each year through the performance measurement program's strategic computations in order to justify the necessity of the performance management system and negotiate funding for its continuance.

COSTS ASSOCIATED WITH EACH OF THE THREE PROGRAMS

For every health care organization the question of how resources will be allocated is challenging. This challenge is made especially frustrating by the turmoil associated with health care reform. Marc Roberts put it this way: "The full meaning of any reform will be uncovered only when it is implemented [and tracked over a period of time.] This means that we had best

design systems and processes that are 'robust'—that can be implemented by real, imperfect human beings with real mixed motives, limited intellectual capacities, and only partial insight. Evidence that a proposed process has actually worked somewhere in the world, that a particular arrangement has functioned as intended, that some experience makes a specific prediction plausible: these are things we should take seriously in our policy choices."[17]

In spite of the various competing visions emerging about how to transform the American health care system, no vision will take root without resource allocations seeding the ground. In other words, without proper funding there can be no performance management system. Figure 17-3 is a pie chart demonstrating the usual method for dividing up monies associated with performance management systems. This chart parallels our three programs of awareness, measurement, and improvement of the performance management system. We have piloted what we believe to be more workable percentage divisions of the costs allocated for the performance management system.

The costs associated with the performance awareness program include those incurred during the initial changes made by reengineering the organization from a hierarchical to a shared leadership management style, the cost of developing standards, the cost of educating every worker to the new system and the three performance programs as well as setting up an organization-wide performance management system and making it operational. Although Philip Crosby considers such costs "appraisal costs" and suggests that they account for more than 15 to 20% of the total performance management system's costs,[6] we consider these as awareness costs and allocate 25% of the performance management system's budget to these awareness costs (Figure 17-4).

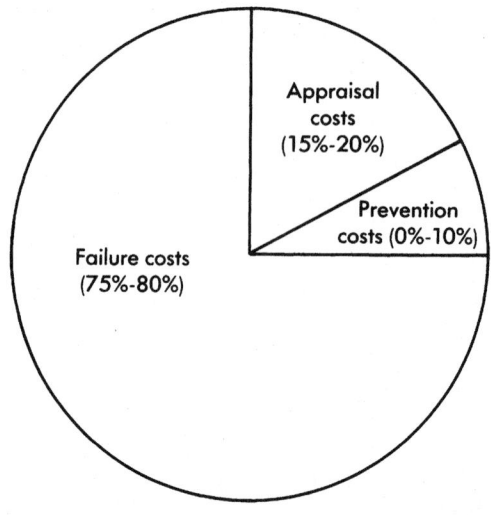

Figure 17-3   The costs of quality.

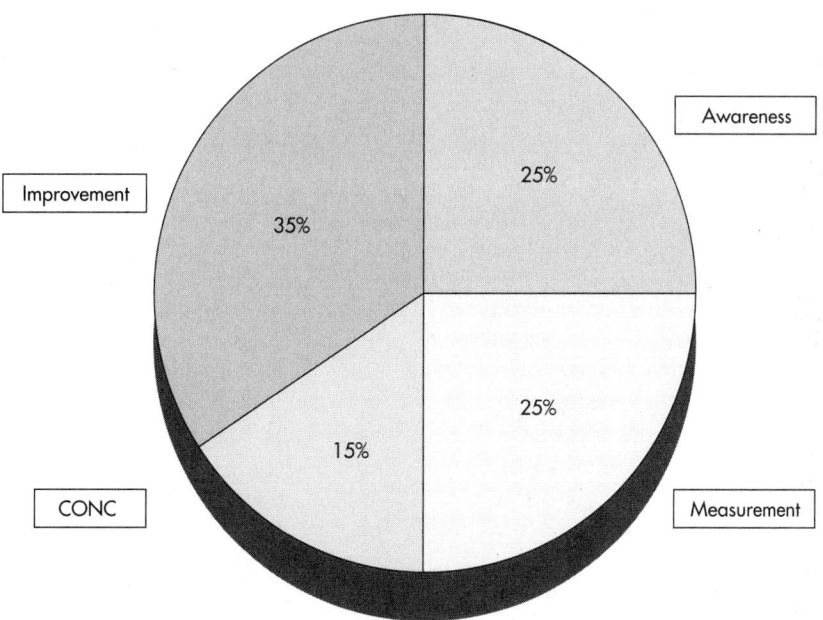

Performance Management System Budget

Figure 17-4   Pie chart illustrating the budget distribution rule.

The costs associated with the performance measurement program include such activities as the costs of staff hours for data collection and analysis for internal and external purposes, the costs associated with turning outcomes data into information, the costs associated with measurements across the continuum of care, and the cost of doing things incorrectly (nonconformance). Israeli and Fisher report that failure costs account for 75 to 80% of the total costs of a performance management system. They state that reducing failure costs will also reduce the performance awareness and performance improvement costs.[12] However, we consider failure costs as part of the performance measurement program. We allocate 40% of the performance management system's budget to the measurement program and devote 15% of that to the cost of nonconformance. This means that 25% of the performance management system's budget is allocated for the operation of the measurement program, whereas 15% is allocated for failure costs or the cost of nonconformance.

Although calculating the CONC is a critical part of the measurement program, it is not the entire program, and we believe that each department should strive to keep these costs as low as possible. However, without a planned methodology for capturing and computing the costs of nonconformance, this vital measurement of nonconformance will be lost. Therefore, as part of the performance measurement program, we address it as a critical aspect of measurement and include a simple method for calculating CONC in this chapter.

The costs associated with the performance improvement program include the costs of organization-wide process improvement teams to resolve the interdisciplinary complexities of opportunities for improvement; the cost of all innovation in service, practice, and governance related to new processes; improved methods, equipment and technology; and the costs associated with risktaking, experiments, and research.

We suggest allocating 35% of the performance management system's budget to improvement activities.

Proof that a health care organization has spent its money wisely will be manifested not only in the 4 indicators of measurement described in this chapter but also in positive outcomes of the 10 indicators of organizational improvement described in Chapter 18. These include top leadership involvement in the performance management system, an adequate budget earmarked for implementing the system, three ongoing programs of awareness, measurement, and improvement, an empowered workforce, continuous education for all employees, unparalleled customer service, information management across the continuum of care, and a culture of happiness. When the 10 indicators of improvement are present, costs may then become part of the budget of each department within the organization. Managers may be vested with the authority to allocate their resources for performance management within their department.

The costs of a performance management system are a critical factor to consider in planning the allocation of the organization's resources each year. Assuring that "the golden touch of Midas" does not become a costly nightmare requires that each individual program within the performance management system be weighed and carefully considered and that the organization benchmark itself against the four indicators of performance measurement. This realistic, organized, systematic approach will permit an organization to examine all costs *by department* that are associated with the performance management system and combine them for a more accurate global figure. Resources for the coming year, accordingly, may be allocated or adjusted organization-wide. Although Philip Crosby estimates that service delivery organizations spend approximately 35% of their total operating budget on the cost of nonconformance alone,[6] many health care organizations today allocate approximately 3% to 5% of their total operating budget on performance management efforts. This amount is not based on research and only time will tell if that amount is adequate.

DETERMINING COSTS ASSOCIATED WITH PERFORMANCE MANAGEMENT

Frequently directors, managers, and process improvement team leaders have no idea how much they spend on actualizing the performance management system. Because a performance management system is composed of three programs, several steps are necessary. Department managers must do the following:

- understand their budgets and allocation of resources
- understand the three performance programs within the performance management system
- calculate the cost parameters of the three performance programs in their department
- share their calculations with the quality management board so that a total organization-wide picture is created

The quality management board decides the range or percent of each department's budget that will be allocated to performance management. It is unnecessary to require every department within the health care organization to conform to a standard percentage of its total operating budget. It may vary, depending on the individual department's needs. However, when *implementing* a performance management system for the first time, we suggest that managers be directed to allocate *no less* than 5% of their yearly total operating budget. Further, this 5% should be allocated to the three programs of the performance management system by the distribution rule of 25-25-15-35.

For example,

- 25% of the performance management system's budget is allocated for the awareness program, which consists of development and education of standards

- 40% is allocated for the measurement program— 25% for the measurement activities and 15% for the cost of nonconformance
- 35% is allocated for the performance improvement program (see Figure 17-4)

We have found that this distribution of resources for performance management activities within each department has proven effective. Occasionally a health care organization must adjust this amount up or down in individual departments, depending on the circumstances. Departments that are unaccustomed to the performance management process might initially need to devote a larger percent of their budget to education and practice of the concepts and activities. As the awareness, measurement, and improvement processes become more familiar and the performance management activities evolve into a part of the daily work experience, the percent devoted to the three programs may decrease.

Using this 5% of the department's total operating budget, here is an example of how it might work. Suppose a department manager of a hospital has a yearly operating budget of $950,000 and allocates 5% of that total to the performance management system. In this example, the performance management system's budget is calculated as:

$$\$950,000 \times 0.05 = \$47,500$$

The next step for this manager is to partition the $47,500 using the 25-25-15-35 distribution rule into the three programs within the performance management system: awareness, measurement, and improvement (see Figure 17-4). These costs include all activities, materials, and wastes associated with the implementation of each program.

This three-part distribution of funds from within each department's budget demonstrates that the performance improvement program receives the largest share of the allocated money. (Note that the 40% allocated to the measurement program has been partitioned into measurement [25%] and CONC [15%]).

The performance awareness program's costs, consisting of money spent developing standards and educating staff, amount to 25% of the department's allocated $47,500, or $11,875. The performance measurement program's costs consist of 40% of the department's allocated $47,500, or $19,000. Within this 40%, 25% is allocated for measurement, whereas 15% is allocated to alleviate the costs of nonconformance that occurs in the department. The performance improvement program's costs consist of the remaining 35% of the department's allocated $47,500, or $16,625.

Using 5% of the department's $950,000 annual operating budget, or $47,500 in this example, and the 25-25-15-35 distribution rule, the cost of the three programs within the performance management system would be the following:

25% of $47,500 = $11,875 allocated for performance awareness

25% of $47,500 = $11,875 allocated for performance measurement

15% of $47,500 = $7,125 allocated for CONC

35% of $47,500 = $16,625 allocated for performance improvement

This calculation should be done by each department as part of its annual budgeting process. It should also be tracked over time to determine if the allocated 5% is adequate to provide a thorough system of awareness, measurement, and improvement in the department and to periodically review the 25-25-15-35 distribution rule to see if it needs adjustment. In other words, each health care organization must create a performance management system tailored specifically to the individual needs of the organization.

Furthermore, these calculations may be used to determine each department's compliance with the organization-wide performance management system. When all departments complete their calculations, compile an organization-wide summary of the performance management system's costs. The average departmental performance management system's expenditures, expressed in dollars and as a percent of the departmental budget throughout the organization, also can be calculated.

It is important to keep in mind that these cost analyses are not organization-wide budgeting allocations for the coming year. These measures are used to identify how budgeted dollars are presently being spent on the performance management system's activities and should provide a basis for adjusting the performance management system's budget up or down for the coming year.

The QMB may then use departmental outcomes compared with allocated percentages and benchmark these results against organization-wide goals to determine if the performance management system is productive and adequately funded.

MEASURING PRODUCTIVITY

Measuring productivity consists simply of developing measures to quantify the use of an organization's resources. Unfortunately, many CEOs' only measurement of productivity lies in a computer printout of staffing patterns compared with census and workers' salaries. This is a very narrow view and the least helpful in measuring an organization's productivity.

Most health care accountants borrow productivity theory from their business schools' curriculum and usually limit productivity to three areas: capital, labor, and materials. Again, this is a very narrow view of productivity, because it prohibits health care organizations from establishing more definitive measures. Definitive measures are necessary because there are many factors that have an enormous impact on the overall productivity of a health care organization. Sometimes top management blames a nonproductive performance management system on the workers, a textbook or consultant, or course of instruction. In truth, there are many factors that act as barriers to a productive organization-wide performance management system. These factors never become visible cost figures and therefore are rarely associated with the success or failure of the organization's performance management system.

For example:

The structure of the organization. Few realize that the very way the health care organization is structured and operated—including chains of command—will produce either a productive or a nonproductive environment for the performance management system. Developing integrated, strategic, and organization-wide mission, vision, philosophy, goals, and policies will lay the groundwork for integrated productivity of the performance management system. In other words, a direction and theme that starts at the top sets the stage for productivity in every department as well as across the continuum of service.

Employee time management. Many managers consider employees who are hustling about their departments are working hard. These managers conclude that labor—working hard—is a productive measure when, in fact, less labor driven by the smarter processes will produce greater productivity. This is where the managers who encourage innovation will shine. Modern technology and improved processes utilized in the workplace ensure enormous strides in managing employees' time and, therefore, increasing productivity. Modern technology is one of the organization's greatest resources to improve employee productivity but is often ignored under the guise of its expense.

One example of valuing employees' time through use of modern technology is the increased use of facsimile machines in each department of many health care organizations. This prevents workers from leaving their departments to hand-deliver interdepartmental reports. The burgeoning field of home care provides another example of wise conservation of employees' time. Many agencies have recognized employees' time as their most precious resource and have learned that increased visits and therefore profits are possible through the implementation of the phone-fax-modem combination and ultimately, telemedicine units for each employee who makes home visits. This investment results in increased and accurate communication with physicians, patients, and the agency as well as providing instant and accurate documentation, thereby raising profit margin. Furthermore, home care employees may telephone the patient before driving miles to a home only to find that the patient has forgotten the appointment and "is away for the day." Additionally, the new technology provides a measure of safety to employees in that they do not have to leave their automobiles to telephone, ask directions, and so on.

Innovation. This is a measure of productivity that is virtually unmeasured by health care organizations because it is undervalued. Drucker defines innovation as "the task of endowing human and material resources with new and greater wealth-producing capacity."[7] Today's managers should seek ways of converting their patients' needs into opportunities for profit if they wish to succeed in the present health care environment. Without continual innovation, profits stagnate. All workers should be encouraged to innovate with proper rewards as recognition for an innovation that is accepted and adopted by the organization.

"The most productive innovation is a different product, process, or service creating a new potential of satisfaction, rather than an improvement. Typically this new and different product costs more—yet its overall effect is to make the [health care organization's] economy more productive."[7]

However, health care organizations do not, as a rule, value innovation that costs money. They lack vision of a future gain from today's investment of resources. For example, "the antibiotic drug costs far more than the cold compress which is all yesterday's physician had to fight pneumonia. The computer costs far more than an adding machine or a punchcard sorter, the typewriter far more than a quill pen, the Xerox duplicator far more than a copy press or mimeograph copier. And, if and when we get a cancer cure, it will cost more than even a first-class funeral. The price of a product is thus only one measurement of the value of an innovation."[7] Often productivity is linked to the bottom line price by VNO managers and is not related to outcomes as a more accurate measure of productivity (see Chapters 4 and 5). For example, the price of a drug for an indigent patient is related to the saving it produces in decreased hospital length of stay.

This requires managers that eagerly seek innovation to embrace improved processes and to not fear change. Alex Markels put it this way in the *Wall Street Journal*: "The future requires a focus on growth . . . you first throw out the old, narrow definition of company goals and aim for the more ambitious one of rapid innovation."[15] This requires you to rethink how your health care organization measures productivity.

Knowledge and expertise. One of the greatest opportunities for increasing productivity is found in the knowledge and expertise of workers. In many health care organizations, the accountant calls productive labor the hands-on performance of tasks to and for patients and other customers. Workers who perform tasks are the least productive labor of the health care organization, because their assessment skills combined with critical thinking skills are poor or nonexistent. By this we mean that they know how to carry out a task without any knowledge of why they are performing it or of the many things that could go wrong while they are performing it. What the accountant calls nonproductive labor—all the workers who contribute to the smooth operation of the organization by exercising their creative thinking skills based on their vast knowledge and expertise—are considered disposable because their contribution is not a visible, direct patient care task. This attitude is seen in those organizations that downsize an expensive employee such as the "supervisor of the house." This higher-paid employee typically troubleshoots the organization-wide problems for his or her shift, resolves these problems, and keeps customers happy. This position is viewed by VNO boards of directors as superfluous, because the supervisor is not performing hands-on care at the bedside.

"Furthermore, learning how to 'flatten' organizations, set up team-based management structures and 'empower' work forces is rarely viewed as the single most critical force behind speeding market responsiveness even though the research is indisputable. This proven management style simply comes up against a wall of tradition that retards progress making health care reform a future dream rather than a present reality."[15]

Staff mix. This measure of productivity is usually made from the bottom line of the salaries and benefits budget sheet with no consideration for service, practice, or governance outcomes. An unfortunate perception is that the least costly staff is the best staff mix. Because there are, as yet, no yardsticks to measure the impact of a poor staff mix on service, practice, or governance outcomes, health care organizations continue to believe they are saving money by decreasing the number of staff members who are the higher-paid "experts" and replacing them with inexpensive "two-fers." "Two-fers" are defined as two lower paid employees for the price of one highly paid, knowledgeable worker with specific expertise. In many organizations, top management believes that this will produce a lower cost of operation while increasing the number of people who can perform the requisite tasks.

For example, anyone can perform the mechanics of taking a blood pressure. In fact, machines can do it without a human operator. So why is knowledge and expertise critical when it becomes necessary to obtain the blood pressure of a sick patient? Blood pressure readings are frequently wrong if the arm of the patient or the blood pressure cuff is positioned incorrectly or the cuff is the wrong size. Hearing normal Korotkoff sounds through the stethoscope during the blood pressure procedure requires little skill for a person with average hearing ability. However, *interpreting* the Korotkoff sounds requires advanced assessment skills and knowledge. Hearing the peculiar thumping of pulsus alternans, one of the first signs of left ventricular failure, or noting the pulsus paradoxus, one of the first signs of tamponade, pericarditis, or severe lung disease and therefore taking immediate action is not a skill possessed by "two-fers." Understanding that a patient admitted for a "rule out myocardial infarction," who complains of severe chest pain along with severe back pain, should have an immediate leg blood pressure performed to rule out dissecting aneurysm or severe vessel blockage from clotting blood are skills that cannot be taught to "two-fers." They do not possess the assessment skills that include a thorough understanding of anatomy and physiology. Data collection can be performed at this level, data interpretation cannot.

Using national database performance measures based on outcomes of health care organizations' practices will be the motivating force to turn around the trend to measure productivity by the bottom-line salary figure. Instead, as mortality figures from downsized health care organizations increase, as many health care professionals are predicting, knowledge and expertise of clinical experts may once again be valued as a critical resource to maintain compliance with national database norms as a measure of a health care organization's productivity.

MEASURING COST BENEFITS

If productivity measurement is to be valuable to the health care organization, there should be a way to measure it in terms of costs. Edwardson[9] describes four benefits of productivity measurement:

1. It measures performance of service, practice, governance, and products.
2. It documents efficiency of performance awareness, measurement, and improvement.
3. It explains whether performance awareness and improvement are due to better design or improved processes.
4. It provides data for resource distribution and prioritization of necessary process improvements.

Measuring cost benefits is useful to demonstrate progress in the domains of service, practice, and governance. It answers questions about whether efficiency and effectiveness are present in the processes of each domain. Are the resources (inputs) necessary to produce the results (outputs) appropriate and cost-effective? Does increased measurement result in increased "progress in goods and/or service,"[9] practice, and governance? Is there measurable "efficiency improvement?" Does measurement show improvements are due to "better design or improved processes?" Does the performance measurement program provide data for "resource distribution and prioritizing of process improvement" activities?[9]

Seidman and Skancke also suggest that measurement be kept simple. Intricate measurement systems can cost more to calculate than the worth of the data they provide.[19] Remember our King Midas story? Traditional approaches to measuring cost/benefits include count and measurement data. Count data are done for comparison. Examples include quality control measures, such as how many studies were done this year as compared with last year, and what was the cost of this data collection. Measurement data analyze the impact of the performance management system on service, practice, and governance performance. In this method, costs are analyzed according to the numbers of resolved problems and/or the cost savings associated with producing the desired results. Effectiveness may be quantified by looking at the number of times the outcome in a specific patient population fell within the predetermined length of stay statistical control limits.

For example, department A measures an outcome for one of the acuity-based care symptom management practice guidelines. Because this outcome relates to the severity of illness index,[11] it is assessed daily for a total of 8 days. Suppose that of the 8 days calculated, outcome performance targets fell within the predefined parameters. The following equation might be used to determine the percentage of time in which a performance target, in this case a specific, predetermined outcome, can be predicted to be in statistical control.

$$100 \times \frac{\text{Number of times predetermined outcome performance target remains in statistical control}}{\text{Total number of predetermined outcome performance targets assessed}}$$

Or, assuming one outcome performance target per day for 8 days:

$$100 \times \frac{8}{8} = 100\%$$

This type of tracking is useful to substantiate a reduction in measurement frequency. The total annual number of measurement events is divided into the number of times the predetermined performance target fell within the statistical control limits. If only six of the eight measurement events fell within the statistical control limits, then the equation would be as follows:

$$100 \times \frac{6}{8} = 75\%$$

In the first instance, the reviewer could say with confidence that 100% of the time, the outcomes fell within the target parameters. However, in the second case, this happened only 75% of the time. By predetermining an acceptable standard for altering measurement frequency, this equation can be used to set next year's measurement schedule. For example, your standard may state that critical processes are measured at least quarterly; however, if over the course of a year, of the four measurement events with adequate sample size, 100% of the data points fall within the statistical control limits, measurement may be decreased to three times per year for the next calendar year. An additional standard must also be written to address readjustment of the frequency upward if the data points are out of statistical control. Why would a health care organization be interested in adjusting measurement frequency? Because the cost of data collection by staff members is expensive and an indirect expense item, resources should be focused on the most critical processes of the organization first! Every organization attempts to control both direct and indirect costs.

Another measure of the effectiveness of the performance management system might be the length of stay. Ideally, a productive performance management system results in reduced length of stay of all patients. Zander describes the impact of the use of the critical path process on anticipated length of stay for Alliant Health System.[22] Measurement of processes revealed the following:

Decreased	*Increased*
Length of stay (ALOS)	*Total discharges*
Charge/cost per case	*Charge/cost per day*
Patient days (relative to total discharges)	*(Greater acuity in fewer days)*
Total charges/costs (relative to total discharges)	

Reduced length of stay expressed as cost savings is an important variable in analyzing whether the benefits of the performance management system outweigh its costs. It is one type of monetary saving that results from improved performance.

Another direct benefit related to the performance management system is the cost saving associated with streamlining the process of providing care while maintaining the efficacy of the outcomes. Zander, for example, projected reduction in charges of over $11 million for three hospitals, primarily resulting from length of

stay reduction. Time, materials, and equipment saved can also be translated into calculable dollar income or savings. Quantifying these benefits makes it easier to compare them with costs and thus easier to make decisions about the allocation of resources.[22]

Patient outcomes may also be measured by calculating costs. A variety of scales are available to quantify patient outcomes.[1,11,13] These scoring systems attach a designated score to each patient symptom, staging it from "at risk," which is stage 0 to mild (stage 1), moderate (stage 2), advanced (stage 3), and severe, which is the worst case scenario (stage 4).[11] Internal scoring systems may be developed based on the stages identified for specific patient symptoms and costs of interventions for the severity of illness attached. These rating scales can then be used to identify the numbers of patients in each category who achieved the desired outcomes for that symptom.[11]

For example, an indicator might be as follows:

$$100 \times \frac{\text{Total number of patients with acquired stage IV pressure sores who progressed to level III or above by discharge}}{\text{Total number of patients with acquired stage IV pressure sores}}$$

These equations are specific examples of a modification of Carroll's productivity calculation:[5]

$$100 \times \frac{\text{Total number of resolved problems}}{\text{Total number of follow-up studies}}$$

This equation focuses only on measurement of problem resolution, however, and does not include the performance improvement aspect (to be discussed in the next chapter.) A more representative approach to outcome productivity related to costs might be as follows:

$$100 \times \frac{\text{Total cost of unexpected outcomes}}{\text{Total cost of all outcomes}}$$

This is a more vivid representation of the importance of controlling outcomes of patient care, including length of stay. It provides a generalized overview of the cost percentage of unexpected outcomes, benchmarked against the costs of total outcomes for a specific patient population. This figure may also be used as a measure of productivity. There may, for example, be many outcomes met, such as length of stay, and only a few outcomes unmet; however, the few that are unmet may cost far more than the many that are met.

For example, one coronary care unit (CCU) admitted and discharged 350 patients who had sustained an acute myocardial infarction (MI) in 1994. In this hospital, the CCU length of stay is 3.5 days. Of the total of 350 MI admissions, 300 were discharged within 3.5 days at an average cost of $12,000 each. This amounts to $3,600,000. Because the patients were within the 3.5-day length of stay, the hospital considered that their outcomes were met, i.e., discharged from the unit within a designated length of stay.

However, 50 of the 350 total MI admissions deteriorated and required various treatment modalities with varying length of stays that averaged $24,000 per patient. This amounted to $1,200,000. Additionally, two of these patients sued the hospital. Both cases were settled out of court. The first case revolved around inappropriately obtained informed consent, and the hospital settled out of court for $5,000,000. The second case concerned a charge of wrongful death and the hospital settled out of court for $1,500,000. The fees surrounding this litigation amounted to $30,000. Furthermore, as a result of this litigation against the hospital, the insurance premiums escalated by $20,000 for the following year. The litigation grand total amounted to $6,550,000 and that is *without* computing the costs of employee time involved in depositions and so on.

There are numerous ways a manager could view this situation in this CCU in terms of costs and productivity. One way would be to look at the grand total and divide by the number of patients treated.

For example:

$3,600,000 cost of 300 patients with met outcomes

$1,200,000 cost of 50 patients with unmet outcomes

$ 30,000 in litigation fees

$ 20,000 in increased insurance premiums

Grand total $4,850,000 (excluding the $6,500,000 paid by the insurance company)

Add the cost of the outcomes within limits ($3,600,000) and the costs of outcomes out of limits ($1,200,000) plus the legal fees ($30,000), and the increase in insurance premiums ($20,000), and the grand total amounts to $4,850,000. If this total amount is divided by the 350 patients treated in CCU, the average cost for each patient with a diagnosis of MI would be about $13,857.14.

Another method for looking at costs might be by acuity-based care.[11] This requires the use of practice guidelines with a severity of illness index built into them. The manager is then able to look at each symptom presented by each patient in the MI population group and tally the number of symptoms and the stages of acuity for each symptom. This information allows the organization to compute costs for interventions of each stage treated. This is one way to see if the organization's charges are capturing the actual cost of care. Costing out care by a severity of illness index is

one way to bill for patient care services. Another way to consider our example might be to figure the percentage of costs going to outcomes that are out of limits. For example:

$$\frac{\text{Out of limit outcomes } \$1{,}250{,}000}{\text{Total cost of outcomes } \$4{,}850{,}000}$$
$$= 0.257 \text{ or } 26\% \text{ of costs going to out of limit outcomes (round figures)}$$

This information provides a manager with a baseline for action. It is a beginning point for staff to develop an action plan for decreasing outcomes in the MI patient population group that are not within statistical control limits.

Defining the outcomes of each of the three programs of awareness, measurement, and improvement enables a health care organization to analyze how much it costs to produce the outcomes it achieves. Once you complete cost-benefit analysis, however, it is then only applicable as an internal measurement to be used for comparison with your historical data. Carroll argues that determining costs related to the performance management system in a health care organization is difficult because of lack of uniformity in cost accounting methodologies related to performance expenses.[5] A standardized measurement program that can be universally adopted to capture health care costs is needed. Although the measurement program provides a concrete perspective on the costs associated with the performance management system, to view costs as the sole determinant of success or failure is economic myopia. Each of the four indicators of measurement as described in this chapter are equally important.

REFERENCES

1. Allen RH: Use of the problem-oriented record to evaluate treatment in a chronic psychiatric population, *Qual Assurance Bull*, 8(3): 13-16, 1982.
2. Bogdanich W: *The great white lie,* New York, 1991, Simon & Schuster.
3. Brown JH, Moore CH: *Process improvement breakthrough: an Rx for health care,* Knoxville, Tenn, 1995, Qualpro.
4. Burda D: Total quality management becomes big business, *Modern Healthcare,* 21: 25-29, 1991.
5. Carroll JG: *Restructuring hospital quality assurance,* Chicago, 1984, Dow Jones Irwin.
6. Crosby PB: *Quality is free,* New York, 1979, McGraw-Hill.
7. Drucker PE: *Managing in turbulent times,* New York, 1993, Harper & Row.
8. Eckkal E: *Solving America's health-care crisis: a guide to understanding the greatest threat to your family's economic security,* New York, 1993, The New York Times Company.
9. Edwardson S: Measuring nursing productivity, *Nurs Econ,* 3(1): 9-14, 1985.
10. Garvin DA: *Managing quality: the strategic and competitive edge,* Glencoe, 1988, The Free Press.

11. Green E, Katz J: *Clinical practice guidelines for the adult patient,* St. Louis, 1995, Mosby.

12. Israeli A, Fisher B: Cutting quality costs, *Quality Progress,* 14(1): 46-48, 1991.

13. Jones KR: Severity of illness measured systems: an update, *Nurs Econ,* 5(6): 292-296, 1987.

14. Juran JM: *Juran's quality control handbook,* ed 4, New York, 1988, McGraw-Hill.

15. Markels A: It's time you became a manager of change, the consultants say, *The Wall Street Journal,* p B1, Tuesday, October 31, 1995.

16. Melum M: The next generation of health care quality, *Hospitals,* 63: 80, 1989.

17. Roberts MJ: *Your money or your life: the health care crisis explained,* New York, 1993, Doubleday.

18. Rodriguez A: Death rate spurs doctor swap, *Chicago Sun Times,* p 1, May 5, 1995.

19. Siedman LW, Skancke SL: *Productivity,* New York, 1990, Simon & Schuster.

20. Tylczak L: *Increasing employee productivity: an introduction to value management,* Menlo Park, Cal, 1990, Crisp Publications.

21. Walton M: *The Deming management method,* New York, 1986, Putnam Publishing Group.

22. Zander K: Estimating and tracking the financial impact of critical paths, *Definition,* 5(4): 1-3, 1990.

Chapter 18

Improving the Performance Management System

Change is the process by which the future invades our lives.
Alvin Toffler

Alice thought she had never seen such a curious croquet-ground in her life: it was all ridges and furrows; the croquet balls were live hedgehogs, and the mallets live flamingoes, and the soldiers had to double themselves up and stand on their hands and feet, to make the arches.

The chief difficulty Alice found at first was managing her flamingo: she succeeded in getting its body tucked away, comfortably enough, under her arm, with its legs hanging down, but generally, just as she had got its neck nicely straightened out, and was going to give the hedgehog a blow with its head, it would twist itself round and look up into her face, with such a puzzled expression that she could not help bursting out laughing; and, when she had got its head down, and was going to begin again, it was very provoking to find that the hedgehog had unrolled itself, and was in the act of crawling away: besides all this, there was generally a ridge or a furrow in the way wherever she wanted to send the hedgehog to, and, as the doubled-up soldiers were always getting up and walking off to other parts of the ground, Alice soon came to the conclusion that it was a very difficult game indeed.

The players all played at once without waiting for turns, quarrelling all the while, and fighting for the hedgehogs; and in a very short time the Queen was in a furious passion and went stamping about, and shouting "Off with his head!" or "Off with her head!" about once a minute.

Alice began to feel very uneasy: to be sure, she had not as yet had any dispute with the Queen, but she knew that it might happen any minute, "and then," thought she, "what

would become of me? They're dreadfully fond of beheading people here: the great wonder is, that there's any one left alive!"

She was looking about for some way of escape, and wondering whether she could get away without being seen, when she noticed a curious appearance in the air: it puzzled her very much at first, but after watching it a minute or two she made it out to be a grin, and she said to herself "It's the Cheshire-Cat: now I shall have somebody to talk to."

"How are you getting on?" said the Cat, as soon as there was mouth enough for it to speak with.

Alice waited till the eyes appeared, and then nodded. "It's no use speaking to it," she thought, "till its ears have come, or at least one of them." In another minute the whole head appeared, and then Alice put down her flamingo, and began an account of the game, feeling very glad she had someone to listen to her. The Cat seemed to think that there was enough of it now in sight, and no more of it appeared.

"I don't think they play at all fairly," Alice began, in rather a complaining tone, "and they all quarrel so dreadfully one can't hear oneself speak—and they don't seem to have any rules in particular; at least, if there are, nobody attends to them—and you've no idea how confusing it is all things being alive; for instance, there's the arch I've got to go through next walking about at the other end of the ground—and I should have croqueted the Queen's hedgehog just now, only it ran away when it saw mine coming!"

"How do you like the Queen?" said the Cat in a low voice.

"Not at all," said Alice: "she's so extremely—" Just then she noticed that the Queen was close behind her, listening: so she went on "—likely to win, that it's hardly worth finishing the game."*

Alice's croquet game left her bewildered, just as today's upheaval in the health care environment is leaving many bewildered. Implementing a performance management system can help turn this bewilderment into progress.

In Chapter 16, we discussed the importance of establishing a new culture in a health care organization in which a performance management system could thrive. In implementing this system, the performance awareness program is developed first, because it is within this program that all standards are created—both internal standards and those to be used across the continuum of care.

Standards, then, serve as benchmarks against which the performance management system itself will be measured—both internally and externally. Adherence to these benchmarks provides the organization with proof that the performance management system's awareness program is functioning properly.

In Chapter 17, we described the measurement program of the performance management system. This program is the second to be constructed. It measures the efficiency and effectiveness of the performance management system, including the costs of nonconformance throughout the organization. Furthermore, this is the program that measures, tracks, and trends critical processes of the performance management system, using the tools of statistical process control.

This chapter focuses on the performance improvement program of the performance measurement system itself. The performance improvement program is the last of the three programs to be implemented, because without the awareness program and the measurement program, this third program cannot function. The performance improvement program incorporates the values from the performance awareness and data from the performance measurement program to determine which critical processes of the performance management system are working and which are not. Armed with the standards developed within the performance awareness program and data from the performance measurement program, employees may, through the performance improvement program, correct the performance management system processes that are not working and refine those that are working but need innovation and improvement.

The performance improvement program offers strategies to assist health care professionals to become change agents for the health care organization by continuous performance improvement. The performance improvement program is designed to foster an environment where successful innovation and improvement is an expectation of every employee.

The old adage "If it ain't broke, don't fix it," is obsolete. For example,

> *Orville and Wilbur Wright would be shocked at the innovations in flight technology today. How stunned they would be to see the current space crafts not only orbiting planet earth but also investigating the others within our solar system and sending pictures back to earth. I'm certain the Wright brothers would be awed by the space crafts that are presently speeding their way beyond earth's solar system into intergalactic space—the scientists at NASA call it 'deep space'—where no object of earthlings has ever gone.[7]*

Without continuous innovation and improvements to the original aircraft at Kittyhawk, North Carolina, there would be no space exploration today. "Without space exploration the world might have missed many of the devices we accept as normal in our everyday lives ranging from the fantastic in medical science such as pace makers and telemetry to the serviceable such as heat repellant clothing for fire fighters."[7]

Continuous progress in performance management requires the same level of improvement and innovation as displayed by NASA and other industries! Shortsightedness in any field of endeavor retards exploration and is a difficult hurdle to overcome. Health care organizations and those that regulate them have, traditionally, had myopic views of progress, which, in part, has contributed to the present health care chaos. Of course, hindsight is always 20-20 and every industry or profession has had its share of myopic visionaries. Consider some past statements that prove the myopic theory:

1. *U.S. inventor, Lee DeForest, in 1926 stated, "While theoretically and technically television may be feasible, commercially and financially I consider it an impossibility, a development of which we need waste little time dreaming."[21] Mr. DeForest was known as the "Father of the Radio," but he was unable to visualize any innovation that could "improve" on what he knew and understood—the radio. Progress in health care, just like progress in the entertainment media, depends on continuous innovation, modification, refinement, and improvement of all processes.*

2. Science Digest, *August 1948, printed these amazing words: "Landing and moving around the moon offers so many serious problems for human beings that it may take science another 200 years to lick them."[21]*

3. *In 1946 Darryl F. Zanuck, head of 20th Century-Fox stated: "Television won't be able to hold onto any market it captures after the first six months. People will soon get tired of staring at a plywood box every night."[21]*

---

*From Carroll L: *Alice's adventures in Wonderland* and *Through the looking glass*, Boston, 1980, GK Hall and Co.

The moral here is this: whatever a health care organization decides to change, improve, or construct, there will always be "side-liners" with myopic thinking, saying "It's impossible," and "This won't work." For that reason, health care organizations need to create a performance management system aimed at overcoming the myopic attitude of its workers. Performance management is designed to overcome myopic employee attitudes. It is designed to foster an environment where successful innovation and improvement is an expectation. Then, through the work of the performance improvement program, the performance management system *itself* may be measured, modified, or improved.

MANAGING CHANGE

In the book *When Giants Learn to Dance*, Rosabeth Moss Kanter suggests that it is getting harder and harder to succeed with traditional corporate methods when technology, customer preferences, employee loyalty, industry regulations, and corporate ownership are constantly changing. And just like Alice playing croquet with the queen, "Instead of simply keeping their own eyes on the ball, they have to watch all the changing elements of the game at once."[9] Survival and success in a health care organization requires "faster action, more creative maneuvering, more flexibility and closer partnership with employees and customers than ever before."[9]

This means that a performance improvement program that is exactly like the one of even a few years ago is obsolete today. A performance management system will be effective only if the QMB plans for change and creates a recognition process for innovation. Creating and managing an effective performance improvement program is a requirement of health care accreditation agencies. However, aside from accreditation requirements, the value to your health care organization of a planned, organized, systematic performance improvement program that functions as an integral part of the performance management system cannot be overestimated.

Chapters 3 through 5 provided information on how to create and implement a performance improvement program. This chapter looks at how to improve the performance management system itself. It focuses on 10 strategies to be used as benchmarks to measure the efficiency and effectiveness of your performance management system. These ten strategies, which form the basis of the performance improvement program, are designed to help health care organizations (a) cope with the constantly changing environment, (b) develop a culture of innovation and continued research, and (c) satisfy external accreditation requirements.

The time has come to relinquish all former ideas of what constitutes *quality* and completely reengineer health care organizations. "It is no secret that health care organizations have reached the 'survive or die' point!"[23] Furthermore, "reengineering can't be carried out in small and cautious steps. It is an all-or-nothing proposition that produces dramatically impressive results. Many organizations have no choice but to muster the courage to do it. For many, reengineering is the only hope for breaking away from the ineffective, antiquated ways of conducting business that will otherwise inevitably destroy them."[8]

The 10 benchmarking strategies will not prove effective until each program—awareness, measurement, and improvement—is implemented and fully operational. Success does not come to an organization that implements performance management system bit-by-bit, piece-by-piece, one tiny, cautious step at a time.

We have observed the floundering of many health care organizations using this piecemeal method of implementation. The staff views this method as slow and frustrating. One staff member, involved in her organization's piecemeal method of implementation, said to us, "We're not doing anything around here about performance improvement! There are some isolated activities going on but nothing of significance. I believe our CEO is just stalling until the surveyors leave our building and then it will be business as usual." Although this unidentified employee obviously was venting her frustration to an outside consultant, it typifies worker attitude about the slow restructuring of the organization.

RESTRUCTURING

Restructuring the health care organization from the hierarchical to the shared leadership management method should take no longer than 18 months. To take longer than this is to see the vision fail from staff discouragement. When implementation of the three performance programs begins, the staff becomes excited and enthusiastic. When staff members fail to see progress, they begin to doubt the organization's intentions, and restructuring often becomes mere downsizing. With a concrete, visual administrative action plan along with a time line for completion of the project, the performance management system will become a reality.

To accomplish the restructuring of the health care organization, change must be embraced rather than shunned. As Alex Markels wrote in an article titled "It's Time You Became a Manager of Change" in the *Wall Street Journal*, "There's an intrinsic need to improve your effectiveness at managing change—whatever form it takes . . . Learning how to 'flatten' organizations, set up team-based management structures and 'empower' work forces will help you bust bureaucracies and speed

10 BENCHMARKING STRATEGIES

1. Top leadership involvement
2. Budgeting for performance management
3. A performance awareness program
4. A performance measurement program
5. A performance improvement program
6. Empowering the workforce
7. Organization-wide education
8. Spectacular customer service
9. Information management
10. Worker satisfaction

the market responsiveness of your company."[11] The health care organization's implementation of the performance management system will be an outstanding success if these 10 strategies for the performance management system's performance improvement are incorporated into its design. They may then serve as benchmarks by which the organization's performance management system can be evaluated. The box above presents the 10 strategies for the performance management system's performance improvement program that will be used to measure the effectiveness and efficacy of the performance management system.

Strategy 1: Top Leadership Involvement

One of the most successful strategies being used by health care organizations today is that of restructuring themselves from the traditional hierarchical management style into one of shared leadership as discussed in Part 2. This should be used as the first benchmark against which the performance management system will be measured.

"No health care organization will thrive any better than its top management will permit; the 'bottleneck' is, after all, always 'at the head of the bottle.'[4] Furthermore, the spirit of an organization is created by the people at the top. Their standards of conduct, their values, their beliefs, set the example for their entire organization. . ."[4]

Along with so many other changes in the health care industry, the role of the CEO also has changed.

This role has become so multidimensional that 'top-management tasks require at least four different kinds of human being: the "thought man," "the action man," the "people man," and the "front man." Yet those four temperaments are almost never found in one person. Failure to understand these characteristics is a main reason why the top-management task is so often done poorly.[4] Whatever the titles on the organization chart, the CEO job in a healthy company is almost always shared.[4]

This team approach has been so successful in the world of business that we created a similar interdisciplinary, organization-wide performance management system that incorporates the same principles. However, it only works if the CEO shares the job. Chapter 5 outlined the concept of shared leadership consisting of a quality management board chaired by the CEO. The details of how this governing body functions and how interdisciplinary councils are organized to carry out the three performance programs are also discussed in Chapter 5. Shared leadership is like a ship and therefore needs a captain. In this role, however, the CEO is not the "boss"; he or she is the *leader.* Some of the most successful companies in the world use such this governance method. We admit it takes one special person—one with confidence and vision—to lead in today's environment. Many leaders think it is worth it.

For example, the president of Du Pont has a governing team, and when a decision is made, he has just one vote and depends primarily on his moral authority for action. At Standard Oil of New Jersey the chairman traditionally did not even have this much legal power; for many years votes, whenever taken, required unanimity. Alfred P. Sloan at General Motors had the legal power to overrule his colleagues on the management team. But he almost never used it. He made a decision after he had made sure that he knew where every colleague on the top-management team stood and that each, in turn, had fully grasped where the chairman and chief executive officer stood.[4] In short, the newly emerged philosophy of the role of the CEO in health care is this: "none of us is as smart as all of us!"[10]

Effective shared leadership by the CEO is demonstrated by the efficiency and efficacy of the performance management system. This sharing of the burdens also promotes employee buy-in to organizational decisions. Without a doubt, restructuring the traditional hierarchical management style of governance into an organized, "flattened" team approach has been a proven successful management strategy since biblical times. One of the most successful CEOs in history was Moses. In approximately 1200 BC, Jethro, father-in-law of Moses, suggested that Moses change his management style and implement shared leadership. The Exodus account reports Jethro as saying, "That will make your load lighter because they will share it with you."[2] A critical indicator of success of the performance management system is the willingness of the CEO to restructure for shared leadership.

Strategy 2: Budgeting for a Performance Management System

"The drive toward health care reform and the spread of managed care have increased the awareness of the critical role of cost measurement and cost management."[6] In the past, costs were considered private information between the accounting department and the CEO. There was no budget set aside for the operation of each department's performance management system, because it was considered part of each employee's job. Occasionally a health care organization would provide a small stipend for the quality management department, but that was often used by those in newly formed "quality" professional roles for seminars and materials to learn about the job. Today an organization-wide budget for the performance management system is necessary. Interacting with national databases cannot be accomplished without planned, budgeted resources. Also, a successful performance management system can not be carried out by *each department* without planned, budgeted resources.

Including a line item in the budget to allot resources for the operation of the performance management system demonstrates the organization's commitment to excellence. Walt Disney spent millions of dollars on the "Disney Way." He budgeted for success and, in the process, created a worldwide standard of customer service unequaled in America. In fact, corporations will continue to measure themselves into the next millennium by Disney's futuristic vision of customer service (see Chapter 6).

> *Granted, everything still comes back to the bottom line:* Can we afford it? *Nothing will derail a program more quickly than lack of funds. Without adequate funding the project will be crippled from the beginning. Taking funds from some other area to finance the newly proposed changes will create a great deal of distrust and unpopularity for the change. Each department needs a budget, and monies must be allocated for aggregate work. Be honest and assess your project's budget using the following three questions:*
>
> 1. *Taking all possible contingencies into account, how much is this change really going to cost?*
> 2. *Do we have that much money?*
> 3. *If not, how are we going to get it?*
>
> *"Never try to implement change on a shoestring budget! It's a little like building a new house without the money for plumbing or electricity. You end up with a shell that is unlivable. Even worse, you end up with visible evidence of your failure."*[22]

This is why

> *all health care managers, not just accountants, are becoming more and more aware of the importance of understanding as much as they possibly can about costs. . . . While traditionally the budget and all cost accounting was considered the domain of the organization's accountant, today's broader perspective encompasses a broad range of financial information that can help managers to manage better. "Cost accounting" in today's health care organizations has become an interdisciplinary process between departmental managers, accountants, physicians, and the top management leaders. From this new perspective of open communication and sharing, organizations find that ultimately they benefit the most because the management of department-level costs are necessary for pricing decisions in negotiations with health maintenance organizations and preferred provider organizations, for purposes of strategic planning, and for profitability analysis.*[6]

However, without a specific budget and concrete guidelines to implement the work of the performance management system at the departmental level, restructuring initiatives will face dismal failure.

Additionally, many health care organizations have learned that crisis management is a far more expensive method of management than is implementing a planned, organized performance management system. Having a budget for performance management means managers are able to focus on costing issues and concepts peculiar to their departments. In fact, most are able to point out areas of waste and nonconformance, which saves thousands of dollars for the organization. Costs may then be used as the baseline factor behind selection of performance improvement projects as well as the selection of process improvement teams. This requires a shared leadership style of management along with a close integration of the measurement and improvement programs.

The information about calculation of the nonconformance costs in Chapter 17 has provided the starting point for the broader planning the organization must do to subsidize the implementation and smooth functioning of the performance management system. When managers become guardians of costs, it will no longer be necessary for the CEO to worry about the bottom line.

A PERFORMANCE AWARENESS PROGRAM

The first program to be developed under the performance management system is the performance awareness program. This program includes tools and techniques to create a thorough understanding of the organization's customers. It further provides a method for delineating and prioritizing the scope of service, practice, and governance of each department. The performance awareness program includes the development and dissemination of organization-wide structure, process, and outcome standards and creating a culture of excellence. Chapter 8 defines these concepts and discusses methods for implementing the performance awareness program. Additionally, a discussion of how to create a standards-based system using structure, outcome, and process standards is provided in Chapter 3. Failure to develop a standards-based system, which forms an integral part of the performance awareness program, will affect the entire organization and cripple the performance management system.

Without a performance awareness program there can be no performance measurement program. This means that critical cost measurements that drive the decisions of the performance improvement program will be nonexistent. In other words, each of the programs are synergistically critical to success.

A PERFORMANCE MEASUREMENT PROGRAM

The national governmental, third-party payers', and accrediting agencies' emphasis in the health care industry on measurement and comparative indicators represent a fundamental shift in the relationship of health care organizations to society as a whole. Gone is the cadre of passive, uninformed patients of yesterday. Today's patients are knowledgeable, informed, street smart, and litigation wise. Health care costs continue to spiral upward and technology is obsolete before the latest gadget is removed from its packing crate. This environment links the performance measurement program with survival. It is one of the most critical strategies for success.

> Many organizations, however, have no theoretical or practical knowledge of what performance improvement really is or how it can help them. There has been little consistent focus on improving processes to improve effectiveness, reduce cost, and increase patient satisfaction. Management typically has not had much education along these lines and simply pays lip service to fragmented efforts, many of which do not even address the most important areas.[1]

A sound performance measurement program is the only defense against fragmentation of performance improvement activities. The answers to when is enough enough? and when does the cost of health care outweigh the benefits? will never be found without a strategic, statistically based performance measurement program. This program provides the framework to determine critical processes of the organization that are out of statistical control. These processes may then be prioritized and targeted for performance improvement. In other words, the performance measurement program of each department exists to provide the measurement data that drive the organization-wide performance improvement program. Members of the performance improvement program then use this measurement data to improve such areas as customer satisfaction with service, practice, and governance, inappropriate and/or unplanned outcomes, as well as decreased costs associated with nonconformance. Wasting resources on a program without obvious measurable benefit to the organization is no longer accept-

able. In today's health care organizations, every penny spent on the performance management system should be accounted for and justified by observable outcomes. This ties outcomes to costs! "Institutions that successfully reduce costs through performance measurement and improvement programs may be rewarded with higher market share (or at a minimum, survival) across the long term."[1]

A PERFORMANCE IMPROVEMENT PROGRAM

A performance improvement program is a successful survival strategy in today's business world. Enter any bookstore and look at the business section. You will see dozens of books on quality, reorganizing, reengineering, and empowerment occupying the shelves. Many health care organizations have been slow to understand how these principles, so beneficial in the business world, can be applied to the service industry of health care. One reason for this is that the accreditation agencies of the United States also were slow to see the benefits and adapt their requirements to the new, successful business techniques of performance management.

Gradually, over the past few years, health care organizations have begun to receive the positive messages of success from the forerunners—brave organizations that were first to launch new performance management systems. Today, many health care organizations are launching performance management systems and benchmarking their success against these visionary organizations.

Unfortunately, some poorly informed top leaders, without any training and direction, leave the development of a performance management system to their direct reports. Few managers have the support or knowledge to know how to go about its implementation. Often, these managers, in the absence of organization-wide authority and with little knowledge of statistical process control techniques, attempt to implement a performance management system in their own "little sphere"—in isolation from the rest of the organization.

This is very unfair to managers. Although process improvement teams are the backbone of the performance improvement program, putting together groups of people to discuss "problems" and calling them "teams" does *not* constitute a performance improvement program. In fact, a performance improvement program cannot work in isolation. It will only work interdependently and in conjunction with a performance awareness and a performance measurement program. The reason is simple: there are *no* processes that involve just *one* department in a health care organization. Many health care professionals have tried to think of one process involving only their department and have been stymied.

This is easy to explain: all processes always involve multiple workers from multiple departments. For example, consider the process of cleaning the department's utility room shelves. This process cannot be accomplished with only the department's employees. Other departments will be involved. For example, medication administration will involve the pharmacy, the physician, the unit clerk, the purchasing department, pharmaceutical vendors, and the nursing department.

A performance improvement program in isolation is analogous to attempting to put a puzzle together when two thirds of the pieces are missing. Although performance improvement is a necessary program of the performance management system, it does not stand alone. Performance improvement is always implemented along with the performance awareness and measurement programs.

EMPOWERING THE WORKFORCE

A shared leadership management style and empowerment of employees go hand-in-hand as indicates success. It is virtually impossible to implement an effective performance management system without empowering the employees. Improvements can rarely be made by one person in a health care organization. This is why shared leadership is such a successful strategy. Because all processes within a health care organization are interrelated, team members are chosen for a process improvement project by identifying those who have a stake in the process. Then, when the process is ultimately improved, everyone involved has had input in the solution. They "own" the improvement decisions, and because they created the solution, they will have an interest in making it work.

"The most distinguishing characteristic of a team is that its members have, as their highest priority, the accomplishment of a team goal. Most nonteam groups, on the other hand, tend to be collections of personalities with their own agendas."[17] Teams, however, may not just appear and begin a process improvement project without a knowledge of awareness and measurement. Potential team members must have education on how to conduct a team as well as a knowledge of measurement techniques *before* they are assigned to participate in a process improvement project.

Shared leadership within an organization means that people who are affected by or involved in a decision have a voice in making it.

The decisions they make may involve problem solving, work scheduling, task assignment, training, or any number of issues that relate to the effectiveness of their operation. People participate in setting goals and in evaluating one another's performance. They may even decide how rewards are distributed. Whatever the decision, the underlying reality is that employees share leadership with their bosses.[17]

Furthermore, people working on process improvement teams will find their work far different from traditional committees. The new management method of shared leadership, involving the use of empowered councils and process improvement teams, makes workers collectively responsible for process results rather than individually responsible for tasks. This means that each worker will use a broader range of skills from day to day. It also requires employees to think "beyond the walls" of their department to consider the big picture.

As work becomes more multi-dimensional, it also becomes more substantive. Reengineering eliminates not just waste but non-value-added work as well. Most of the checking, reconciling, waiting, monitoring, tracking—the unproductive work that exists in health care organizations because of departmental boundaries and to compensate for process fragmentation—is eliminated by reengineering, which means that people will spend more time doing real work.

In organizations that use the shared leadership management style to empower the council members, work becomes more satisfying, since workers achieve a greater sense of completion, closure, and accomplishment from their jobs. They actually create improvements that yield visible results that people care about. Council members share many of the challenges and rewards of a CEO because they are empowered to act! They are not just trying to keep the CEO happy or to work through the bureaucracy. It is little wonder that an empowered workforce has become one of the key indicators of success.[8]

ORGANIZATION-WIDE EDUCATION

On November 22, 1963, John F. Kennedy stated, "Leadership and learning are indispensable to each other."[18] If the performance management system of a health care organization is to prove successful, all employees need sufficient education so that they can discern where the organization is headed and how they fit into the new environment. Traditionally, health care organizations primarily stressed education and competency assessment in the division of nursing with scant attention to workers in the rest of the organization. In a reengineered health care organization the emphasis shifts from education and competency checks for all workers. Competence ensures that employees know the 'how' of a job. Education increases their insight and understanding of the total process and teaches the 'why'."[8]

Health care organizations that offer their people career-long education and an environment in which to use it, are investing in the future. Employees that are constantly learning and incorporating new ideas and techniques into their jobs become a vital and dynamic force. This type of staff can assimilate constant changes and possess the personal power to deal with ambiguity that often accompanies change."[24] Many VNO managers consider money spent on worker education a waste of resources. They reason that the workers should have obtained their education prior to applying for a job. These managers fail to consider the rapidly changing information technology and equipment of all areas of health care. "Education is as necessary to the employees of a health care organization as a road map in an unfamiliar place. Providing employees with the best possible education will get them where they need to be quickly, accurately, and with pride."[18]

Many methods are available for ongoing employee education. Some of these methods include classroom instruction, cross-training, small projects, team activities, mentoring, job rotation and enrichment, films, books, journals, and seminars.

Education is not free, in any sense of the word. It takes commitment of time and money. And time *is* money when you are taking people away from their work.

But there is a payoff. Education benefits both the front and bottom lines. How else can a health care organization bring out the talents in the staff and prepare them and the health care organization for tomorrow and years to come? Education provides a more proficient work force, improves performance awareness, measurement and improvement, and cements loyalty.

Rosenbluth presents these education tips for health care organizations to consider as they reengineer for the future:

- Consider education as an essential part of the health care organization. It means the difference between success and failure in the service industry.
- Make learning fun. People retain more when information is presented in a creative, interactive, and interesting manner.
- Education must be attitudinal as well as technical, and must be perpetual. Culture and attitude are as important to service as is skill.
- Offer education that benefits the personal as well as the professional lives of the staff members. You will be pleased with the results.
- A leadership development program can be an excellent way to groom future leaders. The individuals, the departments, and the health care organization all will benefit.
- Always provide staff education for new products or methods you plan to employ in the health care organization.
- Daily coaching of staff members by their leaders will strengthen the skills of both. The coach orchestrates the play of the game to bring out the talents of each individual for the success of the team as a whole. That's leadership.

- Commit the educational resources necessary for your health care organization—both financial and in terms of time. It is a long-term investment that you'll never regret.[18]

Implementation of a successful performance management system requires education of all employees in every facet of their employment. The extent of a health care organization's educational program for its employees is one of the indicators of success.

SPECTACULAR CUSTOMER SERVICE

A guest approached the doorman at a major hotel and complained that his radar detector had been stolen from his car in the hotel's garage. The doorman, empowered to perform customer service, asked how much it cost, took the guest to the front desk, and commanded "Give this man $150.00" to the clerk. Everybody gulped, but the customer was satisfied. Two weeks later, the general manager received a letter from this customer that stated he had found his radar detector in his trunk. In the envelope was also a check for $150. The postscript to the letter added: "By the way, I will never stay at any other hotel chain for the rest of my life."[8]

This is an example of a service organization that understood that spectacular customer service provides the competitive edge. In a service delivery business, without customers, there is no business.

For the performance improvement program to function, spectacular customer service is necessary. However, many health care organizations suffer from complexity and consider this an acceptable excuse for poor customer service. These organizations are multidimensional, large, sprawling over several acres of land, and sometimes disjointed by two or more campuses. In such health care organizations it is sometimes difficult to remember why the organization is in business. Sometimes the customer gets lost in the busyness of the daily organizational operation.

The hard truth is that spectacular customer service does not happen by accident. Unfortunately, health care administrators cannot hire people to fill customer service jobs, tell them what to do, and then hope that everything will be all right. It doesn't work that way. Delivering spectacular customer service requires knowledge, forethought, and a great deal of concentrated effort. Chapter 6 provides tools for creating a profile to understand the customers of the health care organization. This profile provides the basic knowledge on which spectacular customer service is built.

According to William Martin, there are two dimensions of customer service: (a) the procedural dimension and (b) the personal dimension.

The procedural dimension of customer service is systematic in nature. It deals with service delivery systems. It encompasses the performance awareness program's standards of how things get done. This procedural dimension provides the rules by which customers' needs are met. The personal dimension of customer service is warm, often irrational, and certainly unpredictable. This is the human side of service. It is interpersonal in nature, and it encompasses the attitudes, behaviors, and verbal skills that are present in every personal service interaction. This side of service is the personal dimension of customer service.[12]

Martin identified seven areas in the procedural dimension of customer service:

1. **Timing.** What are the timing standards for delivery of service to customers in your health care organization? How long should the service take? Are there several processes that require different timing standards? Does timeliness equate with promptness? Or can service at times be too fast, causing the customer to feel rushed?
2. **Flow.** How do the various components of the service delivery system coordinate, cooperate, and/or mesh with each other? How do you control the flow of services to the customer? How can you avoid backups and log jams? What are the indicators of this that can be seen or measured?
3. **Accommodation.** How flexible are your processes? Can this flexibility be adapted to varying customer needs and/or requests? How convenient are your processes for customers? How do they make the customers' service experiences easier? Are your service processes designed around your customers' needs? What are your observable indicators of accommodating processes that can be measured?
4. **Anticipation.** How well can you anticipate customer needs? How can you be one step ahead of customers in your service delivery? How do you know when you have anticipated correctly?
5. **Communication.** How do you know when messages are communicated thoroughly, accurately, and in a timely way? How do you know when communication has broken down? What measurable processes reflect effective communication in your service?
6. **Customer feedback.** How do you find out what your customers are thinking? How is customer feedback used to improve service? What are your observable indicators of customer satisfaction?
7. **Organization and supervision.** Efficient procedural service requires organization, and organization, in turn, requires supervision. How are all the parts of the service delivery system kept coordinated with each other? What are the signs that can be seen or measured that tell you all is going well?[12]

William Martin further outlines seven areas in the personal dimension of customer service:

1. **Appearance.** A customer's positive or negative reaction to a given customer service interaction is strongly influenced by what he or she sees.
2. **Attitude: body language and tone of voice.** Because we can't see the attitude of service personnel directly, we see it through their body language and tone of voice. Attitude is exposed for all to see.
3. **Attentiveness.** Attentiveness involves tuning in to customers' unique needs and wants. It is being sensitive and treating each customer in a special, unique way that recognizes his or her individuality.
4. **Tact.** Tact involves not only the way messages are sent but also the choice of words. Certain language can turn customers off and, therefore, should be avoided.
5. **Guidance.** Guidance involves individual coaching and counseling to customers.
6. **Selling skills.** Selling is an integral part of a health care organization's service delivery business. Employees "sell" their skills and expertise to patients and families. Therefore, it is necessary to cultivate and facilitate selling skills.
7. **Gracious problem solving.** Problem solving involves handling customer complaints.

Without both the procedural and personal dimensions of customer service being ingrained in every employee, the performance management system will not be effective.

INFORMATION MANAGEMENT

An information management network is necessary to the implementation of a successful performance management system. For example, Leland Stanford, founder of Stanford University, won his riches not by discovering gold in the West, but by selling supplies to gold miners. "A physical marketplace, such as Stanford's store, or a computer-based trading system like the New York Stock Exchange, simply brings together—efficiently—information to aid buyers and sellers."[15]

Two of the most critical resources in a health care organization are people and information. These two essential resources must be brought together in a way that will raise the probability of positive outcomes and productivity.

All managers are clear on their responsibilities for obtaining the best people they can, motivating them, and organizing them to do the work of the organization. Managers are far less conscious of their responsibilities regarding the information resources used in their work. Even where they know that information is important, they are unaware of the available data on how people get and use information and of what can be done about managing the information-communication processes in their organizations.[19]

In general, the work of health care professionals consists of transforming information from one state to another. The few exceptions include the surgeon, the nurse, the respiratory therapist, and others who need not only cognitive skills but also motor skills to translate what they perceive and interpret into physical results in the form of direct patient care tasks. The Pelz and Andrews (1976) studies of productivity paint a picture of professional productivity being enhanced by frequent exchanges with other professionals. It is a picture that is directly in contradiction with that of the traditional "silent worker" production management view that "If they're talking, they ain't producing."[19] In a study of 2,000 managers and professionals Pelz and Andrews found that "they spend well over 80% of their time in information-communication activities."[19]

This study indirectly emphasizes the importance of interdisciplinary teams within a health care organization. The interaction among professionals from various departments of the organization will enhance the productivity of teams. "In fact, a strong case can be made that *anything* that improves the quality and quantity of information available to health care professionals or improves their ability to receive, process, apply, and transmit information will improve that professional's productivity."[19]

Information per se—the ultimate intangible—is playing an increasingly important role in the world of health care. However, many leaders of health care organizations see neither the importance of interdisciplinary performance improvement teams nor the linkage of computer information networks. They see both as questionable, costly expenditures. They do not view teams or the installation of computers as an asset to the organization, much less as the most critical resources available to shape the future of their organization. The VNO managers just see the dollar signs when teams and electronic information management systems are suggested.

Furthermore, some health care organizations are uncomfortable with the world's shift from isolated, primitive countries with no modernity to instant communication. The world has become one global shopping mall as well as communication center. Via computerization people may order goods and services and converse with friends and strangers from most places on earth. Today the role of electronic information is highly visible and affordable and the knowledge base of the average citizen about computerization has progressed to an astonishing degree. Even children have mastered the fine art of the computer and modem communication.

It is no surprise, then, that computerization—the ultimate in information management—is emerging as critical to the advancement of the health care industry. For example, computers have transformed and enhanced the science of diagnosing disease states of patients. The value of computerized machines, such as the MRI, the CT scan, and telemetry, hardly can be estimated in terms of productivity and patient, staff, and system outcomes. Technology has transformed the world by making it possible for a physician to sit in a hospital in North America and direct a surgical procedure in another country on the opposite side of the world.

Health care organizations today, however, who are struggling to survive the day-to-day, rapidly changing environment, are loathe to find funds for computerization of their entire health care system. Even if computerization is the driving force behind the twenty-first century's Information Age, organizations perceive that day-to-day survival takes precedence over long-term planning. For many, the future is now—and now is all they can handle.

But, ready or not and like it or not,

> the U.S. has become an almost totally brain-based economy, where information manipulation is the basis for advantage in every job and industry, old or new. The fact is, until the computer came along and its dramatic impact became clear, there was little talk about information processing not only in health care organizations but also in the world of manufacturing and business. That was always a mistake. In some sense, information has been "everything" since long before William Scheckley invented the transistor or Steve Jobs and Steve Wozniak emerged from Job's garage with the Apple I.[15]

The big difference today, then, is that the role of information management is becoming more visible and vital as it unites the world economically, socially, medically—just to name a few areas.

Computerization of health care organizations is being driven further into dominance by two of the JCAHO's functional accreditation requirements: Information Management and the Continuum of Care, as well as the rise of several national databases with a focus on organizational outcomes and comparison data. It will be impossible to have a significant involvement with any national database or research project along *the continuum of care* without organization-wide computerization.

Furthermore, outcomes management as well as the conservation of resources will be possible only through an electronic networking mechanism. Outcomes data is necessary not only within the walls of the health care organization but also beyond its walls. The feasibility of tracking long-term patient outcomes beyond the walls of the acute health care organization—a feat that could take years—can not be accomplished without computerization. In addition to the acute care sector of health care, it will be necessary for home care agencies, who will provide the outcomes data from the field, to be computerized so that the data may be forwarded directly into the acute care facility's information system to be routed to one of the national data banks.

In addition to these advantages of computerized health care organizations, "information-communication abilities and actions are relevant to a wide range of managerial activities in a professional organization and affect all of the following:

Hiring
Individual performance
Individual growth
Team capabilities and growth
Dealing with subordinates
Dealing with other parts of an organization
Dealing with vendors
Dealing with clients
Dealing with banks, insurance companies, other professionals from other health care organizations
Dealing with the government payment systems, data banks, and so on."[19]

Suffice it to say that no health care organization "can operate a twenty-first-century economy without a twenty-first-century electronic infrastructure, embracing computers, data communications, and the other new media."[15] That is why the extent, efficiency, and efficacy of a health care organization's information management infrastructure say a lot about its commitment to performance improvement. The sum of this commitment may be used as a measure of the organization's performance management system.

WORKER SATISFACTION

Respect, trust, recognition, and empowerment are the key ingredients to worker satisfaction in a health care organization and, therefore, to the success of its performance management system. Does anyone ever begin a new job with a bad attitude? No. They are filled with anticipation, excitement, and ambition. But health care organizations with little regard for the satisfaction of their employees find that their enthusiasm and open-mindedness are soon replaced by apathy and bitterness.[18]

Rosenbluth and Peters tell this story in their book *The Customer Comes Second:*

I was once discussing the concept of happiness in the workplace with the CEO of a company during a luncheon. We agreed that it's vital to a healthy work force and to providing good service. But we disagreed on one important point—that it's the company's responsibility to ensure the happiness of its people. When I told him some of the things we do to encourage happiness he said, "If they're not happy in our company, we fire them." I didn't take him literally, but at the same time, his message was clearly that companies shouldn't coddle their people.[18]

In our consultations with health care organization administrators, we hear them lament a lack of motivation in the workplace, absenteeism, turnover, apathy, lethargy, and a host of other evils that prevent satisfaction in the workplace. Without satisfaction in their daily work experience, employees will not cooperate with the implementation of a performance management system, regardless of how well-planned, how many posted slogans, and how much in-service is provided. Without satisfied workers, all programs implemented by management will be sabotaged and processes will break down. The productivity will suffer and profits will drop. Patient complaints will soar and litigation will rise because a health care organization is only as good as its employees. A critical benchmark, then, of a health care organization's performance management system is the satisfaction of its employees; this revolves around respect, trust, recognition, and empowerment.

Respect

Respect is necessary to the required indisciplinary nature of a performance management system. Respect, though a nebulous word, is nevertheless the basis for satisfaction in the workplace. Employees within a health care organization want not only to respect their first line and top level leaders but also to receive respect themselves. The golden rule may be old and almost forgotten, but, nevertheless, it is true: Treat every human being as you want to be treated—with respect. In a health care organization, respect forms a circle: employees must respect leaders and leaders must respect employees, who in turn, respect the organization's customers. When this circle is understood and implemented, it will automatically give the health care organization what it desires—patient satisfaction, employee satisfaction, and an increase in profits.

Respect is manifested in many ways in a health care organization. Some of them are:

- showing regard for the feelings of others
- behaving courteously to everyone
- considering the privacy of others
- avoiding workplace gossip
- ignoring workplace rumors
- maintaining equality with everyone in the workforce

Ken Iverson, president of the Nucor Corporation of Charlotte, North Carolina, has learned how to demonstrate all of these qualities to his employees. Nucor, the seventh-largest steel company in the United States, has not had a losing quarter in twenty-five years. Iverson, as CEO, deserves some perks. Nevertheless, he still drives his own car, carries his own bags on business trips, and flies coach on commercial airlines. There is no company plane. There is also no executive dining room or reserved parking places, and any executive who considers himself too good to answer his own phone isn't good enough to work at Nucor. Out of fifty-five hundred employees, only twenty are at headquarters.

> *No employee at Nucor has been laid off for lack of work in more than twenty years, and when the company hits a bad patch, the first people to suffer are Nucor's eighteen officers. When the return to shareholders is less than 8 percent, they get no bonus. In one year, Iverson and his officers took in effect a 60 percent pay cut, but no employee was laid off. In return, the employees are just as loyal to the company as it is to them. Employee turnover is all but nonexistent.[4]*

Respect for each individual worker produces a high level of worker satisfaction. That is why the degree of respect shown to the employees of a health care organization is an indicator of worker satisfaction.

Trust

The old adage, "Trust begets trust," is true. There can be no worker satisfaction without trust. "No trust equals no process improvement team equals no removal of layers of middle management equals no willingness to share strategic information equals no multiskilled training equals no self-management (team or individual) equals no intimate "outsider" (customer, vendor, patient) involvement—equals no dice."[15] Trust is the glue that renders the entire health care organization cohesive and ensures worker satisfaction. Consider how Ralph Heath, president of Ovation Marketing, addressed this issue of trust with his employees.

Employees were told to approve their own expenses. Until this managerial edict, all travel budgets and expense vouchers and purchase orders required approval from middle management and then from Ralph S. Heath, III, himself. The employees did not believe Heath was trusting them to turn in honest expense reports without managerial oversight, so they ignored the new edict and continued turning in their expense reports for approval. Several staff meetings were necessary for Heath to explain that each employee would be trusted to handle the company's money as though he or she was the president. To impress upon employees that he was serious, Heath set fire to all purchase orders that had been turned in by disbelieving employees. The demonstration was effective. He has not received a purchase order to countersign since.[15]

This change has had a dramatic effect. Six months after the beginning of the experiment, Heath found:

- Ovation's travel expenses down 70%
- Entertainment expenses dropped 39%
- Car mileage costs declined 46%
- Office supply expenses reduced by 18%

Additionally, Ovation's business is up 16% in this same period.[15] Worker satisfaction is reported at an all-time high.

There is no such thing as half-trust. Secretary of War Stimson said, "The only way to make a man trustworthy is to trust him."[15] But trust, like respect, works two ways: it is important not only for managers to trust employees but also for employees to be able to trust the managers and top leaders as well.

Without trust the performance management system cannot function in a health care organization, because all workers must be trusted to gather accurate data and all teams must be trusted to perform each step of the performance improvement process. This is why the level of trust in a health care organization plays such a critical role in the measurement of employee satisfaction.

Recognition

Recognition is a critical aspect of worker satisfaction. Tom Peters states, "Farmer, senator, salesperson, engineer, janitor, CEO, you, me, and the kid who mows your lawn—everybody loves being recognized, in any way, large or small. Mary Kay knows! Tupperware knows! And if you're wise, you'll join the parade. Appreciation, applause, approval, respect—we all love it! Balloons, badges, prizes, our picture in the company newsletter—wonderful! Can't get enough!"[14]

Recognition is used to retain workers and to motivate them to achieve their personal and organizational goals.[2] There are two kinds of recognition available to health care workers: intrinsic and extrinsic. "Extrinsic or financial recognition consist of bonuses, merit pay and incentive pay and so on."[2] To some workers, money is a major extrinsic reward and they will perform consistently to obtain it. However, to many other workers the opposite is true; unless these workers see a direct connection between money and performance, it has little effect on them.

"Intrinsic or interpersonal recognition include such things as completion, achievement, autonomy and personal growth."[2] People who want to start and finish a process value task completion more than money. When the task is finished, they achieve a high-level form of self-recognition. On the other hand, employees who are motivated to make decisions and work without being closely supervised value recognition for autonomous productivity more than money. Additionally, many workers want to increase their knowledge and expand their skill potential, so they value recognition for continuing education and training more than money.

Recognition happens when management acknowledges employee achievement. "Put simply (and somewhat coarsely), giving credit costs you nothing, and nets you big-time."[14] Personal recognition, then, serves as a powerful motivator of individual performance and increased job satisfaction.

Effective employee recognition programs share five key elements:

- **Recognition symbols**—by selecting a logo, the firm establishes a focus and gives continuity to the program.
- **Display options**—whether jewelry, pens, keychains, or desk accessories, it is important to get the service symbol out where it can be seen.
- **Meaningful presentations**—managers need to sincerely express appreciation.
- **Program promotion**—health care organization bulletin boards, house newspapers, and personal letters from management hierarchy generate interest.
- **Review and updating**—as needs and values change, the recognition rewards can be modified.[16]

Recognizing length of service, attendance, safety, productivity, and customer service can be a very cost-effective way to improve the satisfaction and productivity of employees. Because an organization-wide process of employee recognition is such a powerful indicator of worker satisfaction, it is used as a benchmark of excellence of the health care organization's performance.

Empowerment

Moving from a hierarchy management style of governance to one of shared leadership is no small cultural change. If, however, the performance management system is to be successful, shared leadership is a necessary organizational change. The extent of the empowerment of the workforce is, therefore, one of the benchmarks of worker satisfaction.

People working in a reengineered health care organization should of necessity, be empowered. "This means that while jobs are more satisfying, they are also more challenging and difficult. Much of the old, routine work is eliminated or automated. If the old model was simple tasks for simple people, the new one is complex jobs for smart people, which raises the bar for entry into the workforce of [a health care organization]."[8] Managerial acknowledgment that a worker must be smart to perform a certain job creates a new focus of empowerment. It permits workers to become experts in their particular job.

What happens when a health care organization reengineers itself? Hammer and Champy have observed eight changes that occur when workers are empowered:

- People's roles change—from controlled to empowered.
- Job preparation changes—from training to education.
- Focus of performance measures and compensation shifts—from activity to results.
- Advancement criteria change—from seniority to ability.
- Values change—from protective to productive.
- Managers change—from supervisors to coaches.
- Organizational structures change—from hierarchical to flat.
- Executives change—from scorekeepers to leaders.[8]

An empowered workforce can transform a health care organization from a struggling quagmire of tradition and status quo into a productive, thriving organization—a leader in the health care industry. This leadership produces great worker satisfaction, because everyone wants to be associated with a winner!

The performance management system described in this book may be used as a catalyst to catapult a health care organization into the future. This conceptually new framework for excellence may be used to cement an entire health care system together so that everyone "sings from the same hymnal." Its three programs of awareness, measurement, and improvement provide the tools and techniques to create and manage an effective performance management system both inside and outside the health care organization's walls.

The pursuit of excellence is, in the words of a popular song, a long and winding road. This book attempts to provide a bridge that connects the traditional, fragmented, hierarchical road of unit-based quality assessment with the new, emerging one of an organization-wide performance management system. It provides the signposts to direct you on a successful journey and should be a worthwhile companion along the way. However, the book alone is merely words on paper. It shares with you our road map for success. The rest is up to you.

In the words of Shel Silverstein,

> *This bridge will only take you halfway there*
> *To those mysterious lands you long to see:*
> *Through gypsy camps and swirling Arab fairs*
> *And moonlit woods where unicorns run free.*
> *So come and walk awhile with me and share*
> *The twisting trails and wondrous worlds I've known.*
> *But this bridge will only take you halfway there—*
> *The last few steps you'll have to take alone.**

REFERENCES

1. Brown JH, Moore CH: *Process improvement breakthrough—an Rx for health care*, Knoxville, Tenn, 1995, Qualpro.
2. Chung KH, Megginson LG: *Organizational behavior*, New York, 1981, Harper & Row.
3. Dobyns L, Crawford-Mason C: *Quality or else: the revolution in world business*, Boston, 1991, Houghton Mifflin Co.

*From Silverstein S: This bridge, *A Light in the Attic*, New York, 1974, HarperCollins.

4. Drucker PE: *Management: tasks, responsibilities, practices,* New York, 1974, Harper & Row.

5. Exodus 18:22. *Bible: New International Version.*

6. Finkler SA: *Essentials of cost accounting for health care organizations,* Gaithersburg, Md, 1994, Aspen.

7. Green LG: Scientist from the National Aeronautical and Space Administration. In a presentation, *Age of the Earth,* at the Frederick Seventh-day Adventist Church, Frederick, Md, December 16, 1995.

8. Hammer M, Champy J: *Reengineering the corporation: a manifesto for business revolution,* New York, 1993, HarperBusiness.

9. Kanter RM: *When giants learn to dance,* New York, 1989, Simon & Schuster.

10. LeBoeuf M: *GMP, the greatest management principle in the world,* New York, 1986, Berkley Books.

11. Markels A: Managing your career, *The Wall Street Journal,* October 31, 1995, p B1.

12. Martin WB: *Managing quality customer service,* Los Altos, Cal, 1989, Crisp Publications, Inc.

13. Naisbitt J, Aburdene P: *Megatrends 2000: ten new directions for the 1990's,* New York, 1990, Avon Books.

14. Peters T: *The pursuit of WOW!,* New York, 1994, Vintage Books.

15. Peters T: *Liberation management: necessary disorganization for the nanosecond nineties,* New York, 1992, Fawcett Columbine.

16. Podsakoff PM, Tudor WD, Skov R: Effects of leader contingent and noncontingent reward and punishment behaviors on subordinate performance and satisfaction, *Academy of Management Journal,* December 1982, pp 810-821.

17. Quick T: *Successful team building,* New York, 1992, AMACOM.

18. Rosenbluth HF, Peters D: *The customer comes second: and other secrets of exceptional service,* New York, 1992, William Morrow and Company, Inc.

19. Shapero A: *Managing professional people: understand creative performance,* New York, 1985, The Free Press.

20. Twersky RS: How to assess quality in ambulatory surgery, *J Clin Anesth,* 4: 25S-32S, 1992.

21. Wallechinsky D: Bad predictions, *Parade Magazine,* September 10, 1995, p 16.

22. Wilson P: *Change: coping with tomorrow today,* Shawnee Mission, Kan, 1992, National Press Publications.

23. Wycoff J, Richardson T: *Transformation thinking,* Atlantic Beach, Fla, 1995, Berkley Publishing Group.

24. Yoder-Wise P: *Leading and managing in nursing,* St. Louis, 1995, Mosby.

Glossary

accountability the obligation to disclose in adequate detail and consistent form the purposes, principles, procedures, relationships, results, incomes, and expenditures involved in any activity, enterprise, or assignment so that they can be evaluated by interested parties

accreditation the act of an official review board granting approval to an organization after the organization has met specific written requirements and standards

acuity a measurement of patient severity of illness that is related to the amount of resources required to care for the patient

administrative action plan a process standard that outlines a critical area for action, desired outcomes, required activities, and a timeline directed at improving organizational performance

aesthetics how a product or service looks, feels, and sounds

Agenda for Change the Joint Commission's 1986 initiative designed to reshape the accreditation process by improving the methods used by the Joint Commission to evaluate and monitor health care organizations

aggregate to combine standardized data and information

aggregate data indicator a performance measure that quantifies a process or an outcome related to many cases, as opposed to isolated cases

AHCPR (The Agency for Health Care Policy and Research) created in December 1989, the eighth agency of the federal government's public health service, designed to enhance the quality of patient care through improved knowledge that can be used in meeting society's health care needs; AHCPR activities include developing clinically relevant practice guidelines

algorithm an ordered sequence of steps or instructions, with each step or instruction depending on the outcome of the previous one, that is used to tell how to solve a particular problem. An algorithm is specified exactly, so there can be no doubt about what to do next, and it has a finite number of steps

alpha testing the initial phase of field testing of indicators

appraisal costs the costs incurred while conducting inspections, tests, and other planned measurement activities to determine whether services, practices, and governance meet their requirements

appropriateness the degree to which the correct service is provided given the current state of knowledge

average cost the total cost of producing a good or service divided by the number of units produced

average length of stay average stay counted by days of all or a class of inpatients discharged over a given period, calculated by dividing the number of inpatient days by the number of discharges

awareness having knowledge of something through information, observation, or interpretation; the first program of the Performance Management System (PMS) in which all standards for the PMS are developed, written, and disseminated throughout the health care organization

bar graph a graphic display of sets of rectangles, each rectangle being identified with a particular classification of data, and the height of the rectangle representing a data value for that classification

benchmarking the search for industry best practices that lead to superior performance

THE BLUEPRINT a comprehensive performance management model that focuses on performance awareness, performance measurement, and performance improvement in three domains: service, practice, and governance

case-mix "Relative frequency of different diagnoses or conditions among patients" (Joint Commission)*

cause and effect diagram a pictorial display drawn to represent the relationship between some effect and all the possible causes influencing it; synonymous terms for this type of diagram are fishbone (named for its appearance) and Ishikawa (named for the creator Kaoru Ishikawa)

chief executive officer (CEO) the individual appointed by a governing body to act on its behalf in the overall management of an organization

clinical action plan a process standard that outlines a critical area for action, desired outcomes, required activities, and a timeline directed at improving patient care

clinical path a process standard that addresses the care of a medical diagnosis

clinical practice guideline a process standard that outlines the care and outcomes for specific patient symptoms

common cause variance a minor variation in performance that is the result of chance occurrence(s) involving the patient, staff, or system that cannot be controlled

---

*Definitions designated Joint Commission are reprinted from Joint Commission of Healthcare Organizations: *Primer on indicator development and application,* Oakbrook Terrace, Ill, 1990, The Commission.

compliance to act in accordance with stated requirements, such as standards; it is composed of those controllable patient, staff, and system factors that affect performance

conformance the degree to which a service meets preestablished industry standards

continuous variable a measurement that is limited to specific options

continuum of care the concept that health care providers maintain consistent patient treatment and service regardless of the health care setting

control chart a run chart with statistically determined upper and lower limits drawn on either side of the process average

control limit a line or lines on a control chart used as a basis for judging the significance of the variation from subgroup to subgroup

cost of nonconformance (CONC) a method for computing cost of variables in a process

cost-benefit analysis the evaluation of the relationship between the resources necessary to complete a project and the results obtained from its completion

council a group of individuals charged with a specific ongoing function within an organization

count data measurements of volume, how many, or how much; used in quality control measurements

critical path the longest sequential series of tasks in a project; minimum necessary tasks to accomplish an objective or meet a goal

critical process a process that is high volume, high risk, problem prone, and high cost

data the collection of material, items, or facts on which a discussion or an inference is based

data collection effort the relative effort required for, and associated cost of, collecting data in relation to the importance of the measure

data trend a type of data pattern on a run chart or control chart that rises or falls in a series of points; attention is given when the points exceed a predetermined number

demographic data service, practice, or governance variables that may influence the results of monitoring a specific indicator

dimensions of performance attributes of organizational performance that are related to organizations "doing the right things" and "doing them well"

discrete variable a measurement that is limited to specific options

discriminatory the extent to which an indicator identifies variation across multiple health care organizations

documentation the information recorded as a result of data collection, planning, and evaluation

durability amount of use one gets from a product or service before it physically deteriorates

effectiveness the degree to which desired results are produced

efficiency the act of producing output with the minimum of waste, expense, or unnecessary effort; the ratio of useful output to the total input in any system

employee development plan a process standard that outlines a critical area for development, desired outcomes, required activities, and a timeline for completion directed at improving an individual staff member's performance

evaluation (1) the mechanisms by which a service will be monitored, including quality assessment, customer satisfaction, and research. (2) "The review and assessment of the quality and/or appropriateness of an important aspect of care for which a preestablished level of performance (threshold for evaluation) has been reached during monitoring activities. The review and assessment may include peer review, pattern analysis, and/or trend analysis and is designed to determine whether there is a problem and/or opportunity to improve care, and if so, to develop a plan of action to address the identified problem or opportunity to improve care."*

extremely important process a process that is any combination of three of the following: high-volume, high-risk, problem-prone, and/or high-cost

features secondary characteristics that supplement a service's basic functioning

fishbone diagram (see *cause and effect diagram*)

flowchart a statistical process control tool that schematically diagrams the steps in a process

frequency distribution the number of times something occurs within a specified period of time

goals measurable end results that individuals, groups, or organizations attempt to achieve by expending resources

Governance Improvement Council (GIC) the council-assigned accountability of the governance domain of the organization; this council functions under the direction of the QMB

governance model a visual representation (paradigm) depicting the type of governance style being utilized by the health care organization's CEO

high risk an important process, procedure, or activity that exposes a patient to a greater chance of undesirable outcomes if not carried out effectively or appropriately

high volume a process, procedure, or activity that is performed frequently or affects large numbers of patients

histogram a statistical process control tool used to depict frequency of occurrence (see Pareto chart)

---

*This definition is reprinted from the *Joint Commission Glossary of Quality Assurance Terms*, which appears in Patterson CH: Standards of patient care: the Joint Commission focus on nursing quality assurance, *Nursing Clinics of North America* 23: 3, 1988.

important process high-volume, high-risk, high-cost, or problem-prone process that directly affects service, practice, or governance

indicator a performance measure that focuses on desired outcomes and/or key processes. It is a valid and reliable process or outcome measure related to one or more dimensions of performance

integrated delivery system a health care system that provides all types and levels of health care services within the same health plan, including primary, secondary, tertiary, community, and home care services

job description a structure standard that outlines the requisite knowledge, skills, attitudes, responsibilities, and scope of authority of a specific position within an organization

Joint Commission on Accreditation of Healthcare Organizations (Joint Commission, JCAHO) a private, voluntary, nonprofit, nongovernmental agency that was founded in 1951 as The Joint Commission on Accreditation of Hospitals (JCAH). It surveys and accredits hospitals and other health care organizations according to its published consensus standards

kaizen a continual improvement process involving everyone in a personal quest for excellence

matrix diagram a flow diagram that places the activities in the diagram under columns representing tasks or performance measures carried out under certain conditions designated in the horizontal headings

measure to collect quantifiable data about a dimension of performance of a function or process

measurement the systematic process of data collection, repeated over time or at a single point in time; the process of quantification

Measurement Improvement Council (MIC) the council that serves as the central clearinghouse for all data generated by the organization; this council functions under the direction of the QMB

mission the overall business in which an organization is engaged

national database an organized collection of data in a standardized format, typically stored in a computer system so that any particular item or set of items can be extracted or organized as needed

nonconformance failure to act in harmony with prescribed practices or comply with an established process

organization-wide throughout the organization and across multiple structural and staffing components

outcome the result obtained through enactment and completion of a service, practice, or governance process

Pareto chart a statistical process control tool used to determine and visually depict frequencies and priorities

perceived quality what the customer thinks is quality

performance the application of inherent and/or learned capabilities to complete a process according to specifications/standards

performance analysis measurement of specific indicators of performance

performance awareness a program that assigns responsibility for performance management, defines key processes, and educates responsible parties about their roles in the performance management system

performance improvement a program of the performance management system that includes the plan to improve the dimensions of performance, the implementation of the improvement plan, and communication of the results of the plan's implementation

performance management a standards-based approach to the reduction of process variability and the improvement of process capability

performance management system an organized system comprising a series of programs designed to define, measure, and improve organizational performance

performance measurement a program of the performance management system that involves collecting performance data and compares actual results with projections to determine process/outcome variance; it includes performance, satisfaction, and technology analysis

philosophy a written statement of an organization's beliefs about customer service, staff practice, and governance

plan a process standard that outlines an intent to act

policy a structure standard that defines the service, practice, and governance rules of an organization; when not adhered to, it creates a legal threat to the customer, employee, or organization

practice guideline a written process standard for symptom management; a written process standard for client care management that has the potential for improving the quality of clinical and consumer decision making; it "includes assessment and diagnosis, planning, intervention, evaluation and outcome" (ANA)*; "a descriptive tool or standardized specification(s) for care of the 'typical' patient in the 'typical' situation" (Joint Commission)‡; "a systematically developed statement to assist practitioner and patient decisions about appropriate health care for specific clinical circumstances" (AHCPR)

Practice Improvement Council (PIC) the council that governs the practice domain of the organization; this council functions under the direction of the QMB

procedure a series of recommended actions for the completion of a specific task; psychomotor tasks

---

*This definition is reprinted from *The American Nurse,* 23: 3, 1991.
‡Definitions designated Joint Commission are reprinted from Joint Commission of Healthcare Organizations: *Primer on indicator development and application* Oakbrook Terrace, Ill, 1990, The Commission.

process the manner in which service will be delivered; procedures, practice guidelines, action plans, and documentation systems describe process

process capability the measured built-in reproducibility of the outcome of a process

process variance the inevitable differences among individual outputs of a process

productivity the process of yielding favorable, desirable, or useful results

quality "the degree to which patient care services increase the probability of desired patient outcomes and reduce the probability of undesired outcomes given the current state of knowledge" (Joint Commission)*

quality control the process by which actual performance is measured, the performance is compared with goals, and the difference is acted upon; the use of statistical methods to measure quality

quality improvement the process of attaining a new level of performance or quality that is superior to any previous level; the attainment of a new level of quality that is superior to any previous level of quality

quality management the process by which people are mobilized to achieve quality goals

Quality Management Board (QMB) the governing board of the performance management system

rate-based event a service, practice, or governance occurrence for which a certain rate of occurrence is expected when state of the art care is provided. Investigation is required when the rate at which the event occurs exceeds a preset target

reengineering the fundamental rethinking and radical redesign of business processes to achieve dramatic improvements in critical, contemporary measures of performance, such as cost, quality, service, and speed

relevance the applicability of an indicator to the services provided by affected health care organizations

reliability the ability of an indicator to accurately identify the targeted events across multiple organizations

run chart a statistical process control tool used to document the frequency with which an event occurs over a period of time

satisfaction analysis the customer's evaluation of the value of the service provided

scope the range of performance that the performance management system controls

scope of service the range of care or service provided by an organization, department, or service, including conditions treated, managed, or prevented, treatments provided, procedures used, populations served, locations where service is provided, times when services are provided, and professional disciplines and specialties providing services. The delineation of the scope of service is the basis for identifying the critical processes of service, practice, or governance

sentinel event a serious service, practice, or governance occurrence that always requires investigation

Service Improvement Council (SIC) the council that governs the service domain of the organization; this council functions under the direction of the QMB

shared leadership an organizational culture characterized by a shared vision, empowered workers, cooperation among organizational units and departments as they work to improve processes; there exists a high degree of openness to feedback and data, and optimization of the organizational whole versus its many parts

special cause variance a variation in performance that occurs as a result of patient, staff, or system variables that can be controlled

staff development plan a process standard that outlines a critical area for development, desired outcomes, required activities, and a time-line for completion directed at improving the performance of more than one staff member

standard a written statement that specifies expectations

standard deviation a measure of the dispersion of a frequency distribution that is the square root of the variance

standard of governance a written value statement that defines the rules, actions, and conditions that direct institutional or departmental functions

standard of practice a written value statement that defines the rules, actions, or conditions that direct the maintenance of professional status and credibility

standard of service a written value statement that defines the rules, actions, or conditions that direct service

statistical control a state in which the results of measuring a process fall consistently within the target parameters but without an obvious trend or pattern

statistical process control the application of statistical techniques to the control of processes

structure the circumstances under which a service will be delivered; the organization's mission, philosophy, goals, policies, and job descriptions define its structure

tampering attempts to fix minor variations in performance that are due to chance; it usually results in wildly fluctuating variations that overcorrect or undercorrect a variation

---

*Definitions designated Joint Commission are reprinted from Joint Commission of Healthcare Organizations: *Primer on indicator development and application,* Oakbrook Terrace, Ill, 1990, The Commission.

target a statistically derived mean that serves as the aim, benchmark, objective, or point for control of a process; the border between performance and nonconformance

target parameters the upper and lower limits of acceptance that establish an acceptable range of compliance or non-compliance

technology analysis the measurement of product performance and research

TEFRA Tax Equity and Fiscal Responsibility Act

trending analyzing the results of numerous studies on the same indicator to identify patterns that may influence the quality of outcomes related to the important aspect of care or service being monitored

trifocus approach a strategy for monitoring and evaluation that considers all three domains of practice: service, practice, and governance

validity evidence that indicator data identify important events and provide a basis for performance improvement activities

variation a difference in performance related to an important aspect of care; it may result from controllable or uncontrollable factors

very important process a process that is any combination of two of the four important aspects of care, i.e., high-volume, high-risk, problem-prone, and high-cost

visible numbers-only manager a manager who considers only the bottom line of the financial report when making a decision

Index